Life on Wheels

Life on Wheels

The A to Z Guide to Living Fully with Mobility Issues

Gary Karp

SECOND EDITION

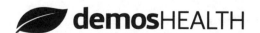

Visit our web site at www.demosmedpub.com

Library of Congress Cataloging-in-Publication Data
Karp, Gary, 1955–
    Life on wheels : the A to Z guide to living fully with mobility issues / Gary Karp.
    — 2nd ed.
        p. cm.
    Includes index.
    ISBN-13: 978-1-932603-33-0 (pbk. : alk. paper)
    ISBN-10:   1-932603-33-6 (pbk. : alk. paper)
      1. Paraplegia—Popular works.   2. Paraplegics—Care.   3. Wheelchairs.
    4. Paralysis—Popular works.   I. Title.
      [DNLM: 1. Disabled Persons—psychology. 2. Disabled Persons—rehabilitation.
    3. Quality of Life.   4. Wheelchairs. WB 320 K18L 2009]
    RC406.P3K37 2009
    616.8′42—dc22

                                                                    2008017421

Special discounts on bulk quantities of Demos Medical Publishing books are available to corporations, professional associations, pharmaceutical companies, health care organizations, and other qualifying groups. For details, please contact:

Special Sales Department
Demos Medical Publishing
386 Park Avenue South, Suite 301
New York, NY 10016
Phone: 800–532–8663 or 212–683–0072
Fax: 212–683–0118
E-mail: orderdept@demosmedpub.com

Printed in the United States of America
08 09 10 11   5 4 3 2 1

To my parents,
Sam and Bette Karp

Contents

Foreword

No one signs up for a disability. We can't choose how or when such a thing might impact our lives. But we can choose what happens next; whether to sit around and wait for the future to happen, or to jump in and *make* it happen.

I chose the second option. And while that may look like the obvious answer, it's not necessarily an easy one. At least it wasn't for me. I worked hard to become knowledgeable about life with a disability. I struggled to overcome fears. I dealt with the seemingly endless challenges of my new life as a person with a disability.

I wish I'd had this book.

Life On Wheels is a unique and invaluable resource for active wheel-chair users ready to jump-start their life's journey or explore new options. Gary Karp has packed these pages with helpful information, personal insights and a triumphant spirit, resulting in a book that takes you by the hand and confidently guides you toward personal mastery.

Being in a wheelchair doesn't mean you can't live a full and rewarding life. The journey toward fulfillment begins when you believe you *can*, and continues as you do whatever it takes to achieve your goals. Let *Life on Wheels* be your "travel guide" along that journey, providing wise and won-derful learning tools to unleash your mind, body and spirit. With this book, the more you explore . . . the higher you'll soar!

Gary has done an outstanding job of taking over a third of a century of personal experiences and research during his own disability journey, boil-ing it all down into user-friendly, bite-size nuggets of practical advice. There's never a dull moment, as he illustrates how exciting life can be when it has real purpose and meaning. Best of all, this isn't a "one size fits all" formula for fulfillment; rather, Gary will help you create a truly customized approach for achieving a life of health, self-sufficiency, intimacy, and fun.

As a wheelchair user with a spinal cord injury since 1978, I know first-hand that overcoming great challenges brings even greater satisfaction.

When the wheelchair industry was content to produce one bland, heavy, institutional chair after another, I co-founded Quickie Designs to challenge the status quo. The result? We innovated a whole new kind of chair that enabled millions of people to enjoy unprecedented mobility, opportunity, and freedom. We "reinvented the wheel" and revolutionized the entire industry, helping wheelchairs evolve from institutional heavyweights to liberating ultra-lightweights designed with cutting-edge materials, full adjustability, modern styling, and a fun personality.

Interestingly, I found myself not only in the business of advancing wheelchairs, but changing broad perceptions about the people who used them. With their Quickie chairs, users were seen as empowered instead of helpless, and by the millions they were able to proudly take their places in every level of society. Today, people with disabilities no longer let their wheelchairs keep them from working, traveling, raising families, and making their mark on the world. And I'm both proud and humbled to have played a role in that.

But society still has a long way to go in providing the environment and resources that make more possibilities available for wheelchair users. Which is why we need *Life on Wheels* now more than ever. Gary has infused these pages with a spirit of self-advocacy, empowering people with disabilities to insist on our innate right to realize our full potential. Here, you'll find inspiration not only for living well, but also for taking a leadership role in knocking down the obstacles that stubbornly stand between you and your dreams. You'll learn not to limit your challenges, but to challenge your limits!

I strongly believe in your potential. I deeply care about your right to the tools you need to reach that potential. I highly recommend *Life on Wheels* for the inspiration and motivation you need to not just survive, but thrive.

Marilyn Hamilton
Paralympic Athlete

Founder
ENVISION (Speaking, Writing, and Consulting)
Winner on Wheels (Children's Nonprofit)

Co-Founder
Motion Designs (Quickie Wheelchairs)
Discovery through Design (Women's Nonprofit)

Preface

Life on Wheels was originally published in 1999 by O'Reilly & Associates. I was proud of the book and especially proud to have received the kind of feedback I had gotten—from readers and reviewers alike. *Life on Wheels* was just the book for people facing changes in their mobility and independence. The late Barry Corbet, editor of *New Mobility* magazine, wrote that *Life on Wheels* was "perhaps the best distillation of the disability experience."

    Life on Wheels was also the right book for family members and loved ones sharing the experience of a recent disability. As I traveled and spoke, people would tell me what a substantial difference the book made for them. It only took one such expression of appreciation to prove to me that the two-plus years of work in the original writing was entirely worth the effort. You are now holding the updated and refined second edition of *Life on Wheels* published by Demos Health.

    I generally write in principle—trying to provide a core understanding of issues and methods so that readers can apply these to their own lives and situations. This book has never been so much about offering specific recommendations or prescriptive guidance (though you'll find a bit of it here and there) but instead is about empowering with information that helps people make the best choices and find their own way.

    At the same time, in the eight years since the book's first release, I've gained a deeper understanding of the disability experience through a wide-ranging involvement in the broader disability community. This was not the case when I first began this project. My connection with the national disability scene has been a tremendous source of insight and information and growth, which I have brought to the updating of this book. So, I have gone through the entire text and refined the language, added a significant phrase of embellishment here and there, struck some material that didn't make a strong enough point, and rounded things out with new paragraphs and sections. As great as *Life on Wheels* was in its first life, it's now truly new and improved.

The impetus for the book, though, has changed little. Thousands of people acquire or are born with characteristics that are objectively impairing. They have a "disability," a word that is increasingly meaningless exactly because it can mean so many different things in so many different people's lives. The prospect of using a wheelchair will always—naturally and understandably—be a prospect one would not choose. The issue remains: once it becomes your reality, what are the choices? What are the options? This is what *Life on Wheels* answers for you.

The Wheelchair—A Changing Paradigm

The wheelchair is widely viewed as a symbol of illness and loss. Becoming a wheelchair user is to be avoided at all costs, even when conditions cry out for an alternative method of mobility. People with progressive conditions such as multiple sclerosis or amyotrophic lateral sclerosis do all they can to delay using a wheelchair, feeling that to do so would be to surrender to their disability. Many people in the early months after a traumatic disability resist the purchase of a customized wheelchair because they insist they will walk again.

Yet, those who have lived with a disability since childhood experience it as a natural state. They don't experience disability as a loss, they have not had to adapt to significant changes in the way they function in the world, or they have not had to redefine their potential in the context of their disability. To them—and to the people who have chosen to integrate their disability into their full sense of self—the wheelchair is a treasured tool. They know it makes their life possible.

Those with no disability (a temporary condition, it is said, for most people) recoil in horror at the thought of being "wheelchair-bound." In their minds, it is a mark of tragedy, of lost dreams, of pity, grueling effort, and regret. One becomes an object of charity—thanks to the ubiquitous image in our culture of the "poster child"—who needs care and lifelong medical management. It is an image fostered in the media in which films and television dramas emphasize the extremes of either tragedy or the heroism of people with disabilities rather than portraying the largely normal daily life that many chair riders experience. Newspapers typically use the phrase "confined to a wheelchair" and write about chair riders as human interest stories rather than as the whole people they are.

These beliefs are simply not true. The wheelchair is a tool that enhances quality of life. Wheelchair users are not always ill and are not condemned to a life of no meaning or pleasure. Even for people with life-threatening illness, the right wheels facilitate their ability to be out in the world, continuing their lives, partaking of the many realms of human experience.

All of this entails a simple choice that everyone must make: to live the potential our life has to offer with our disability, or not. Most people arrive at the choice to live, to figure out how it works, to reach out—or fight—for the resources that make it possible. They become accustomed to a new public identity and learn to base how they feel about themselves on their own view rather than adopting the prevailing social view, which they ultimately come to learn is simply wrong.

The human spirit in each of us gives us a remarkable capacity to adjust to traumatic change. We learn that our spirit is whole and unaffected—and has nothing to do with the ability to walk. Or use our hands. Or speak clearly. We learn that we can survive and thrive on wheels, just as well as we could on our feet. Thousands and thousands of people prove this point every day, but the wider society still has a way to go to take full notice.

There is a huge gap between the way our culture views disability and the truth of the experience. More than 54 million Americans are thought to have a disability that significantly affects their lives. There are 1.7 million regular wheelchair users in the United States. Disability awareness and advocacy are extending throughout the world, as people everywhere choose to be active and independent. People with disabilities of ranging degrees of impairment are getting on with having a life—working, marrying, traveling, playing sports, being full members of their community. They have various limitations to deal with, but most will tell you that any difficulties they would ascribe to their disability are more about misguided cultural attitudes and a political and architectural environment that places unnecessary obstacles in their way.

People with disabilities are not "broken"; neither are they heroes. Like everybody, people with disabilities are simply human.

What This Book Offers

This book offers an initial road map to the lifelong, complex, and fascinating road of the disability experience. This book is primarily a guidebook for those with a mobility disability, with practical information about how to adapt the home, choose a wheelchair, explore sexual identity, optimize health, and more. This book is designed to help people make their adjustments sooner and more completely by explaining how one adapts to disability, and by addressing misconceptions that only delay one's ability to adapt. Throughout it I have tried to foster the principles of choice, of control, and of everyone's right to pursue their interests and convictions.

Life on Wheels is also an effort to explain that inclusion is an innate right for everyone and that people with disabilities are excluded for reasons not based on a balanced or realistic understanding of what is possible. It's time our world caught up with the reality, closed that gap, and allowed millions of people with disabilities to play their full role in society. A modern disability movement of spirited advocacy on the part of people with disabilities has already made tremendous progress toward that end. The disability movement has become increasingly sophisticated and accomplished; the future will only continue to brighten for those of us living a *Life on Wheels*.

Why I Wrote This Book

I've been living the experience since I fell out of a tree and injured my spinal cord in 1973 at the age of 18. After 13 weeks of hospitalization and rehabilitation I went on to college, obtaining an education in architecture; I have had an active professional life as a graphic artist, manager, and consultant. Since the original publication of *Life on Wheels* in 1999, I have devoted myself to being a communicator about disability issues, having published a total of four books and speaking extensively across the U.S. at rehab centers, universities, and a wide array of conferences, meetings, and businesses. I have kept up my sidelines as a musician, juggler, and performer. I have traveled, moved to California, married and divorced, married again and together with my wife raised an incredible yellow Labrador retriever puppy, pursued spiritual interests, developed enduring and deep friendships, and given and received support from my family.

Well, you get the idea. It's been a full life, marked by the whole range of experience that is the nature of being human—ups and downs, successes and failures. Not being able to walk has really been a pretty small part of it, in a way. In other ways, my paralysis essentially defines who I am.

This book comes from my desire to use my skills as a writer to convey the truth of the disability experience, but it has also been a personal process of facing my own disability identity. I was a "mainstreamer." On a certain level I knew that I was not comfortable being seen in the world as having a disability. I wanted to appear as "normal" as possible, perhaps understandably because I had eighteen years of nondisabled identity still inside me. I pursued my personal interests and goals, and had little interaction with other chair riders.

But writing this book has deepened my sense of just how much I have in common with this large population of people with disabilities. We are not seen fully for who we are, but are excessively defined in the world's eyes by a mistaken conception of the meaning of our disabilities—rather than the deep and universal truth of our souls. In the years since beginning this book, and the wide range of experience I've had since as a writer, speaker, and advocate, my own relationship to my disability and how it is integrated in my life has changed dramatically. This is exactly the effect I hope this book will have on you.

Acknowledgments

These pages come all the more to life thanks to the many personal stories and experiences included throughout. Some are in response to questions posted on my web site and others were drawn from online discussions, all used with kind permission for them to be quoted here. My sincere appreciation to the following people for sharing their heartfelt insights: Blane N. Beckwith, Blaze Henry Birinyi, Chris Bourne, George Buckner, Steven Edwards, Michelle Gallagher, Rebecca Gavin, Annette Hanna, Steve Hegg, Gary Hervey, Pauline Horvath, Paul and Jill Jacobs, Erika Jahneke, Jesse Kaysen, Dawn Kellman, Warren King, Douglas Kruse, Emmett S. Land, Constance Laymon, Linda Janine Lipe, Leeya Lowe, Kimber Mangiafico, Tracy L. Mankins, Francois Matte, Bob Mauro, Stan Melton, Carol Swedberg Meyer, Anet (AMARIS) Mconel, Lois Klesa Morrison, Tamar Magenta Raine, Dylan Ryall, Gary Schooley, Gale See, Gary Shakerdge, Marjie Smith, Viki Solomon, RN, Michael Warner, Holly Waters, Chester M. Worwa, and those who wish to remain anonymous.

Those unfortunate enough to be included on my email list got a recruiting request to be on the "Tricks of the Trade Team" for *Life on Wheels* II. The following generous souls took the time to contribute their unique insights and experience which are also to be found throughout the text. Much appreciation goes to Cheryl Angelelli, Bart Brophy, Anthony Tusler, Bruce Cameron, Art Blaser, Adrian Dieleman, Erin Ryan, Santina Muha, Jaehn Clare, Jack Osborne, Patrick Kenneally, Paul Tobin, Rosemarie Rossetti, Judi Rogers, and Yvette Cenerini.

A number of very gracious souls took time from their busy schedules to lend support throughout the writing process. Special thanks to Ron Cohen, Barry Corbet, Tim Gilmer, Carol Gill, Deborah Quilter, Sam Maddox, Stephen Rosenbaum, and Mitch Tepper, with particular appreciation to Dr. Wise Young, for their ongoing and extremely generous help as the book evolved.

One of the most satisfying parts of the work was the process of interviewing people, including healthcare professionals at the forefront of their particular domain of the disability experience. For their openness and willingness to be quoted throughout these pages I thank Alex Barchuk, MD; Cynthia Bishop; Michael Boninger, MD; Mary Lou Breslin; Doe Cayting; Jim Cesario; Dennis Choi, MD, PhD; Paul Church, Ron Cohen, MD; Marcel Dijkers, PhD; Saunders Dorsey, Esq.; Jeff Ewing; Ann Marie Fleming, MFCC; Carol Gill, PhD; Sheldon Ginns; Jody Greenhalgh, OTR; Bob Hall; Deborah Kaplan, Esq; Naomi Kleitman, PhD; Sandra Loyer, MSW; Ron Mace; Linda Mona, PhD, Providencia Morillo; Edward Nieshoff, MD; Linda Noble, PhD; Margaret A. Nosek, PhD; Richard Patterson; Uli Salas, PT; Marco Saroni; Michael Scott, MD; Bonnie Sims; Denise Tate, PhD; Louis Tenenbaum; Mitch Tepper, MPH; and Janie Whiteford.

Special thanks to my colleagues in the National Spinal Cord Injury Association, for whom I gained even more experience as a writer and editor through my stewardship of the NSCIA newspaper, SCI Life. I treasure the partnership of Marcie Roth, Eric Larson, and Tari Susan Hartman-Squire (who also pitched in early with promotional efforts for *Life on Wheels*) and the irreplaceable Harley Thomas, whom we lost in 2007. They also saw fit to honor me with induction into the Spinal Cord Injury Hall of Fame in 2007 as a Disability Educator. The work is all about service to people with disabilities, but it sure felt great to get this incredible affirmation from my community of professional peers.

Much appreciation to Joe Canose, director of the Christopher and Dana Reeve Paralysis Center, who has so generously provided sponsorship for me to speak around the country at rehab centers and to students in university programs of occupational and physical therapy since 2002, and to the PRC's Angela Cantillon, for handling so many important details of this great program.

And to Jeff Leonard, publisher of *New Mobility* magazine for his cosponsorship of the Reeve program and for his partnership in my other book project, *From There to Here: Stories of Adjustment to Spinal Cord Injury*.

I am, as always, deeply blessed by the enduring love and support of my family and friends: Margi and Morry Opperer, Carolynn and Stacey Karp, Iris and Glen Goldstrom, Sylvia Baker, Mark Glasgow Johnson, Peter Winchell, David and Kate Downey, Bob and April Garrity, Dieter, Lynne, Sophie, and Lena Gloeckler, Jessica Jones, Alan and Elena Woontner, Frish Brandt, Richard Knight and Judith Lynch, Lawrence Elkus, Daya Waldman, Laurie Brown, the Malls, the Reveres, the Cassidys, Rob Robb, Lori Simon-Rosinowitz, Patricia Gleeson, Katherine Halsig, PT, Sherrie Foster, OT, and Oscar and Sarah Ichazo. And, above all, my wife, Paula Siegel.

This book would not exist without the patience, experience, wisdom, and support of my original editor at O'Reilly & Associates, Linda Lamb, who sought me out as a writer, and campaigned within O'Reilly to produce the original series of Patient-Centered Guides. She skillfully guided me through the mysterious straits and whirlwinds of first time authorship, and I am much the better writer for it. To the degree that this new edition has risen to an even higher level, it owes to how I have continued to grow as a writer and editor myself thanks to Linda's mentorship.

For this new edition, Noreen Henson deserves my deep appreciation for her belief in the great value of this book and for her desire to see it reach the wider audience that the first edition had yet to find. Thank you, Noreen, for your commitment, for keeping me going on the updated manuscript, and for the vanilla latte at Starbucks as it rained down in Manhattan.

Despite the inspiration and contributions of so many, any errors, omissions, misstatements, or flaws in the book are my own.

Lastly, to people with disabilities everywhere, please accept this work with my prayers that it make a positive difference in your lives. I hope, at least, to have given you cause to consider that your boundaries are a little farther out than you thought.

Chapter I

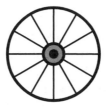

Rehabilitation

Because you are a wheelchair user, optimizing your physical capacity and learning independence-enhancing skills are the keys to reaching the full life potential that your body and medical condition allow. After your having acquired a traumatic disability, a rehabilitation hospital or clinic is the place where you develop these abilities. It is also a place with which you establish and keep a relationship for maintaining your health, receiving specialized medical support, or possibly, where you participate in a research study. It is a place of hard work, unique relationships, and challenges and opportunities at every level of your life—emotionally, physically, intellectually, socially, and, for some, financially.

The rehabilitation process is designed to reduce the restricting effects of disability so that you can enjoy life again and adapt to physical changes. Do your best to make the most of it. Your time there is brief, and you may not get another chance to work with a group of highly trained professionals assembled to help you adapt to your disability.

Hope and Adjustment

Rehab is a place of safety, where you have the benefit of a controlled environment in which to do the work of returning to your life on the outside. Being in rehab is also a challenging process of considerable adjustment and emotion.

This woman with an L1 spinal cord injury expresses the dichotomy:

*The whole experience was valuable. I could never have pro-
gressed to being so independent without it. However, I found it
unpleasant because living in the rehab unit for four months
was like being in prison. The schedule of therapies was stringent. No freedom whatsoever.*

Rehab is a chance to explore possibilities. A person who has experienced a paralyzing stroke, spinal cord injury, or traumatic brain injury, for
instance, might walk out with braces and crutches or using a walker. Or
you might wheel out. You and your medical team should carefully consider
what is physically possible and set your goals accordingly—with a little
room left for that occasional miracle.

Dr. Michael Scott of the Rancho Los Amigos Center in southern California tries to be realistic when people with brain or spinal cord trauma ask
him the "cure" question:

*I think we're on the road to a cure. But I tell people that cure
doesn't necessarily mean that you're going to be up and running around again. A cure probably means we're going to find
a way for you to be a little better and able to do more.*

Dr. Wise Young, Director of the Neuroscience Center at Rutgers, State
University of New Jersey, is concerned that some rehab centers are too pessimistic when it comes to recovery from spinal cord injury:

*I certainly agree that rehab is a place of safety, but many
places are still discouraging the hopes of people who are
interested in recovery. Most rehabilitation centers, in my opin-
ion, are unnecessarily pessimistic. They emphasize that the
goal of therapy is to make the most of what they have, and
many people are told that they should not expect much recovery. This is applicable only to a minority of severely injured
patients. The vast majority of patients with spinal cord injury
recover substantially.*

Use the rehab experience to keep yourself in optimal condition. By
waiting for recovery rather than working with what you have, you risk robbing yourself of motivation to gain skills that might contribute to your
degree of independence. Do the work available to you, adapting as much as
possible to your condition while working to foster your recovery. Learn skills
being taught, even if you don't expect to be using them for long.

*Believing I would walk really didn't affect my participation
in rehab. I guess it goes back to my being an overachiever or
something. I've always been the best at whatever I've done in*

many ways, so I set the hospital record for getting out with
my level of injury.

How Rehab Has Changed

The rehab experience has changed much in the past 20 or so years. You generally are admitted to rehab sooner, and the "length of stay" has gotten shorter. You no longer have the luxury of many months of adjustment and training, which means that you will go home with less than your full ability—your inpatient stay is just a beginning.

There are plenty of things about rehab that are far better than 20 years ago, including the following:

- The evolution of wheelchair design has advanced so far that rehab professionals are now able to fit people to their ideal chair and extend their independence in ways that had not previously been possible.
- Bedding and cushion technology have significantly reduced the risk of decubitus ulcers (skin breakdown), which have often interfered with being able to participate in the rehabilitation process.
- Assistive technology has evolved that gives people with limited arm use much more control over their environment. Rehab centers increasingly have dedicated staff who identify such solutions and provide training during the rehab stay.
- Psychological, sexual, family, financial, and political dynamics of disability are addressed in ways that they were not in the past.

Shorter Stays

Stays of several months in rehab were once common. Longer stays allowed people more opportunity to develop strength, gain skills, and make psychological adjustments and for family members to prepare for the return to home.

Stays of several months are now very rare, given current insurance coverage. There are exceptions. Veterans Administration rehab hospitals have achieved a much higher level of quality than you might remember from the film *Born on the Fourth of July*. Veterans are more likely to be sent home when they're ready instead of when the clock runs out on insurance. Those covered by workers' compensation also sometimes fare better; some rehab centers are able to exert more influence on funders. Some succeed at getting funded for an optimal length of stay by the sheer force of strenuous advocacy, often asserted by a family member or friend. A person's claim must generally demonstrate that he or she is continuing to make gains in order to be allowed to stay. However, much rehab work is slow and small gains are the natural pace. The pressure to show progress can cause great stress.

Longer periods of acute care in a hospital before transferring into a rehab program were once the norm.

> *I spent six weeks in a contraption called a "circle electric" bed, which was used to alternate me from my back to my chest so I wouldn't develop pressure sores as I recovered from my surgery. Having had my broken spine fused, I had to lie straight while it healed.*

The common practice now with spinal injuries is to mechanically stabilize the spine with surgically-implanted "Harrington rods" and get you up. There are often secondary injuries in traumatic accidents, such as broken bones, injured organs, or even a brain injury. There might not be a full commitment to optimal medical stability before heading to rehab. Some people arrive less than fully prepared to benefit as much as possible from the intensive work of inpatient rehabilitation.

For people who find themselves in rehab only days after a disabling injury, it can be very difficult to commit emotionally to the rehab process—assuming they are even medically stable enough for the hard work of rehab. Says Dr. David Chen of the Rehabilitation Institute of Chicago:

> *There was a time when we would never see an IV pole on a rehab floor. Now it's common.*

The initial, acute period of medical recovery can be an important opportunity to make the emotional adjustment to disability and find out more about what your degree of impairment will actually be. Some people do regain function, after all, and this informs choices made in the rehab program.

A person with a traumatic injury needs more than medical stabilization. The psychological shock and its social implications can be massive, but the short rehab periods that are now typical barely allow people to begin these adjustments. Dr. Marcel Dijkers, a rehab researcher at the Mt. Sinai School of Medicine in New York City, observes:

> *The compression of length of stay forces us to treat people as "patients" rather than being a socio-emotional development center where people can take time and think about what has happened to them. In Europe they still have lengths of stay of four and five months with a very low-key treatment program. It might look like they are just hanging around, but they talk*

*and interact and have the opportunity to adjust. Here, we
essentially kick them out just as they are starting the mental
change process.*

Short stays also put the squeeze on patient services staff who are
trying to organize equipment, modifications, support resources, and financial coverage you will need when you leave. Bonnie Sims directs the
Patient Services Group at Denver's Craig Hospital. She says: "Resources
may be out there, but the challenge is to call them into play within the
time allotted."

Despite shorter stays, rehab can become comfortable and safe compared to the outside world, which can seem quite scary to someone about
to return to that world on wheels. Rehab staff are very aware of the danger
of allowing people to get too settled into rehab, where they are in a largely
obstacle-free setting, are taken care of, don't need to discipline themselves
thanks to a built-in schedule of activities, and are generally surrounded by
people who understand their disability. At some point, it is time to move
on. And it is important to not delay that time unnecessarily.

Those with high quadriplegia have a number of unique issues to deal
with. They might use a ventilator to breathe and might rely more on others
to get dressed and get in and out of their chair. They are unable to do their
own pressure-relief lifts and have more extensive muscle atrophy, so they are
at greater risk of developing pressure sores. Sores limit the ability to participate in therapy and might make a longer stay necessary.

Rehab practitioners must squeeze much more treatment into much
less time. Many mourn the fact that they know they are unable to accomplish as much as they want and that people are not being given sufficient
time to adapt to what has happened. Since rehab now begins so soon after
injury, the focus is placed more on medical stabilization. Says Dr. Alex
Barchuk, physiatrist at the Kentfield Rehabilitation Hospital in northern
California:

*Basically all rehab is doing is providing a good environment
for the body to heal. There are so many things that can go
wrong—blood clots, pressure ulcers, things like that—which
really can affect the long-term rehab of an individual.*

Sandra Loyer, clinical social worker at the University of Michigan
Rehabilitation Unit, sees that, rather than helping people to complete rehab,
staff must teach people to do it for themselves after they leave:

*All we can do is get them medically stable, teach them basic
skills like bowel and bladder management, help them attain*

what strength they can in that time, and then they're gone. We
have to help them be able to advocate for themselves because
we just can't follow through for them.

In other words, having made the best possible effort to ensure you get
to rehab only when you're good and ready, once there it should be recognized as a precious opportunity that will last for only a limited time. Even
if psychological strain is telling you to resist, do all you can to keep moving
forward with the guidance of the rehab team. You don't want to look back
on this period with regret that you didn't make the most of it. Your rehab
stay, no matter how long or short, will make an inestimable difference in
the quality of life you ultimately achieve.

Not All Bad

It can be beneficial to initiate the rehab process sooner so you can begin to
develop strength and skills. The goal of early rehab is to make the healing
process more efficient—which saves costs and also speeds your return to
independence. This early rehab approach can also head off certain risks associated with extended bed rest, including progressive weakening, pressure
sores, contracted muscles, infection, or falling into a depressive or angry
state. Any and all of this can interfere with your eventual commitment to the
rehab process.

Shorter stays have also motivated rehab providers to tighten the efficiency of their programs. The luxury of longer stays did not require them to
design a rehab stay so that a person made the most progress in the best possible time span. The pressure from insurance companies has motivated
providers to tighten up their systems, as well as to pursue more detailed
research into what really works. Dr. Scott of Rancho Los Amigos states:

I don't know that shorter stays are all bad. I think we've
learned to become more efficient, working at how to be
more critical about what we do, about what works and
what doesn't work. There's a lot more attention being paid
to functional outcome.

Different Approaches in Response to Short Stays

At some centers, it has become common practice to send a quadriplegic
home with a halo on and discontinue therapy until it is time for the halo to
come off. Rich Patterson has C5 quadriplegia and directs the peer support
program at the Santa Clara Valley Medical Center in northern California.
He says:

They will send people home with a halo on because they feel
that their therapy has stopped. Once equipment can come off,
they come back for therapy. People have to use their own
equipment or rentals and loaners. Most of those people come
back with pressure sores or are very dejected, confused,
and frustrated.

That does not have to be the case. A quadriplegic man in his 20s states:

I was happy to be sent home until my halo could come
off. I got to be with my family and spend time with my
friends. They would take me to restaurants, and we had a
great time. I was in a much better mood by the time I went
back into rehab.

A greater emphasis has been placed on outpatient services. Once your time as an inpatient has reached its coverage limit, then the rehab process can—in fact, must—continue by regularly returning to the rehab center for therapy and support. Outpatient services are also sometimes limited by insurance funding, so you might require yet another round of persistent advocacy.

An example is the Do It! program at the Mt. Sinai Rehabilitation Center in New York City. The program includes components such as aerobics, computer education, community integration, a psychotherapy group, a technology group, weight training, and wheelchair mobility. Not only do the staff members deliver outpatient services, but they foster continued contact with others going through the same adjustments. They provide an opportunity to address specific issues—and skills—involved in community reintegration, as well as the internal adjustments of being in the world as a person with a disability for the first time. Says Mt. Sinai's Jim Cesario:

The Do It! program's philosophy is to emphasize health
promotion, wellness, and advocacy rather than disability,
injury, and dependency. Trained peer mentors empower the
participants by sharing their knowledge and experience.

Do It! is an example of a day program—sometimes called a "bridge" program—where overnight stays are no longer necessary, but one spends a full day in rehab activities on an outpatient basis. The full range of services, including occupational therapy, physical therapy, psychology, and nutrition are available, all with an emphasis on community reintegration. These have become an increasingly common feature of rehab programs.

Telerehab

The advent of the Internet, the low price and small size of video cameras, and the presence of high-speed Internet in almost everyone's home have fostered the growing field of telemedicine. Certain kinds of therapy and information gathering can take place through a videoconference without having to go to the rehab center at all. Some centers will send a client home with a camera and connections needed for teleconferencing in order to help manage the reentry process, to answer questions as they come up, or to assist with the continuing process of home modification.

Diagnostics can also be performed in situations such as the appearance of a pressure sore. Clearly it is far more effective to be able to see someone's home or skin or posture in a wheelchair to help resolve such issues. This is likely to be a dramatically emerging and more common technology, although some people have had difficulty being comfortable using it.

Too Far from Home

An appropriate rehab program might not exist within range of where you live. Many people travel to major regional rehab centers, such as Craig Hospital in Denver or Shepherd Center in Atlanta. The inevitable discharge from the inpatient facility to a location too far away for a day program means that a primary focus of the inpatient rehab plan should be the design of a great home rehab program.

Community-based rehab has arisen from the short-stay issue, personified by Rehab Without Walls, a service of Gentiva Health Services, Inc. A rehab team, including many of the same types of therapists who work at the inpatient and outpatient centers, designs a continuing rehab program that can be performed at home and in the community. A therapist will visit and identify activities that can be performed in the home, as well as at a local facility, such as a local health club or university athletic center.

Simulating What You'll Go Home To

An increasingly common feature found at rehab centers is an apartment unit where one can spend a few nights—potentially with a family member or spouse—to closer approximate some of the issues that will arise once home. Usually very basic—with a bedroom, bathroom, living room, and kitchen—an on-site apartment is where you can regain control of how you spend your own time, prepare your own meals, choose your bedtime, get in and out of a regular bed instead of a hospital bed, and so on. There is still the security of rehab staff being at hand if needed, with emergency pull cords at hand.

Some larger centers have a separate building where someone approaching release from an inpatient facility can spend weeks. Family members can spend a significant time getting trained in what kinds of assistance they might be providing—or helping to train a hired assistant to perform.

On the Street Where You Live

Rehab is a very controlled environment. Everything is accessible, the floors are smooth and level, doors are wide, and so many of the elements of a daily life—from the ATM machine to bank or hotel counters that are above eye level—are completely nonexistent.

Some rehab centers have built areas that specifically simulate these elements. During the inpatient stay, it is possible to encounter common obstacles and conditions of the outside world, with the consultation of therapists and experienced chair users on hand to improve skills before discharge from the program.

Magee Rehab in Philadelphia has built such a resource on the roof of their building—which means that those who are inpatient at the facility during the winter get the extra gift of dealing with snow and slush before going home! It includes typical sidewalks—where joints are commonly raised up by tree roots—and the kind of not-so-smooth-and-level surfaces one might encounter at a door or near a parking space.

Adaptive Technology

Technology has made a tremendous contribution to the range of options for people with disabilities, especially for persons with more significant disabilities such as high quadriplegia. As these technologies have become more advanced, smaller, lighter, and less expensive, rehab centers have been able to equip themselves with training rooms where clients can be exposed to options, be assessed for what works best for them according to their goals, and get trained in their use. If returning to an existing job is a priority, access to adaptive technologies in rehab can move that process along much more quickly.

Computers contribute in four areas.

- Control of mobility. Power wheelchairs have evolved in quality and flexibility. Speed and acceleration can be finely controlled. Voice-controlled wheelchairs are not far off. Digital controls for vans are also making driving an option for more quadriplegics.

■   Control of the environment. Commercial products allow remote con-
     trol of doors, lights, telephones, or almost any electrical device from
     the wheelchair. The remote controller might be a keypad similar to
     the television remote control or a puff-and-sip device for people with
     limited arm use.
■   Communication. The Internet connects people to the world. It has
     discussion groups and is a powerful resource and research tool. For
     those with limited ability to get out of the home—however tempo-
     rary—the Internet can become a place of community and support. It
     can extend the rehab process by helping people discover possibilities
     they didn't know existed.
■   Vocational possibilities. Research has shown that computer skills erase
     the pay gap that people with disabilities otherwise experience in the
     job market. Adaptive keyboards and voice control systems provide full
     computer access and thus access to jobs that have nothing to do with
     physical labor. Many rehab centers with fully equipped computer labs
     include computer training during the inpatient rehab experience.

Nontraumatic Disabilities

Someone in an accident who acquires a spinal cord or brain injury will find
himself in a medical facility and will generally be transferred to a rehabilitation services program. But what of people with a condition from birth,
such as muscular dystrophy or spina bifida, or with a progressive condition
that appears later, such as multiple sclerosis (MS) or amyotrophic lateral
sclerosis (ALS)? How are they helped to adapt to a disability, particularly
when the progressive nature of a condition demands continuing adjustment?

Organizations dedicated to specific disabilities sponsor services at
major medical centers or sometimes finance their own facilities. The
National Multiple Sclerosis Society is very active in making support available nationwide, as are the Muscular Dystrophy Association, American
Syringomyelia Alliance Project, United Cerebral Palsy, and the Spina Bifida
Association, among others. If you are facing a late-onset progressive disability, your doctor should refer you to such sources. However, doctors are not
always well informed about what options are available for you. You might
need to research such programs on your own. These groups and services
may be able to help you adapt to the condition in ways that your present
doctor might be unaware of, and may possibly even reduce the progression
or impact of the condition by informing you of recent advances in research.

For example, Shepherd Center in Atlanta has established an MS
center—one of 32 in the US—that provides both inpatient and outpatient

services. Shepherd Center is a medical unit with staff members who are capable of diagnosis and treatment and who participate in research and clinical drug trials, at the option of the client. A study published in the *Archives of Physical Medicine and Rehabilitation* found clear benefits to a period of inpatient rehabilitation for people with MS. People in the group with intensive treatment learned greater degrees of adaptive skill and came out with better attitudes about their ability to function with MS than did the group who came as outpatients.[1]

People with MS or ALS typically establish a working relationship with a neurologist. However, if the neurologist is attending to many people with other conditions, she might not gain the same detailed experience as someone working in rehab who spends her time with people with a given condition. Cynthia Bishop of Shepherd's MS center notes:

> *Neurologists may have a very small percentage of patients with MS. The patient might be getting good medical treatment from her neurologist, but the doctor is not able to be completely current in the many developments happening in MS and its treatments. We might see patients and notice that they're starting to experience foot drop and will refer them to our brace clinic and help them with their gait in therapy. A neurologist might not notice that. A person with MS commonly has issues with bladder or bowels. A neurologist is not an expert in that type of thing. You really need someone who knows rehab.*

Transition from Childhood Disability

The rehab system discussed in this chapter is largely targeted to adults, many of whom already work or are educated. Many disabilities are work related; conditions such as MS typically occur in adulthood. Children with disabilities such as cerebral palsy, spina bifida, or muscular dystrophy are serviced under a different system.

With the passage of the Individuals with Disabilities Education Act in 1975, children began to be integrated into public schools, and those systems were required to provide services to those children. In effect, rehab for children gets delivered through the school system—although parents and schools sometimes find themselves in conflict over the extent and nature of these services. Physical therapists work with children with disabilities at the schools. Equipment and medical services continue to be supplied by charitable organizations.

The difficulty with this delivery system is what happens when children become adults. For some, the transition is not smooth. This man with muscular dystrophy is angry about what happened once he became an adult:

> Throughout my childhood and adolescence, these agencies were very good about providing various things I needed such as wheelchairs, orthopedic shoes, braces, clinics, etc. Unfortunately, when I became an adult, they forgot I existed. I no longer fit their marketable, "dying child" image.

Once children with disabilities leave the school system where they were receiving medical and therapeutic services, they need to establish a relationship with physicians and facilities qualified and equipped to address their needs. New issues also appear in adulthood, such as weight gain, the start of sexual activity, living independently, driving, or alcohol use. People in such transition need a specialized set of services, and the family doctor is not in a position to provide them. As Stanford Hospital's Jody Greenhalgh describes the transition:

> When they turn 18, where do they go? Hopefully the children's services doctors refer them to a rehab doctor, but it doesn't always happen. If they get a job and go on an HMO program, they get assigned a primary physician who may not know much about their disability. The physician may not know their equipment needs or that they need ongoing therapy.

Dealing with Insurance

Many medical professionals believe that insurance companies have gained excessive control of medical treatment. Spending limits tie the hands of physicians, whether limits are set by a health maintenance organization, private insurance, or government programs like Medicare. Medical professionals chafe at decision-making control being out of their hands. Insurers complain of cost pressures, rising prices, shrinking profits, and a healthcare system too expensive for many people to afford. Business owners trying to provide coverage with minimal employee contributions to premiums also add pressure to insurers. Because the insurers are demanding lower costs, we, as a result, receive less coverage. The issue is too complex to simply demonize insurers.

Alex Barchuk of the Kentfield Rehabilitation Hospital in northern California states:

> All these new products coming out are great, but no one can afford to buy them. Insurance doesn't pay for them. We've all

transitioned into managed care. We get reimbursed at a per diem rate. No matter what we do in the hospital, the insurance company doesn't care—they pay us a certain amount. Somebody can cost us $2,400 a day, and the insurer pays $750 a day. In that situation, you have to go with cheaper medications that have good efficacy. You can't compromise somebody but, a lot of the new wheelchairs—the ones that stand or recline—the insurance companies don't want to go with. We have to really fight for those.

Cynthia Bishop of the MS center at Atlanta's Shepherd Center knows that inpatient stays are very effective in certain situations for people with MS:

We have all the research articles about the value of inpatient stays for people with MS, because the difficulty we have is getting insurers to pay. Since MS is a progressive disease, the insurer's position is, "What's the point? You can rehab them now, but they'll only be worse later." It seems ridiculous, but that's what they say. The insurance people can see that if you have a spinal cord injury, there's a major life change and you need rehab. It's one time, and then they're done with it. But, with MS, a person might need rehab five different times. It's a hard sell.

The new insurance environment has affected a critical piece of equipment for Bob Mauro, a writer and disability activist with significant postpolio syndrome. His Medicare coverage—now administered by a private HMO—has begun to deny coverage for a second ventilator, which allows him flexible mobility by use of one by his bed and the other on his power wheelchair. More importantly, the second ventilator is a backup in case the primary ventilator breaks down—which they inevitably do.

I cannot express the terror these routine denial letters give me. I only have two ventilators, and both are vital. I must have two ventilators to stay alive! I am permanently disabled, will not get better, and will probably get worse as I age.

By the Book

The services and coverage you get are increasingly defined by manuals and policies developed at hospitals and insurance offices. Managed care can lead to cookie-cutter classifications and treatments, with some danger of not seeing the case or person as a whole. According to Jody Greenhalgh:

*Insurance has disability ratings, and people get plugged in.
"This is how many days you're going to be seen; this is
where you should go." But not everyone fits the mold of
the way insurers see these cases. There might be other conditions along with the one they've rated, and it makes a big
difference in what someone really needs. There's a lot of
education [needed] to get insurance to look at the bigger
picture.*

There can be advantages to these automated, modular approaches to
care. Once you have been given a disability rating, any member of your
healthcare team might recognize a certain condition. By reporting it, they
will initiate a trigger that automatically leads to a pathway of treatment.
When these triggers and pathways are clearly defined, the doctor is spared
having to diagnose and prescribe every last detail of treatment. It makes her
job more efficient and can get you into the treatment process sooner, keep
you from losing strength, and get you back to your life sooner. In the
process, the insurer saves money, which helps.

Managed care has attempted to improve the efficiency of a medical
system laden with immense demands and expense, while trying to ensure
that care is appropriate for the individual. Your medical care cannot be
entirely automated. There needs to be flexibility to adjust to changes.

The Rehab Team

You have arrived at rehab, which means that a group of dedicated and highly
trained professionals are at your service—the rehab team. The team consists
of a case manager and others in patient services, a physician, and a range of
therapists, depending on your needs. The team is committed to helping you
reach the highest possible level of function with your disability.

Dr. Gary Yarkony of the Rehabilitation Institute of Chicago observes:

*The foundation of a comprehensive rehabilitation program is
an interdisciplinary team. The staff must be willing to work
together while breaking down the boundaries of individual
disciplines for the betterment of those they serve.*[2]

Jody Greenhalgh of Stanford University Hospital notes that the respective roles of team members are important:

*Regardless of what discipline you are from, when you go in to
assess rehab needs, you find yourself advocating for the*

patient's needs. Although I'm an occupational therapist, I'll
point out a physical therapy need, when I see it.

You, your family, and peer supporters will also function as part of the rehab team.

Patient and Family Services

Patient services—often referred to as the social work department—will deal with finding resources, determining insurance coverage, and making sure you get all the benefits to which you are entitled. Even before you arrived, your case manager was looking into insurance policies and participating in the admissions process. Case managers deal with insurance adjusters; bureaucrats at federal, state, and local levels; charitable agencies; and the team at the facility who will serve you.

The people who do this work might have a social work degree or not. Bonnie Sims explains:

> *We have counselors with varied degrees in our department,*
> *but all have a master's degree in their field. We hire with an*
> *eye to experience as well as a degree, which gives us differing*
> *viewpoints.*

Your case manager or social worker is a key member of the team with whom you might develop a close relationship. Sandra Loyer, clinical social worker at the University of Michigan Medical Center in Ann Arbor states:

> *I am often one of the first people to make contact with the*
> *patient and the family. That is a chance to develop a close rela-*
> *tionship from the start. I try to make them comfortable enough*
> *to ask me whatever questions are on their mind, and then I get*
> *the chance to find out more about their needs. I often discover*
> *important details that I pass on to the rest of the rehab team.*

It is a challenge for a case manager or rehabilitation counselor to spend as much time as they'd like on each person's case. With the pressure to contain costs and the complexity of the job, there is only so much time available to be a good listener. Many times case managers feel they can do their best for you by getting back on the phone to explore services and benefits to meet your needs. Bonnie Sims observes:

> *The counseling relationship can be very supportive to some*
> *people. However, the opportunity to create this relationship*
> *has become limited. Counselors spend so much time on the*

financial and discharge issues that it becomes difficult to
spend quality time with patients.

You might be unaware of some of the benefits you have. For example, you might have credit card insurance or a policy for your mortgage or auto loan that makes payments if you become disabled. A case manager should ask these questions and help you research all possible ways to ease your financial burden.

Unfortunately, much of the case manager's time is spent trying to make up for coverage you don't have. Sims notes:

When people buy insurance, they assume they have coverage
for all their needs, including healthcare. This is usually
not the case, and so much of their care ends up falling to
the family.

Often people must take extreme measures to qualify for state Medicaid to fill the gaps left in home care or equipment. They are required to spend their savings and assets before they qualify for assistance. Basically, they become paupers to get the care they need. There is a huge array of details involved in government programs like Medicare, Medicaid, workers' compensation, or vocational rehabilitation; in the particulars of any given policy from any of hundreds of insurers; in the offerings of charitable groups like Easter Seals or the local Rotary Club; and in programs offered by centers for independent living (CILs), and so on. Sims says:

We have to spend almost as much time researching as we do
working on the actual cases. I spend an inordinate amount of
time just keeping up with changes and what programs are out
there, trying to keep current and keep my staff current. I don't
have time as a supervisor to actually take cases. We've got so
many resource listings, packets, and handouts—it can be
overwhelming just keeping up.

There are many preparations to make for the day you leave rehab and return to your daily life in the outside world, a process that begins even before you arrive. Patient services might arrange transportation, set up the relationship with a home healthcare agency, or assist you with finding personal assistance services, as necessary. Sims finds that discharge is often difficult:

The transition out to the community is always chaotic. We
never know why everything breaks down at the last minute.
You get the whole thing set up, you get the home health
agency ready to come in, then the patient gets sick and you

have to cancel everything. Or when you implement discharge,
you forget something, so the transportation goes awry, and so
forth. Some chaos is typical.

Take good advantage of the patient services staff. Get to know them early and learn all you can. Start planning for departure as soon as possible, and you'll have a better chance of making a smooth transition from rehab.

The Physician

The physician—most often a "physiatrist," who is a specialist in physical medicine and rehabilitation—is the leader of the team. The physiatrist coordinates the members of the team, is responsible for maintaining clear records that everyone on the team will share and contribute to, and oversees the common strategy. The physiatrist relies on input from other team members who are spending time with you. Dr. Scott explains:

The physician is the team leader, but the leadership shifts
depending on the topic on hand. For instance, if a psychologi-
cal issue is at hand, then the psychologist takes the lead.

The doctor's goal is to help you be in the best possible health so you can get the most out of rehab. There is a tremendous amount of research and information for a doctor to keep up with to bring the latest resources to bear in supporting your rehab effort. The quality of your relationship with the doctor has tremendous impact. In the past, doctors were likely to play a very strong leadership role, taking little stock of the personal experience of their clients, making unilateral decisions, or at least making it difficult for someone to disagree. To this day, many people find themselves intimidated by their physicians, afraid to speak up, hesitant to challenge them. But this attitude is changing, both on the part of people who now prefer to be "clients" or "consumers" rather than "patients" and on the part of some doctors exploring a more holistic approach.

With restricted budgets and pressure for hospitals to work efficiently and profitably, doctors' schedules are very tight. As much as they might want to be good listeners, or take time to learn more about your life and experience, they are hard pressed to be able to devote the kind of time you might prefer. You can help by being prepared with questions and being informed. Take advantage of therapists, nurses, other rehab consumers, and a rehab center library, if one exists.

Doctors are human. They aren't perfect. The nature of your relationship with them should not be one of absolute trust but one of respectful cooperation. If you suspect someone is not competent or fully committed to your needs, pursue your right to ask for someone else. If you are not getting what you need, or if you can tell that something is not right, speak up. Statistically, mistakes are far more the exception than the rule, but they do happen.

> *When my halo was removed, I was told it would not hurt.*
> *There were originally two people removing my halo, but*
> *one got called away in the process. He had only unscrewed*
> *half of the screw on the front left side before he left, and*
> *the other doctor pulled on it thinking it was completely*
> *unscrewed.*

Rehabilitation Nurses

Perhaps more than any other team members, the nursing staff will be the people with whom you have your central relationship. Rehabilitation nursing is a certified specialty, supported by organizations such as the Association for Rehabilitation Nursing and the American Association of Spinal Cord Injury Nurses. The associations provide continuing education required for certification. Rehab nurses are trained in being able to recognize and attend to the unique needs of people with disabilities. Nurses in a general hospital might not ever see autonomic dysreflexia, deal with pressure sore management, or understand the respiratory needs of someone with postpolio syndrome, for instance.

Rehab nurses play many roles. They treat. They advise the client, the family, and the physician. They teach. They interact with and support the rehab team. They are crucial to the rehab process, since they have regular contact with you and because they are generalists, able to recognize any of many different needs you might have. They also direct the nursing aides who do much of the hands-on daily work, such as assisting you with bladder and bowel care, washing, or dressing. The rehab nurse might also achieve the most trust and connection and, so, be a source of emotional support, possibly fielding personal questions the client is uncomfortable asking.

The family dynamics and emotional experience of early disability are best supported by professionals experienced with the complex set of adjustments you are called upon to make in rehab. Nurses can be a source of tremendous emotional support.

> *I was in rehab to have a large sore closed surgically. After*
> *weeks of not sitting while it healed, I was at last allowed to*
> *start to sit for brief periods in preparation for going home. It*
> *turned out that the sore had not healed properly beneath the*
> *skin, and it broke down again, leaving another large, open*

wound. In that moment, when I realized that I was about to
spend another several weeks there, having the rehab nurse
just sit with me after showing me the sore and explaining
what had happened was a great comfort. She knew she didn't
have to say anything. I could tell she understood how upset I
was. It meant so much to me that she would commit her time
to me and not leave me alone.

Therapists

Therapists who specialize in rehabilitation must strike a balance between driving you to work hard and keeping an upbeat and friendly atmosphere. Their job is to encourage and support you in applying yourself as fully—and enjoyably—as possible to the process of rehabilitation.

There will always be some people who don't connect or a therapist who is difficult to work with, as this paraplegic woman found.

The only trouble I had was with one of my physical thera-
pists. I ended up firing her because we had no rapport at all.
She was patronizing and mean.

But the following view is probably more typical.

My therapists made a huge difference in the process of getting
back to my life after my injury, and I think I have been more
successful because of it. I bless them for their contributions to
my life.

Your therapy will be customized to your needs and the issues of your disability. Someone with MS will have a very different program from someone with a spinal cord injury, as explained by Cynthia Bishop.

With MS, the problem is not inability to walk; it's a combina-
tion of gait difficulties and severe fatigue. MS causes very,
very severe fatigue. Physical therapy for MS has to take this
into account, along with the problem of overheating. Even a
core temperature increase of .5 degree in an MS patient can
affect his or her ability to function. It's not anything like
spinal cord injury where you just work, work, work, work,
work 'til you drop!

The ranks of specialized therapists include physical therapy, occupational therapy, respiratory therapy, recreation therapy, and speech therapy. These people are experts who have worked with other people in your situation and have seen them master the skills they will be teaching you.

When you first enter rehab, some goals might seem unattainable—whether lifting yourself easily in and out of a wheelchair or becoming accustomed to breathing with a ventilator. These doubts are a common and normal reaction, particularly to people with sudden trauma, with its dramatic change in physical capacity.

Your rehab program will be based on goals developed by the team along with your input. Members of the team are unlikely to suggest a course of rehab work unless they think that your medical status allows for it. They will have seen others in situations similar to yours and know from past experience what is possible. They might know that you can go beyond limits that seem unreachable to you. They will ask you to put a certain amount of faith in them—and in yourself.

Therapists must set reasonable goals for you, day by day, and let you know what to expect. You might make very gradual progress that seems too slow to you but is expected for a person in your situation. The better you understand the expected pace of your rehabilitation, the more you will be able to celebrate your advances, instead of pressuring yourself and feeling that you are failing because things are going too slowly. As you give your therapist honest feedback about your experience, you can work together to adjust your program as you go.

Your Roles

The hard work you will do (read "be driven like a slave to do") while in rehab makes a tremendous difference in your range of options and degree of independence, but rehab only gets part of the credit. Its contribution is of no use unless you choose to make the most of the experience, use the tools and skills offered, and continue your own process of growth and evolution after you leave. This woman with C6/7 quadriplegia observes:

> The public approaches me with the attitude I was "taught"
> independence in "therapy." Nothing could be further from the
> truth. It took years of personal exploration and peer examples
> to get where I am.

Many rehab centers will include you in team reviews of your case. How much you participate is up to you, but it is your right to ask questions and have your say. Of all the members, you are the most important person on the team.

Your main role is the hard work you will do, which offers you the chance to reach your optimal ability and, in the process, gain a sense of the range of possibilities open to you. People often discover that those possibilities reach much further than first imagined. Novelist Reynolds Price, after being paralyzed by cancer, describes his rehab experience in his book, *A Whole New Life*:

> *Few sessions passed without my learning at least one skill,*
> *and soon I felt surprising new strength in my arms and*
> *chest—more upper-body strength than in my past life.*
> *Throughout that summer, my chest size went from forty-two*
> *inches to forty-six, and my arms and wrists thickened pro-*
> *portionally. Best of all, the new skills produced in most of us*
> *a heady sense of control and choice. Those physical choices*
> *are obviously more limited than the almost limitless array*
> *that's offered to the able bodied. But in time I was skilled*
> *enough in the homely detours and reinventions to put myself*
> *through almost all the motions I needed for the necessary*
> *work of my life.*[3]

You will also need to advocate for yourself to make your hospital/rehab stay as humane as possible. If you find yourself faced with a staff member who won't or can't take the time to listen, choose an ally who has time to campaign for your needs. It can be helpful to talk to patient advocates, social workers, peer support volunteers, psychologists, or simply someone who has taken a personal interest. Any one of them might prove to be your most effective champion.

The Role of the Family

Your family plays an important role in your rehab experience and influences your attitude. It is of inestimable value for you to have regular visits and to know that family members are seeing to personal business outside of the facility and that they are sharing the emotional adjustments of the rehab process. Your disability, in fact, has happened to them, too. Rehab staff know the importance of family involvement. Rich Patterson Peer Support Coordinator at Santa Clara Valley Medical Center notes:

> *It's important for us to get to the family as soon as possible,*
> *to help them make sense out of the situation, explaining*
> *how rehab is going to help, what physical and occupational*
> *therapy are about. In general they know what those people*
> *do, but they don't know how it's going to apply to their*
> *family member.*

Family members also need to learn the line between reasonable expectations and hope. This is a delicate line, says Patterson:

*It is more common than not that people think they're going to
walk out. You have to tread lightly on that one because you
can easily upset the family and the person by saying they
won't walk out. Their denial is a coping mechanism.*

A disability experience is a potent test of the quality of family relationships. It reveals the depth of commitment and ability to adapt to a crisis.
Family response can express itself in extremes. Christopher Reeve's wife,
Dana, was a model of being entirely involved in his support. She affirmed
from the start that she would stay with him for the rest of his life. On the
other hand, according to Margaret Nosek who researches women with disabilities at Baylor College of Medicine:

*It could be a very minor injury and the spouse is out the door.
This is not related to the level of severity. It has more to do
with the quality of the marriage before the disability.*

Peer Support

While in rehab, you are likely to get a visit from someone who had an experience similar to the one you are going through or be invited to attend peer
support meetings. Although everyone's experience is different, the chance to
talk with someone who has a similar condition can be very powerful. Janie
Whiteford, peer support coordinator in Santa Clara, California, explains:

*Though doctors and therapists talk about these things, some-
times it is more validating to hear it from a peer. Sometimes
there are things going on in the hospital that the client needs
to talk about, such as relationships with staff.*

Not everyone is ready to meet someone who has made the adjustment
to disability. It is very common to operate on a belief in recovery during the
acute stage after an injury or to feel committed to resisting a progressive
disease. This quadriplegic man describes his first visit from a peer supporter:

*I remember somebody coming to visit me, and he was in a
chair. He was talking to me about life in a chair and what had
happened to him, and I just refused to accept that I was anyone like him. I kind of resented him being there, although I
realized it was a nice gesture on his part and he was trying
to help.*

After rehab, some people participate in outreach programs sponsored
by the rehab hospital. Rancho Los Amigos has a program called Teens on
Target, which also exists in other communities. Says Dr. Michael Scott:

*Teens on Target is a violence-prevention program for adoles-
cents. They meet on a regular basis and go out to talk to kids
in schools. It is an effort to do proactive outreach to prevent
injuries. It has a rehabilitative effect for the people going out
to speak, too.*

Peer support doesn't have to happen in a formal, organized manner.
People build relationships as they encounter each other in rehab, whether
inpatient or outpatient. Cynthia Bishop has seen people create close bonds:

*We have formal support groups, but I think a lot of the best
peer support is the informal stuff that happens at the aquatic
classes, or in physical therapy, or in our waiting room! It gets
to be a social thing, too. People make their appointments
together so they can hang out with their friends while they
do it.*

One benefit of a specialized rehab center is the chance to share the
experience with others who are facing the same challenges and process. This
bonding is encouraged by rehab staff, who are often surprised by the deep
friendships that develop. Friendships are also a source of some fun in rehab,
particularly during an inpatient stay. This quadriplegic man was injured at
the age of 14 in 1977:

*I made some great friends. Most days after training classes,
we would get together and party a little. Just off the corner of
the rehab property was a place we called "The White House"
where we would party in the front yard. A few times, in the
fall when it started getting cold, we would build a small fire.
During the cold months, we would sneak in some orange juice
and rum and party in a friend's dorm room.*

Not all rehab centers allow people freedom to come and go from the
property, but people have a way of finding places to meet. Bonnie Sims notes
that Craig Hospital has a Friendship House where families, friends, and
patients meet, away from the hospital atmosphere.

Physical Therapy

Our strength and mobility are the main concerns of physical therapists. The
physical therapist will work with you in areas such as:

■   Exercising specific muscles and muscle groups
■   Stretching and range-of-motion exercises
■   Developing balance

- ■ Wheelchair skills
- ■ Transfer training
- ■ Bed mobility
- ■ Aquatics
- ■ Standing programs
- ■ For some people, gait training

As a wheelchair user, you will need a certain level of strength for many activities. For people with paraplegia or quadriplegia who have sufficient upper body function, your arms will take on much of the work that you used to do with your legs. Not only will you push a wheelchair, but you will also do "transfers"—lifting your body into and out of the wheelchair.

The strength you have will substantially influence how much you can do on your own, without assistance. A sufficient level of strength will allow you to perform daily functions with less fatigue, handling your body and the wheelchair with less exertion and strain.

Muscles and Stretching

Physical therapists know your anatomy and what muscles allow you to move or balance. Based on the nature of your disability and an evaluation, the therapist will know exactly what muscles you have control of, and will design exercises and use equipment to make the most of what you have.

Physical therapy is a precise process. To exercise a certain muscle in your arm, you need to apply resistance to that muscle in a particular direction in order to make it work and become stronger.

Each person and each condition involves some special need. Many wheelchair users will need to develop strength for pushing wheels and for pressure-relief push-ups in their chair. Someone with quadriplegia might have control of only some muscles in the upper arm that can be strengthened enough to lift the forearm at the elbow. Someone with a traumatic brain injury and resultant cognitive difficulties needs to have a simply designed program that he can remember. Someone with a lower limb amputation will need a program for the residual limb, so that the muscles do not contract or get weak. (The muscles in the limb are not getting used for walking during the acute and rehab stages; if a prosthetic leg is to be fitted, it cannot happen until later so that healing of the socket can take place and swelling can be reduced.)

In rehab, you will need to do some serious stretching. Your muscles, tendons, and ligaments have a natural tendency to shorten when they are not used. The initial period after a traumatic injury is marked by very limited physical activity during which your tissues tighten up and become weak. You might not have been in great shape before the injury. The physical therapist will do stretching work with you, to soften up these tissues and increase the range of movement of your joints. Stretching is also part of the strength program. Elastic muscles that can travel a greater distance during a contraction are stronger.

Balance

Being immobilized for a period of recovery compromises your sense of balance. The physical therapist will help you recover and increase your sense of balance, strengthening the muscles that will help you achieve greater upper body stability. An activity as simple as playing catch with balls of various sizes is a common physical therapy technique for improving balance:

> *I remember how surprising it was to sit up in that bed for the first time in six weeks and find that I had to hold on to something to keep from falling over. My upper body was just dead weight. Sitting up was now foreign to my body. My center of balance was entirely different, given the loss of weight from muscle atrophy below the waist and from the fact that I no longer had the use of my legs to stabilize my upper body.*

After you have had a paralyzing injury, the map of your body changes. Your new center of gravity depends on the level and type of injury. Lower-level spinal disabilities leave more trunk muscles in contact with the brain. Use of the hips and abdominal muscles makes a big difference in your ability to maintain balance and stability while sitting and while engaged in any physical activity. With the loss of control of trunk muscles, more support is required from the wheelchair, and you will rely even more on arm strength to move your upper body. Strengthening can make the difference between independence and reliance on support.

Wheelchair Skills

In addition to building the muscles you will use when you propel your chair, you also need to gain experience using the chair. Your body learns from doing, and your nervous system and muscles adapt. At first, using the chair will feel awkward and foreign. You will have to think carefully as you wheel, whether by pushing on wheels, operating a joystick, or using breath control. It will not feel natural because you are unaccustomed to it.

The physical therapist's goal is to help you develop expertise in your chair. There are some refined movements that you'll have to think about at first, but, eventually, it will become second nature. For instance, when you turn a manual chair, you might either pull back on one wheel or else hold one wheel in place as you push the other, depending on the turning radius you need to achieve. You will apply just the right pressure in the right direction on a joystick, letting go to allow the precise time the chair needs to decelerate.

If you have sufficient strength and balance, you are likely to be taught to do a "wheelie," to negotiate curbs or single steps, going up and down. The technique is also helpful on uneven terrain. These skills extend independence and are worth learning to the degree you are able. Safety is the first priority.

Your therapist should prepare you for falling out of a wheelchair. If you play a sport like wheelchair basketball, hockey, or rugby, you can count on falling out. Even if you are careful and have excellent wheeling skills, accidents can happen. The therapist will teach you how to fall, practicing it with you so you will not be afraid. You can develop a natural, habitual reaction that protects you by properly breaking your fall. The therapist will teach you techniques for getting back into the wheelchair. If you have the strength, you'll be able to learn to transfer into your chair directly from the floor or by lifting yourself onto successively higher surfaces. If you don't have the strength or balance to perform such transfers on your own, it is still extremely valuable for you to learn to guide the people who will be assisting you.

Is a Wheelchair Necessary?

It is not always clear that someone should be using a wheelchair or for how long. Someone with MS might need one during a severe exacerbation or in the later stages of progressive MS. A person with brain injury might need one early on but, later, might reach a stage of needing wheels only for trips and when away from home. Viki Solomon is a rehab nurse who works with brain injury clients:

> My concerns are for the ones who have cognitive problems
> and who make strides in physical rehabilitation. I find they
> are often kept in the chair as a primary mode of transporta-
> tion because it is a way to restrain a person who has poor
> cognitive abilities. In other words, the wheelchair is used for
> staff convenience. What happens next is the person "learns"
> that he is wheelchair bound and so do the therapists and other
> professionals who treat the person.

The process of rehab should be about determining your proper relationship with a wheelchair, not to make you dependent on it when it might serve you best as a part-time tool. Therapy in that case would be to develop skills for using wheels, while at the same time working to optimize your walking abilities.

This woman in her forties has spinal cord quadriplegia, but she has limited ability to stand and walk. For her, the wheelchair proved to be the better solution, despite the beliefs of rehab staff:

> I'm an incomplete quad. It's a funny disability because it does-n't fit any of the categories. When I got out of rehab, I started off walking with a cane, which I still use in the house to some extent. This was back in the early '70s when the goal was to get you up on your feet if at all possible. My balance was very poor. I was just tottering around. The rehab staff thought it was great, but it was really dangerous. Eventually, I changed to using a chair. That was liberating because then I could cross streets by myself.

Gait Training

In the initial stage after onset of a mobility disability, it is entirely natural to want to walk, even if by means of some assistive devices. Based on the rehab team's assessment, you might be considered a candidate for gait training with braces and crutches. There is undeniable value to be gained from stand-ing and gait training: reaching high surfaces, interacting with other stand-ing people at eye level, or being able use an inaccessible bathroom. Weight bearing on your legs helps maintain bone health, warding off osteoporosis, a common secondary deficit that occurs with mobility disability. It also helps keep the tissues throughout your legs stretched, limiting the tendency towards contracture—chronic shortening of tendons and ligaments—which is another typical effect of paralysis.

Yet, standing takes some effort; balance has to be maintained much of the time with your arms using the crutches. It can be awkward to reach for things on that high shelf when you have to maintain your balance or to enjoy that conversation at eye level if you're getting tired from supporting yourself upright. The work it takes to develop the strength and skills to use braces is intensive. It is not for everyone. Dr. Michael Scott of Rancho Los Amigos describes how he approaches the option of gait training:

> We definitely motivate people with incomplete injuries who have gait potential, to maximize their locomotor ability. We evaluate complete paraplegics on an individual basis. We explain what it would be like walking with long leg braces with locked knees and crutches, and how it's not like walking

*before. We show them videotapes of what that would look
like, talk about the tremendous energy expenditure, and how
it's not really practical. For those who are motivated and have
enough upper body strength, we proceed.*

Uli Salas, of HealthSouth Rehabilitation Hospital, states:

*Standing is very motivating for some people. The chance to
get on their feet helps involve them more in the rehab process.
Then there are people who find very quickly that it is more
effort than they care to make and are satisfied with using a
wheelchair.*

Gait training involves being fitted for braces to keep knees from buck-
ling and feet from dropping as you propel yourself using crutches or a
walker. Some braces provide support for the hip as well. Most are made of
metal or plastic. Braces in general have become lighter in weight, and some
can be worn discreetly underneath clothing. If you have little strength in
the buttocks and upper leg muscles (which lock the knees), walking in this
way relies almost entirely on your arms and shoulders. Generally, people
with injuries above T12 are typically not considered candidates because of
lack of enough stability in their waist and abdomen. If you experience muscle spasticity, this is likely to exclude you as well. Gait training is not for
everyone, but, if you really believe it is possible for you and you want to
give it a shot, advocate for your chance to try:

*I think that the leg braces actually help to strengthen your
core. They did for me. My physical therapist is the one who
recommended that I get them, and I was terrified! All the doctors I'd seen told me I would not get any return, but she
believed in me. Don't ever let a doctor tell you that you can't
do something. Every injury is different.*

As compared to this person who didn't experience much success:

*I found gait training very painful. I could not tolerate it
for very long. It made me tilt my pelvis, and, even when I
was totally stretched, I couldn't handle it for more than
three minutes. I was afraid of falling, and it never seemed
practical.*

Since walking with braces is tantamount to being on stilts, there is a
risk of falling, breaking a bone, or developing a sore if you accidentally
bump yourself or are forced to sit on a hard surface; if you have atrophied
buttock muscles, you will have trouble finding properly cushioned surfaces.

Most people find that using a wheelchair is easiest and safest for their daily activities, but some like to be able to stand and walk, perhaps maintaining the skill to be used in certain situations—such as walking down the aisle at their own wedding.

There are a number of programs that offer intensive walking therapy employing braces. They typically involve months of work and considerable expense not likely to be covered by your insurance and are not associated with a formal rehab center or hospital. Check out walking clinics carefully, and talk to others who have gone through the program. People give mixed reactions to these programs. Some say they were drawn in by a desire to stand, based on elaborate promises that did not come to pass. Others say they were urged to have reasonable expectations from the start and gained functional abilities beyond what they were able to achieve in rehab.

You might be a candidate for FES (functional electrical stimulation) walking, in which electrical impulses make your muscles contract to reproduce the movements of walking. This technology is still developing, but some people are using it in their daily lives. It can be used by some people with injuries higher than T12, although it still involves intensive training and sufficient strength. FES is discussed in Chapter 6, Spinal Cord Research.

There are a number of patent applications in place for power-assisted gait orthotics. Motors and batteries have all become smaller and stronger, and microprocessors are able to read information, such as the amount of force on your leg or foot, as well as the position of your knees and hips. One particular design has buttons on the crutches that the user presses to cause one leg or the other to swing forward. Clearly, researchers, inventors, and entrepreneurs are not going to give up lightly on helping get people with paralysis back on their feet. The trick will always remain to balance emotions and desires against practical value and the investment of your time and money.

Occupational Therapy

The occupational therapist is primarily concerned with the practical activities of your life known as activities of daily living (ADLs). The occupational therapist will condition and train you to optimize self-care and your ability to work and perform typical daily tasks. The therapist's expertise is in techniques and tools to increase your independence. Occupational therapists will teach you methods for making transfers and for performing bowel and bladder management. The occupational therapist is usually the person involved in wheelchair selection, often in cooperation with the wheelchair vendor (see Chapter 4, Wheelchair Selection).

Jody Greenhalgh compares occupational and physical therapy:

*Occupational therapy (OT) adapts people to their disability
to be functionally independent or to optimize their function.
Physical therapy is more purely about physical capacities.
OT is physically oriented, but we focus on functional skills
so people can perform daily activities. There is definitely
overlap.*

In occupational therapy, you might find yourself making cookies or
doing a craft project like stringing beads. Some people make the mistake of
thinking they're being trained to perform a menial job, but this is not the
case. Such tasks are used therapeutically as a way to improve your dexterity and your ability to recover cognitive skills (especially in the case of brain
injury) and to retrain muscles that might have become weak or lost coordination. Making cookies might help you pursue a career as a medical technician. Don't judge the task. Consider the goal.

Sometimes the occupational activity is also exercise, as a man with
spinal cord injury recounts:

*I worked on a special loom designed by an occupational ther-
apist. As I made a rug, I was also lifting weights.*

Occupational therapists are very involved with orthotic devices. They
might fabricate splints or braces, working with an array of materials they can
shape to your body. Occupational therapists might make a functional brace
that gives you greater leverage for a task or keeps your hand and fingers
from curling with muscle contracture.

Focusing on activities of daily living is perhaps the greatest portion of
the occupational therapists' work. Every rehab facility has a kitchen, a bathroom, and often a bedroom or other areas of a home where they can simulate conditions, helping you learn to function in these spaces. Activities of
daily living address such activities as:

- Grooming
- Bathing
- Dressing
- Feeding
- Housekeeping
- Using of automated environmental controls
- Driving (this might also fall to the physical therapist or a specialist)

In the bathroom, you might have sufficient control to transfer from
the wheelchair to the toilet for bladder and bowel activities. Transferring
from the chair involves body strength, dexterity, and balance. Some people

will always empty their bladder from a catheter or leg bag. Your bowel program might be more easily performed in bed with a bedpan. You may never need to transfer to the toilet. If your abilities and program make transferring appropriate for you, the therapist will have you try the transfer from a variety of positions, since, in public places, you will encounter restrooms with limited space near the toilet.

You will explore the best method for getting dressed, which might be done lying down, possibly using assistive devices such as extended shoehorns, button pullers, and grabbers to help pull up your pants. Getting into and out of your clothes is another task that some people will need to perform in the bathroom, a task that is very doable with sufficient arm strength. You might have no need to undress in a public restroom, reserving your bowel program for home, using a leg drainage bag for your bladder, or doing intermittent catheterization that only requires that you open your pants rather than get them down altogether.

More adaptive methods and devices come into play in the kitchen than perhaps anywhere else in the home. You can use a grabbing device to extend your reach to high shelves. There are utensils for quadriplegics that require no grip strength to use. There are lap tables for cutting and other tasks that are awkward at typical counter heights. The occupational therapist will teach you to be extra cautious of handling hot items, since you cannot move away from a sudden spill as easily. If you lack sensation, you are at greater risk for burns.

John Hockenberry, a journalist with spinal cord paraplegia, tells of making stuffing for a Thanksgiving turkey in his book *Moving Violations*. The turkey was in a dish that had been refrigerated after cooking on the stove. The handles of the dish were cool, so he set it on his lap to work with. After a time he noticed unusual spasms. It took a while to realize he had set a hot pan on his lap. He writes:

> *Removing my trousers revealed the place where the hot dish*
> *had sat for perhaps two full minutes. The skin was gathered*
> *into a leathery, shrunken depression on the top of my thigh.*
> *The hairs had all been cooked into a blistered white wound.*[4]

Occupational therapists are concerned with more than techniques and tools. Their task is also to train you to change your habits and views. Hopefully you will not have to suffer burns, falls, or urinary slips before you build an awareness of these risks into daily life. Your therapist will tell you that new habits will seem unnatural at first. But, if you make a point of doing them, they gradually become transparent, part of your daily routine and lifestyle.

Activity-Based Rehabilitation

Christopher Reeve was unique in a number of ways, but, aside from his ability to be an international figure and advocate for disability, he was able to commit to an ongoing regimen of therapy. No one before—for lack of financial resources, time, or sheer persistence, all of which Reeve had in spades—had devoted themselves to this kind of extended therapeutic effort to regain function.

Then, amazingly, seven years after his injury, Reeve began to regain sensation below the shoulders and, most incredibly, was able to voluntarily lift a finger. He also worked doing supported walking in a pool, clearly contributing to some of the movement with his own leg muscles. No one with quadriplegia had ever before achieved such gains.

These startling events reinforced a recent line of research: the notion of a patterned response, suggesting that walking was not entirely dependent on nerve impulses traveling up and down the spinal cord. Reeve's proof accelerated the way to an entirely new milieu of rehab and research—activity-based rehabilitation. Not only does activity help muscles to stay in touch with the nervous system, and support an individual psychologically, but is suspected to actually contribute to the very healing of the spinal cord and its search to restore the neuronal connections necessary for walking.

The Christopher & Dana Reeve Foundation has been funding research grants in a number of rehab settings through the NeuroRecovery network. Therapeutic techniques being employed include:

■ Locomotor training, in which an inpatient is supported upright with a sling above a treadmill where walking motions are simulated
■ Direct electrical stimulation to elicit movement from select muscles
■ FES bikes, which uses electrical stimulation to pedal a stationary exercise bike

Neurologist Dr. John McDonald—now at Baltimore's Kennedy Krieger Institute, although his initial exploration of this new territory took place at Washington University in St. Louis—was Reeve's physician and is now the standard bearer for activity-based rehab. Quoted in the *Baltimore Sun*, McDonald said, "In this new world, the nervous system is much more capable of change than we ever thought. Old ideas are starting to fade away."

This avenue of research can be applied easily in rehab, since it involves no pharmaceuticals or surgical intervention. The Food and Drug Administration does not have to approve it as a form of physical therapy, so treadmills and FES bikes are increasingly becoming standard equipment in therapy gyms across the US.

Recreation Therapy

While in rehab, you are removed from your daily life in the outside world. You face considerable psychological adjustments, do hard physical work in the therapy gyms, and possibly live with pain. A little fun is an important element of successful rehab. Recreation will also be an important aspect of your life after rehab, so the recreation therapist will help you begin to identify—and maybe try—those options. And, like other forms of therapy, recreation therapy helps you develop and optimize your strength and skills.

A recreation therapist is a trained professional. Recreation therapists understand the physiology and psychology of your disability and what physical and cognitive capacities are necessary for a given sport or activity. By bringing that information together, recreation therapists help determine athletic options and are aware of adaptations that make a sport available to you, such as the mono-ski or sip-and-puff controls for target shooting. They will work with the occupational therapist and physical therapist to design supplemental activities that give you the chance to use the strength and skill you will develop in the therapy gym and once you're back home.

There is a remarkable and expanding set of sports and recreation options that are increasingly open to wheelchair users, discussed in great detail in Chapter 8, Getting Out There. Choices include wheelchair basketball, quad rugby, snow skiing, kayaking, waterskiing, archery, billiards, Ping-Pong, tennis, shooting, and many other sports accessible to chair users, often by means of adaptive devices. Many sports are available to people with limited arm strength, including swimming, archery, bowling, camping, sailing, and even throwing a Frisbee, thanks to the Quad-Bee designed by Foster Anderson, a man with quadriplegia in northern California.

The recreation therapist will discuss what interests you and what you did before your disability and will then point you to organizations that sponsor events where you can observe activities that interest you. You could even set your sights on devoting yourself to an event enough to compete on a world-class level at the Paralympic Games.

Rancho Los Amigos uses sports as a way of finding out what interests people have. The center offers hockey and wheelchair basketball games, as described by Dr. Michael Scott:

> We have a very active recreation program. We introduce people
> to various sports to make them aware of options. We have
> developed a highly competitive sports program. The recreation
> therapist also takes them on outings in the community.

Many rehab centers take you on field trips, organized and overseen by the recreation therapist. Therapists know the value of contact with the outside world, to help you through those early moments of feeling conspicuous as a wheelchair user and to give you a taste of an accessible recreational activity. The outing might just be a stroll around the block or going to a movie, but recreation therapists do their best to get a little fun into the experience.

HealthSouth Rehabilitation Hospital's Uli Salas takes people to local wheelchair basketball games:

> People might just sit and watch, or join in, depending on their ability. It is a good way for us to get them out and thinking in terms of still being athletic.

Outings show the recreation therapist your reactions to disability and help you learn how the world will react when you begin to appear in the world as a chair user. Dr. Scott explains:

> Based on how they do when they go out, we give them counseling about how to handle certain situations. The first time they go out they might come back and say, "People were staring at me!" or "People were much nicer to me!" It really depends. Everyone has a little different experience.

How much exposure you'll get to various options depends on the facility and the space and resources it is able to devote to recreation. Some smaller rehab hospitals will not have a space devoted to recreation. Your room might become the principle gathering place. Visitors will have to come to your room—usually shared with one to three others—and you might feel like there is nothing much more to do than be in bed. Recreation therapists in such settings will try hard not to let that happen, being as creative as they can by renting videos and setting up an evening "theater" in the therapy gym or throwing parties around a holiday. Their goal is to keep you active and, to the degree they can, give you a taste of available athletic options.

Respiratory Therapy

Oxygen is essential to all metabolic processes and to life. Breathing is particularly an issue for people with postpolio syndrome or high-level spinal cord conditions. The muscles that cause the lungs to expand and contract are often weakened by these conditions, limiting the amount of air you can draw in. People with higher level paraplegia can also face breathing difficulties from limited use of trunk and abdominal muscles and a reduced ability to cough and clear mucus.

The respiratory therapist's job is to ensure that you are getting sufficient oxygen into your lungs. Respiratory therapists determine the efficiency of your breathing by measuring "vital capacity," based on body size and age. Therapists can measure oxygen saturation in the capillaries of the ear or finger. They listen to your lungs with a stethoscope to judge air movement and the presence of secretions. If your oxygen saturation levels fall below a certain percentage, the therapist will take measures to improve your breathing.

Doubts about your ability to breathe are often a source of deep fears and insecurities. Respiratory therapists are acutely aware of the anxiety associated with breathing; part of their job is to reassure you. If you have respiratory issues, the respiratory therapist is one of the first people you will meet and one of the first to spend significant time with you.

Respiratory therapists will work with occupational and physical therapists to select activities that help strengthen muscles in the chest and diaphragm used in breathing. Respiratory therapists interact with other rehab team members, advising them how your respiratory status needs to be considered in the work they are doing on your behalf, instructing them about respiratory issues, and, in some cases, teaching basic methods, such as use of a resuscitation bag.

If your vital capacity is low, respiratory therapists might recommend a stretch program. A ventilator machine literally inflates your lungs to stretch them out—hyper-expanding them—to increase their capacity. Pressure is increased gradually, taking your comfort level into account. This is usually done for 10 to 15 minutes, four times per day.

In some cases, breathing needs to be assisted with a ventilator. Not all centers are equipped to work with ventilator-dependent quadriplegics; this requires special skills and facilities. During initial rehab, the goal is always to work toward getting off the ventilator, which many people ultimately achieve with hard work.

Volume Ventilation

One of the strongest images associated with the polio epidemic of the '40s and '50s was the iron lung. It was the assistive breathing device of the day, using negative pressure to create a vacuum that would cause the lungs to draw in air. Now the most common approach is positive-pressure ventilation, in which a machine delivers a measured volume of gas into the lungs. The machinery has become very advanced. There are a number of portable products that can be installed on a wheelchair. Many more people are familiar with this equipment thanks to the broad public exposure of Christopher Reeve. The machines are equipped with alarm systems that indicate either volume or pressure drops; the sensitivity can be adjusted. Machines even have the ability to simulate a sigh and to recreate the normal pattern of breathing as much as possible. Settings control respiratory rate, humidity, and pressure.

Assisted breathing settles into a routine part of life for those who rely on it, as this ventilator user notes:

> I have had my trach and vent for a couple of years now, and it just seems like it has been part of me for a long time. But I do remember when they took me off of the hospital vent and put me on my personal one that I coughed and choked a lot until they got the vent settings adjusted correctly. When you get used to it, using the vent is no more traumatic than brushing your teeth!

Successful use of a ventilator depends on good training provided by a respiratory therapist, not only for yourself, but for people who will be assisting you:

> When I first got the permanent trach and vent over four years ago, the respiratory therapist and doctors were excellent in training my partner, me, and my personal assistants in trach cleaning, suctioning, vent settings, etc. I was not allowed to go home until both my partner and my [personal assistant] were taught CPR. I must say that the training was excellent.

The Tracheal Tube

With a ventilator, breathing occurs through a tube inserted through the neck, nose, or mouth. An inflatable cuff tracheostomy tube is often used in the neck to maintain pressure into the opening and prevent respiratory gases from escaping around the outside. The cuff precludes the user from being able to speak, although it can be deflated for periods to allow speech.

After the acute stage, some people pursue the goal of using a Jackson tracheal tube, which allows speech. The tracheal opening requires greater care to prevent infection and drainage of secretions than when the inflatable cuff is used.

The acute period in rehab when a cuffed ventilator user is unable to speak is very frustrating for the user and family. Communication options are reduced to smacking the lips or clicking the tongue to get attention. Lip reading, eye blinks, or a spelling board are sometimes tried. You might be afraid of not being heard over the sound of the machine. Experienced rehab nurses are very aware of these issues and will teach various options. They will do their best to be readily available and responsive and to encourage the presence of family to help reduce everyone's level of anxiety.

The tracheal tube needs to be changed, depending on the sensitivity of the opening to infection and the amount of secretions. Some people change the tube every two to three weeks, but each person finds a pattern, as does this woman with postpolio syndrome and quadriplegia:

> *Trach changes depend on what both patient and doctor agree on. I have gone as long as six months without a change. I was checked by myself, doctor, and partner for signs of infection. If cleaning the trach area occurs daily, the tube can be kept in for months. My doctor doesn't like me to change a lot, due to irritation of the tracheal wall, which could cause bleeding.*

Ventilator users are generally unable to cough up secretions on their own. The respiratory therapist or rehab nurse might use a technique of assisted coughing, in which pressure is placed in an upward motion at the base of the rib cage to release mucus from the deep sacs of the lungs. Suctioning secretions is part of the ventilator experience and is done as often as every eight hours for some people. It is important not to do suctioning more than necessary, since it irritates the trachea and can increase secretions, as well as the risk of infection. A suction machine is usually kept near the bedside, and portable models are also available. Family and assistants can be trained in suctioning. At first, suctioning is a scary thing—having the air sucked out of you to try to get mucus up. But as time goes by, it's just a way of life.

Weaning

Some people will always need to use a ventilator 24 hours a day. Others wean from mechanical ventilation and are able to breathe on their own, even if for portions of the day. Whether you are expected to breathe on your own or not, the respiratory therapist will develop a weaning program for you.

Using a ventilator at all times allows respiratory muscles to atrophy. Even five minutes of breathing on your own several times a day helps maintain some tone. A typical goal is to achieve the ability to breathe unassisted for 10 to 15 minutes. In the case of a mechanical disruption, the ability to breathe without the ventilator for a brief time until assistance arrives obviously means the difference between life and death.

Since depression is a very common feature of the acute stage of high quadriplegia, the rehab team will typically suggest that you wait until you are stable psychologically to begin the weaning process. It takes a certain degree of motivation to participate in the weaning process, which can be frightening. A respiratory therapist will always be present during any weaning session, and all staff members are trained in the use of a manual resuscitation bag, which should be kept with you at all times.

Psychotherapy

The goal of the psychologist is to work with you as an ally to help change mental patterns that can limit you. In the past, you would only have been referred to a therapist if you were considered a "problem patient" or in such deep despair that staff was concerned for your safety. Present-day rehab therapy takes a different view. Powerful feelings, confusion, or rebellion are widely recognized as understandable reactions to sudden disability. Rather than stigmatize people who experience extreme emotion, now psychologists work with everyone to help them deal with their feelings, understanding that the feelings are adaptive reactions and part of your survival process.

There are many possible emotional responses to a disability. Many factors come into play, including age, degree of injury and impairment, financial and class status, cultural expectations, and so on. How the disability occurred is also crucial, as peer support coordinator Rich Patterson explains:

> *Whether it was an accident, someone else's fault, or gang-related—this makes a big difference in how everyone responds. It's hard enough to feel that you made a stupid mistake but, when someone does something to you and puts you in a chair, that tends to be pretty hard to swallow.*

Depression and suicidal feelings are common during acute rehab—although not everyone experiences them. The staff is trained to recognize behavioral signs of these feelings. Depression and suicidal feelings are treatable and generally temporary.

The overall work of rehabilitation depends on commitment—an attitude that promotes full participation and cooperation with the process. In these times of relatively short rehab stays, it is especially important that you not be unnecessarily limited by manageable emotional burdens. The psychologist helps you sort out what drives your behavior in ways that limit you, cause you unhappiness, or compromise the potential you can reach in the rehab process. Types of behavior that could interfere with your ability to gain from rehab include:

- Passive-aggressive behavior, in which one is indifferent to the value of what is being offered and places responsibility on others' shoulders
- Extreme dependency, in which one fails to participate proactively and surrenders the opportunity to feel personal accomplishment

■ Severe antisocial behavior, in which one possibly represents a danger
   to self or others

Rehab doctors and therapists know they must adapt their approach to
each person according to how that person is coping. Says Dr. Michael Scott:

> Everyone copes in a different way. Some people are more ener-
> getic, gung-ho and motivated. Some are depressed. Everyone
> does their best, and we try to motivate them and get them
> going. Some are able to do a little more early on, and we try
> to adjust for that. If someone isn't up for a vigorous weight-
> lifting class or tires out, we try to space things out to accom-
> modate what they can and can't do.

The fact that someone is depressed or angry while in rehab does not
mean he will fail to adapt to disability. Saunders Dorsey was a young attorney in Detroit when an angry client attacked the office with a rifle. Saunders
jumped out of the third-story window and became spinal-cord injured:

> I was extraordinarily dependent. I needed 24-hour attention. I
> wouldn't do anything. I was virtually helpless. It was obvi-
> ously more emotional than physical. I was so angry; I laid
> there for two years and wouldn't do a thing.

Dorsey has since returned to a thriving law practice, established a
successful accessible transportation company after seeing the flaws in the
services he was receiving, and is living in a comfortable home with his wife
and children.

Violently Acquired Spinal Cord Injury

Violently acquired spinal cord injury (VASCI) has been on the rise since the
1990s. The vast majority involve firearms. The incidence, understandably, is
higher in urban areas. Automobile crashes remain the number one cause of
traumatic spinal cord injury. Violence has been moving into and out of the
number two spot in recent years, trading places with falls. The incidence
has been growing; between 1973 and 1977, violence accounted for approximately 14% of all spinal cord injuries. Data from the National Spinal Cord
Injury Statistical Center (1994) indicate that during the 1973–1978 time
period, violence accounted for 13% of new spinal cord cases. By 1994, this
figure had increased to 30%, and ethnic minorities accounted for 72% of
this group. The greater emphasis is on African American and Latino men.

Statistically, victims of VASCI tend to have fewer financial resources,
so VASCI places more demands on the resources and dollars in the system

in the form of emergency medical services, rehabilitation, home modification, and so on. They also tend to draw family members away from work—and preciously needed income.

A unique set of issues arise in the context of VASCI. Features unique to people with VASCI include early anger at being a victim and the impulse for revenge, a "macho" type of personality that tends to resist participation in rehabilitation (especially when small white women therapists attempt to direct them), and the challenges of returning to the very environment where they were at risk in the first place.

The Disabling Bullet Project is a program out of the University of Illinois in association with Schwab Rehabilitation Hospital in Chicago, the National Rehabilitation Hospital in Washington DC, and Oak Forest Hospital in Cook County, Illinois, where there are notable populations of patients with VASCI. The Project aids these young men in the process of reintegration into their community through a peer-mentoring strategy. They get the benefits of the experience of other young men who have made the transition back into the community—and achieved a better quality of life. Mentors go through a rigorous training process that starts by taking the young men through their own initial experience with VASCI and reviews topics, including disability awareness and etiquette, the various emotional stages one might go through as they adjust, dynamics particular to their particular minority status, and how to establish an optimal peer-mentor relationship based on trust and strong communication.

Working with a Psychotherapist

The rehabilitation period is recognized as an important time for psychological support. Psychotherapists are typically included on the rehab team. Many rehab clients have the opportunity to spend time with a therapist as part of their daily schedule, where they are free to ask questions and explore their feelings confidentially.

Many people who find themselves in rehab will never before have met with a therapist. Those persons might feel as if therapy is being forced on them and is an invasion of privacy. Psychologists expect that some people will be unwilling to participate at first and will have negative ideas about the psychotherapeutic process.

Meeting with a psychologist means revealing intimate facts and exploring deep and often troubling emotions. Although the process can seem threatening at first, the therapist's job is to be an ally—not a friend, because this is not a personal relationship—who listens openly and explains what he or she has to offer. Psychotherapists can affirm the validity of what you are going through and help you begin adapting.

Jeri Morris, PhD, of the Department of Rehabilitation at Northwestern University Medical School in Chicago, writes:

> *The immediate goal of the psychologist is to encourage a willingness by clients to think about the long-term effects of their injury. The psychologist must get on the side of clients rather than make himself or herself their adversary.*[5]

Thinking about long-term effects can be especially hard for people with progressive conditions, such as MS or ALS. People with MS fight hard to maintain their health. One of the most difficult moments is when it is time to begin using a wheelchair, as explained by Cynthia Bishop:

> *A lot of people see using the wheelchair as giving up, as giving in to their disease. We hear that over and over, "I'm not giving in to it; I'm not using a wheelchair." We have to do a lot of talking. "How does it affect your day-to-day life function? If using a wheelchair would make it possible to go to your child's Little League game, would you rather go or would you rather stay home? How about using the wheelchair at work so you still have the energy to stay up with your family when you get home, as opposed to walking at work and becoming so tired that you just come home and collapse in a heap?"*

Generally speaking, it's not something that people receive warmly. We have to continue the process over several visits. We have to gently bring them to the point where they say, "Okay, I'd like to do that, I think it might be a good idea."

Most rehab centers emphasize education, offering programs on an array of topics to enhance your sense of control and sense of self. Dr. Michael Scott describes the offerings at Rancho Los Amigos:

> *We have a program that all patients go through called Starting Out class. Every day of the week there's a different topic. One is called Take Control, basically an assertiveness training class. It's given by one of our former tetraplegic patients, who does a great job with it. Other topics are Attendant Management, Funding and Resources, and Learning Your Rights, which is an introduction to the ADA. We let them know what the resources are and how to stick up for themselves.*

Sexuality

The confidential relationship with the psychotherapist is an opportunity to safely discuss this crucial topic. You might be hesitant to bring up questions as personal as what kind of sex life you might be able to look forward to. Dr. Michael Scott describes his approach to helping people ask about sex:

> Most patients are reluctant to bring up sexuality initially. They're definitely thinking about it. We use the approach of giving them permission to talk about it. I'll say, "You've had a spinal cord injury, things are different for you now, you probably have some questions, and one thing people usually want to know about is sexuality and sexual function. If you have questions about it, then please let me know." Usually they'll say, "Oh yeah, I've been wondering about that, doc."

The priority of sexuality to the person depends on many factors, including the type of disability, age, and sexual experience. Dr. Ed Nieshoff of the Rehabilitation Institute of Michigan, himself a chair user with quadriplegia, talks about younger men with a spinal cord disability:

> They're still in the grip of their raging hormones like any teenage guy, and all that energy is hard to redirect. It is very hard—and often angering—for them to have to redefine their sexuality. It adds to the pain. People think that walking again is the most important, but I'd say for most people it's about number five on the list. For a quad, first of all you want your hands back, second you want to be able to urinate, third you want to control your bowels, and then your sex life, and last of all walking. When you're nineteen, you'll take the sex before the walking!

Much of the information offered in rehab is about male sexuality. Since women with disabilities are generally not prevented from having children, the emphasis often falls on male fertility. And since maintaining erection is an issue only for men, this also tends to weigh the discussion in their direction. There is a lot of information about penile implants or injections, and harvesting sperm is now possible.

Yet women also face questions regarding vaginal lubrication, positions, bladder control, and how to attract men in a culture that doesn't encourage women to be the pursuer. Women need to hear about birth control, pregnancy, and gynecological care. Margaret Nosek of the Baylor College of Medicine Center for Women and Disabilities has been researching sexuality in women with disabilities, and says:

> *I've heard from women who said they were put in groups with*
> *men and were very uncomfortable with that. They felt it was*
> *introduced at a time when they didn't feel ready to deal with*
> *it. It's just that rehab centers have people for such a short*
> *period of time now that they try to cram all this stuff in.*
> *Women need more time to adjust.*

Women might have underlying issues of abuse. Their disability might even be the result of spousal abuse, which is sadly responsible for a share of brain injury and spinal cord injury from gunshot, for instance. A past history of sexual abuse will certainly be aggravated by becoming a woman with a disability. Women become more attractive targets for abuse by being in an increased position of vulnerability.

It is common for women's menstrual cycles to be interrupted for up to six months to a year after a spinal cord injury.

This raises psychological issues about the desire to have children—the loss of a feature that is a matter of feminine identity for some women—and anxiety about whether the cycle will return, despite what rehab staff says.

A skilled psychologist can help women begin to address these and other issues in order to achieve success in their sexuality. Nosek again:

> *The key is self-esteem. Our studies have shown that when*
> *women feel good about themselves, disability has no effect on*
> *the quality of their relationships. But there is so much more to*
> *study. We want to find out more about what makes women*
> *have high self-esteem.*

Sexuality is discussed in more detail in Chapter 5, Intimacy, Sex and Babies.

Vocational Rehab

A primary goal of rehab is for you to be able to work, if at all possible. Rehab staff want to foster your opportunity to return to your previous or some other kind of job. The anticipation of returning to a productive role in the world can increase your appreciation for how the rehab process is a path to an integrated, fulfilled life with your disability.

You will work with a vocational rehabilitation counselor who might be employed by the rehab center, assigned by the insurer, or representing your state vocational rehabilitation agency. Vocational rehabilitation (Voc Rehab) is a government program that exists at both state and federal levels. Legislation dating as far back as 1917 has authorized money to help injured workers get back to work. Your insurer might also have vocational rehab services and funds to offer you. If you get back to work, they figure you will not require as much expensive continuing healthcare or long-term disability benefits.

Counselors you work with will have varying loyalties, depending on who employs them. Those loyalties can limit their effectiveness, as attorney, quadriplegic, and disability activist Deborah Kaplan, former Director of the World Institute on Disability notes:

> The Voc Rehab system is sometimes helpful, often not. And very frustrating, very bureaucratic, very rigid. These days, they don't want to spend much money per client. You have to be a fairly sophisticated user of government entitlement services to get anywhere with rehab, unless you happen to luck into a good counselor who is genuinely trying to facilitate life. Counselors usually want to put you into a community college, get you a trade and say that they rehabilitated you. If you get a job, they have succeeded, whether you keep it or not.

The hard truth is that your state vocational rehab agency will generally work with you only when they consider you employable. How that gets defined might be up to the particular case worker you encounter. This man with advanced muscular dystrophy reports:

> I went to their office, did the entire intake process, interviewed with a case worker, but nothing ever came of it. They said they would call me, but never did. I talked to other disabled people more familiar with the workings of the California rehab system, who told me the reason they probably didn't follow up is because they considered a person with [muscular dystrophy] in his late thirties a "bad risk." That is, I would probably die before I would work enough to make the money spent on me worth it. As cold as this may sound, I believe it to be true. I've heard about this type of thing many times before.

State vocational rehabilitation services are getting tighter these days. There has been greater demand on these programs, in part due to the increasing number of repetitive strain injuries resulting from computer use in offices. In some states, legislation limits the money that can be spent for a given case—this limited amount can be small if you need an education and adaptive tools such as a computer or a modified vehicle. Voc Rehab funding is also sensitive to the economy. State budget cutbacks following the burst of the "dot.com bubble" in the 1990s had a negative impact on Voc Rehab money.

You always have the chance to advocate for yourself. For instance, you don't have to accept the first counselor who is assigned to you. If there is someone in the rehab facility to organize your vocational rehab, she might work harder on your behalf because she has no association with the funding source. When a counselor is doing her job well, she does the following:

- Takes a history of your past job experience and skills
- Learns about your medical status and prognosis
- Considers how your disability affects your ability to return to previous work
- Evaluates new career possibilities and makes suggestions to see what interests you, if your previous work is not possible
- Surveys the job market to help identify realistic options
- Explores sources and means of funding, if you require training or education
- Coaches you on job-seeking and interview skills
- Advises you and your employer on possible modifications and accommodations that make it possible for you to perform the job

Vocational counselors want to make the most of your physical and psychological rehabilitation, accomplished with hard work by you and the rehab team. They want to make a smooth transition to work or to education and take best advantages of your accomplishments in rehab.

Research Programs

Many of the major rehab centers—including but not limited to Craig Hospital near Denver, Colorado; Shepherd Center in Atlanta, Georgia; Rancho Los Amigos near Los Angeles, California; The Rehabilitation Institute of Michigan in Detroit; Jackson Memorial Hospital, which is closely associated with The Miami Project to Cure Paralysis in South Florida; the Kessler Institute for Rehabilitation in New Jersey; Drake Center in Indianapolis; and Mt. Sinai Rehab in New York City—have research programs. The types of projects in which these groups engage include data gathering or measuring such things as quality of life with a disability or public attitudes toward disability. Or they might be involved in basic science, such as spinal cord regeneration or pain management.

This means that your connection to one of these centers could contribute to knowledge and understanding about disability, which the center will disseminate to others working to be of service to people with disabilities. Beyond participation in various kinds of research studies, there are increasing opportunities to participate in human clinical trials, should you fit the criteria that are always very clearly defined for such procedures.

Beyond Rehab

There is not always time for you to make full adjustments before leaving rehab. States Dr. Michael Scott of Rancho Los Amigos:

> In the past when there were longer stays, people had the support of staff to go through some of the psychological adjustment issues. Now they're going through them in the community. It's probably more difficult.

Once you are out of rehab, how can you find out how much more progress is possible in gaining strength and skills? How do you make that progress on your own? This is the challenge of shorter stays.

Rich Patterson of the Santa Clara Valley spinal cord unit notes:

> It is very tough to see people who don't get the chance to make adjustments while they're in rehab, though it depends a lot on where they were at socially, their communication skills, and level of education. If they don't have these skills, then they run into some serious difficulties dealing with all facets of life, from family and neighbors to doctors and equipment suppliers. They need to learn how to develop these skills. We try to help that by matching them to a peer supporter, but we run into the problem of people who, when they are released after three months, don't want to talk to anybody. They're still very insecure about their disability. They don't think that other people have the same problems they do. They're still in the denial stage.

Your rehab experience might be unpleasant for you. You might resent the controlled environment or feel you just want a break from all the hard work. But the resources there exist for you, and it is a mistake not to take advantage of them while you have the precious opportunity. Don't wait until you find out how limited you are by having stopped short of gaining your optimal strength and skills. Even people who hated rehab reconsider. Bonnie Sims says:

*I am sometimes surprised when people who seemed so
dissatisfied during their rehabilitation return for treatment. I guess it's true that we look a whole lot better
looking back!*

It is much harder to achieve your optimal level of function without
the support and regulated schedule of a rehab facility. Nonetheless, take
advantage of outpatient services your rehab center offers, find similar services nearby if you live too far from your inpatient center, or at the very least
be sure that you have a home program designed for you when you leave
rehab and do your best to stick with it. There is always more you can
achieve. Once you are home, don't let the rehab process stop. It's only just
begun, and the quality of life possible for you lies ahead—if you choose to
remain on that path.

The Transition to Home

The question of what you will go home to comes up quickly once you arrive
in rehab. There is a lot to do to get ready, so the process should begin as
soon as possible.

The first question families have is usually about the adaptation of
their home. As discussed in Chapter 7, Home Access, this may not be a
simple matter of adding a ramp or putting in grab bars. Contractors may
need to get involved, doors might need to be widened, lifts installed, or
full additions built onto the house. Some people find they must leave their
existing homes and find another more accessible place to live. These things
take time—and money.

Equipment is another key to the discharge process, but the task of
identifying a wheelchair is difficult to accomplish early in the rehab process.
As Bonnie Sims explains:

*In the first weeks of rehab, most people plan on walking out.
The last thing they want to do is order a chair when they
believe there will be no need for it. Power chairs can be
especially complex. There isn't sufficient time to prescribe,
fund, order, and fit the chair prior to discharge. We do have
a loaner system that makes timely discharge possible in
most cases.*

Many major rehab centers have special apartments designed as transi-
tional living locations, but most insurers will not pay for a stay at such
a facility.

Building a Support System

You want to create an environment for yourself that helps you continue cop-ing. The choice of people you interact with makes a big difference.

Your relationships will change with some people. A disability has a way of flushing out relationships, of showing who is really committed to you as a true friend or even a family member, and who is unwilling or unable to accept you on new terms. There is both heartbreak and joy in this. You will find a deeper connection with some people in your life, and you will be disappointed in others, facing the loss of their presence because they are unable—perhaps only for now—to face their fears raised by your disability:

> *I found out years later that some of my closest friends felt my life was over once I had become paraplegic. A couple of them did not see me for years, and when we reunited later, they said that, at the time, it was just too painful for them.*

You will also meet new people and develop friendships in ways you might not expect. You have control of who you interact with and in what ways. You have new priorities for maintaining your health and redefining an active, satisfying, and meaningful life. You have to choose how you need and want to live, give people you've known the chance to understand your new terms, and try to have enough people in your life who inspire you and support you.

Relationships take work. Expressing emotions to each other is part of the process of deepening your connection. Even if others grieve about your disability or tire of the caregiver role, keep communication open. The rela-tionship can grow, so long as people are expressing themselves.

In her book, *Coping with Limb Loss*,[6] Ellen Winchell, PhD, describes aspects of a successful support system:

- Our lives are enriched by emotionally nourishing relationships.
- We are innately social beings who turn to each other in times of need.
- Knowing people love and care about you reduces your sense of isola-tion and the burden of the experience.
- One "best friend" is not a complete support system, but is an over-whelming responsibility for that person.
- You are not a burden to people who care enough to want to contribute and will find meaning for themselves by doing so.
- Accepting support is not a matter of shame—everyone needs support in some way at some time in their lives.

Family Caregivers

By speeding the date of discharge, insurers have placed more responsibility for care on families. Coverage for home nursing and personal assistance is also limited, so families end up carrying much of the load. For a person with quadriplegia who is ventilator dependent and must have someone nearby at all times, this is a large task indeed.

According to a June 1998 article in the *San Francisco Examiner*:

> *Managed-care companies and hospitals conscious of the bottom line have weighed in, pushing to get clients home faster and, many critics contend, sicker. The result has been an explosion in family caregiving. A poll by the National Alliance for Caregiving found that the number of people providing free care to a family member grew to 21 million, up from 7 million in 1987.[7]*

Some families have a great deal of trouble with the caregiver role. It is, at the least, a financial strain. Often at least one family member must leave a paying job to perform a caregiver role that produces no income. Caregivers take on medical responsibilities, such as assistance with a bowel program or suctioning secretions for a ventilator user, but might not have received sufficient training. They might have an emotionally difficult time performing such intimate and invasive tasks.

Many people who use personal assistance say that they would not recommend a family member playing the role of primary caregiver, especially a spouse. It alters—sometimes seriously strains—family relationships. When a parent assists an adult child, the quality of the relationship can revert to when the adult child was young, as the protective instincts of the parent resurface. Even when a parent-as-caregiver relationship succeeds, parents will have increasing difficulty with the physical tasks as they age.

Some families succeed by sharing the caregiver tasks among parents and siblings. No one person is overwhelmed, they learn to perform tasks and procedures effectively, and everyone knows the first priority is preserving the disabled family member's rights of decision-making and control—and dignity. People can discover that tasks that they considered unpleasant—like providing bowel assistance—become more accepted with experience:

> *I know a family with a son who has significant cerebral palsy. He is unable to walk or speak. He has deformities in his spine and arms and is spastic, yet with the support of his large family, he has graduated with high grades from high school, uses*

*computer technology by means of a mouth switch, and trav-
els often with the family in a specially outfitted recreational
vehicle. They even developed a special system of communication in which he clicks with his mouth in response to a
system of prompts. The father says that he wouldn't change
a thing, that the experience has been a remarkable gift for
his family.*

When the caregiver role falls to a family, there are choices about how
to approach it and what to make of it. With appropriate training and support, a family can settle into a routine that is not burdensome and makes a
full life possible for their loved one. Chapter 2, Healthy Disability, contains
information about personal assistance services.

Use Outside Resources

Rehab is only the start of the process: there is more to accomplish. You might
not be a resident at a rehab hospital anymore, but your insurance might
cover continuing therapy on an outpatient basis. Even if you live in a different city from the major rehab hospital where you stayed, there are an
increasing number of small rehab hospitals or therapy groups that can work
with you closer to home.

There is likely to be a Center for Independent Living (CIL) in your
area. Although not a rehab hospital, a CIL can help in many ways. If you are
struggling with your insurer about coverage for continued therapy, the CIL
might be able to offer you advocacy training and support to gain funding for
your needs, possibly even for home adaptation. Many CILs conduct support group meetings that give you the chance to meet others who share your
circumstances. You get to learn from the pros, who will gladly share their
"tricks of the trade." Of course, each CIL has its own programs. Offerings
vary widely.

Just because the insurance industry calls the shots on how long you
get to stay in rehab does not mean that you are denied the chance to be as
strong and active as you can be. It just means you have to do more of it on
your own.

Janie Whiteford of Santa Clara Valley Medical Center notes:

*When you're discharged, you are definitely not what you're
going to be a year from now. We really push people not to
think in terms of where they are now. Consider where you
might be a year from now, because it will be a totally different
picture.*

Rehab is inevitably a sheltered environment where you can begin adjustments. Once you get out, there will be new stresses, even for the person who has good coping skills. Kentfield Rehabilitation Hospital's Dr. Alex Barchuk comments:

> *Psychological adjustment is very, very, very, very individual.*
> *People who don't have a history of depression and usually*
> *have felt okay about things will go through a period in*
> *the beginning of not knowing what the heck's going on.*
> *Then, they realize, "Oh boy, this is a whole new life!" But*
> *it isn't until they get out of the hospital that it really hits*
> *them hard.*

Ongoing Healthcare

Your disability will need continuing medical management. Maintain a relationship with your physiatrist. If you traveled to a regional rehab center, identify a place that can offer ongoing physical medicine services. Ask your rehab doctor for a referral.

You are also going to have general medical needs. You'll get the flu, sustain a deep cut, deal with allergies, and so on. Don't neglect your standard healthcare. Get checkups and have a relationship with a family practitioner.

You'll have to educate these doctors about your disability. There is much they will not understand, since they do not deal with disability on a daily basis. You will have to ask whether their office has an accessible bathroom, for instance. Believe it or not, the office itself might not have room for the passage of your wheels.

Even if you have been living with your disability for many years—whether you had a formal inpatient rehab experience or not—the rehab community still has something to offer you. Says Margaret Nosek, PhD, researcher at Baylor College of Medicine in Houston:

> *There are a lot of people in this world who got their rehab a*
> *long, long time ago and have never made contact again, so*
> *they don't get the benefit of current knowledge. Despite all of*
> *the setbacks due to managed care, rehab has improved and*
> *learned a great deal over the years.*

References

1. Di Fabio RP, Soderberg J, Choi T, Hansen CR, Schapiro RT. Extended out-patient rehabilitation: its influence on symptom frequency, fatigue, and functional status for persons with progressive multiple sclerosis. *Arch Phys Med Rehabil* 1998;79(2):141-6.
2. Yarkony GM. Overview of spinal cord injury rehabilitation in the acute phase, the rehabilitation team, and classification of spinal cord lesion. In: Yarkony GM, ed. *Spinal Cord Injury: Medical Management and Rehabilitation*. Gaithersburg: Aspen Publishers; 1994:3.
3. Price R. *A Whole New Life: an Illness and Healing*. New York: Plume/Penguin Books USA; 1994:101-2.
4. Hockenberry J. *Moving Violations: War Zones, Wheelchairs, and Declarations of Independence*. New York: Hyperion; 1995.
5. Morris J. Spinal injury and psychotherapy. In: Yarkony GM, ed. *Spinal Cord Injury: Medical Management and Rehabilitation*. Gaithersburg: Aspen Publishers; 1994:225.
6. Winchell E. *Coping with Limb Loss. Coping with Chronic Conditions: Guides to Living with Chronic Illnesses for You & Your Family*. Garden City Park, NY: Avery; 1995:225-26.
7. Fisher I. Families Struggle to Care for Loved Ones. *New York Times/San Francisco Examiner*; June 7, 1998.

Chapter 2

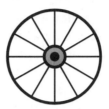

Healthy Disability

Our culture broadly equates disability with "sickness." Your mobility impairment might indeed correspond to a medical condition for which you are being treated or from which you are recovering. Many disabilities, however, are relatively stable conditions. This is generally true for spinal cord injury (SCI), cerebral palsy (CP), amputation, brain injury, and others once medical stability has been reached if there was a traumatic cause.

All of which is to say that there is such a thing as health in the context of disability and that putting your attention and priority on optimal health is a worthy choice. Especially if you are in treatment or recovering, being as healthy as possible in all other ways will only help the process. In any case, being healthy means having the greatest independence and less emotional burden. It could even mean feeling great as you get out there and live well.

Your disability might entail the risk of certain medical complications. You'll need to be aware of those that could affect you so that you can take preventive actions, recognize early warning signs, react promptly, and capably participate in treatment decisions.

Medical Concerns

General Concerns

Being a person with a disability who uses a wheelchair entails additional health risks, and you must work harder to maintain your overall well-being. That said, the better you maintain your general health, the less prone you will be to secondary conditions pertaining to your disability. If you lack sensation, you must be alert for other signals from your body. Primary care doctors might not understand specialized needs you have; specialists in a particular condition or body system might not understand how your disability changes how they would normally treat a condition.

The 2004 National Organization on Disability/Harris Survey of Americans with Disabilities[1] notes that those with disabilities are less likely to be able to afford healthcare, get insurance, or have special needs covered by insurance.

- Slightly more less one out of five (18%) adults with a disability did not get medical care that they needed on at least one occasion during the past year, compared to one in 14 (7%) adults without a disability.
- Thirty-nine percent of adults with disabilities postponed getting healthcare they thought they needed in the past year because they couldn't afford it.
- One in four (26%) adults with disabilities report having trouble finding a doctor who understands their personal healthcare needs, compared with only one in ten (10%) of adults without a disability

It is wise to learn all you can about healthcare and advocate for yourself before an emergency or serious health threat arises. General precautions you might want to take to prepare for potentially serious medical situations include the following.

- Educate yourself about insurance options and your coverage.
- Know your medical history.
- Know your medications. Be familiar with all types of medications you are taking and which ones you're allergic to. Before you accept a prescription from your doctor, let her know what medications you are presently taking, and ask her to check her *Physician's Desk Reference* for any possible conflicts. Establish a good relationship with your physician.
- Tell others about particular health risks. Inform those closest to you and most likely to be present should an emergency arise about particular health risks. For example, if autonomic dysreflexia is a possible complication for you, give close family and friends enough information so they know how to recognize it and how to respond.
- Become a MedicAlert member. Consider getting a MedicAlert bracelet or necklace to help alert emergency medical services personnel and others in case of an emergency, particularly if you have difficulty communicating or have a nonobvious medical condition. The initial mem-

bership fee for MedicAlert is a minimum of $35, depending on the style, metal, and size of the bracelet or necklace you order. After that, the annual renewal fee is $15.

■ Execute a durable power of attorney document. A durable power of attorney for health care (DPAHC) is a legal document that must be signed by a competent adult. It allows you to transfer medical decision-making authority from yourself to a person you designate as your agent. Obviously, the person you select to be the agent of your DPAHC should be someone you know and trust and someone you feel is capable of making decisions based on your wishes. The DPAHC guarantees that your healthcare choices will be carried out according to your wishes, values, and beliefs. Once signed and witnessed by either a lawyer or a notary public, the DPAHC can only be executed if you are unable to make the decisions yourself, for example, if you are unconscious, comatose or cannot speak for yourself.

Autonomic Dysreflexia

Autonomic dysreflexia (AD) is also called autonomic hyperreflexia or paroxysmal hypertension (among other names). Autonomic dysreflexia is particular to people with spinal cord lesions at or above the sixth thoracic vertebra, although it has been reported with injuries as low as T8. It is marked by an increase in blood pressure and should be taken very seriously. AD can cause stroke or seizures and can be life threatening.

The nervous system tries to send a message to the brain when it perceives an irritant to the body, such as a full bladder or a wound. Since the message can't get past the spinal cord lesion to the brain, and since the brain can't respond by sending inhibitory agents down the cord past the injury, a "hyper reflex" occurs. The body keeps trying to send the messages, and blood vessels tighten below the injury level. Above the injury level, vessels open, which causes the typical red, blotchy skin seen with AD.

Stimulations that can produce this response include:

■ Urinary tract infections
■ Impacted bowel
■ A full bladder
■ Pressure sores
■ Bladder, kidney, or gall stones
■ Hemorrhoids
■ Deep vein thrombosis
■ Burns to skin, including sunburn

- Open wounds
- Ingrown toenails
- Sexual arousal
- Fractures
- Labor and childbirth
- Some surgical or diagnostic procedures
- Tight-fitting or wrinkled clothing

As you can see from the list, you have control over most causes. Bladder distention is the most common cause of AD. Users of indwelling urinary catheters need to manage the catheters well to make sure they do not become clogged or bent into a kink that blocks the flow. Fecal impaction is the second most common cause. A well-managed bowel and bladder program is very important, not only to decrease the chance of an occurrence of AD, but to prevent secondary conditions like infections and stones, which can also cause an event. When blood pressure rises, any of the following symptoms might occur:

- Pounding headache
- Red, blotchy skin above the lesion level
- Profuse sweating above the lesion level
- Cool, clammy skin below the lesion level
- Nausea
- Blurred or spotty vision
- Nasal congestion
- Goosebumps
- Slow pulse
- Anxiety

Many people learn to recognize the signs of high blood pressure early and find they can manage episodes of AD. However, if signs persist, it is very important to get immediate medical attention. There might be a fracture you are unable to feel or a urinary infection of which you are unaware.

If symptoms appear, the first thing to do—after removing the offending stimulation, if possible—is to sit up. Elevating the body helps reduce blood pressure by encouraging pooling of blood in the lower extremities. Check if your leg or bedside urinary drainage bag is full. This could indicate a distended bladder that is backed up and causing the event. Empty your bladder if you can, but empty no more than 500 cc at a time, since this can cause spasms, which would exacerbate the situation.

If you need to go for medical attention, the first thing a physician should do is check your catheter or take measures to empty your bladder. You might need to be catheterized. The act of catheterization itself could increase stimulation to the nervous system. The treater might use an anesthetic jelly such as lidocaine to minimize sensory input and relax the urinary sphincter muscle to avoid exacerbating the problem. A physician should also check for fecal impaction. A physician might gently clear some stool at the opening of the rectum. Again, an anesthetic agent might be used. In some cases, the physician might give you an antihypertensive drug to quickly bring your blood pressure under control while he continues to work to identify the cause of the AD.

If you are being treated in a general emergency department or by your family physician, it might be necessary for you to educate the staff about AD, since they will probably not have treated AD very often.

During medical treatment, your blood pressure will be monitored closely, since it can change quite quickly during an episode of AD—as quickly as every two minutes. You might be watched for as long as two hours to ensure the episode does not recur. It is necessary to be certain that the cause is removed, rather than simply improved by short-term treatment. If the episode of AD is serious enough, you might be admitted to the hospital for closer observation.

A medical alert card for autonomic dysreflexia is available from the Paralyzed Veterans of America. The card includes instructions for how to help if someone needs to assist you in an emergency. Information on how to contact the Paralyzed Veterans of America is given in the Appendix.[2]

Bladder Cancer

Bladder cancer is not widely seen in the general population, but its incidence is slightly higher among people who rely on catheterization for bladder management. In a study of 2,660 records at Craig Hospital in Denver of people with SCIs, only 13 cases of bladder cancer were found, or less than 1%. Still, it is worth knowing what measures you can take to reduce the chances further.

Bladder cancer is more likely when there is repeated irritation to the bladder. Tumors have been seen inside the bladder at the point where a catheter makes regular contact. Indwelling catheters and suprapubic catheters are thought to be the greatest potential risk. People who use intermittent catheterization are less vulnerable. Infections are also an irritant— whether you are a catheter user or not—as are the presence of stones.

Smoking is also thought to contribute—carcinogens from smoke can be carried in urine.

Some physicians feel the risks of bladder cancer are already lowered by the development of modern antibiotics and safer nonrubber materials now used for catheters. Anticholinergic drugs such as oxybutynin (Ditropan®), propantheline (Pro-Banthine®), or oxyphencyclimine (Daricon®) are bladder relaxants that are sometimes prescribed to aid a bladder program and that can secondarily reduce bladder irritation.

The most common symptom of bladder cancer is blood in the urine. Blood in the urine does not mean that cancer is necessarily present. Blood can also be present with urinary tract infections (UTIs) or other causes. But take the symptom seriously and get examined soon by a urologist.

The urologist might suggest a cystoscopy, a diagnostic procedure in which a scope is inserted into the bladder allowing the physician to visually search for tumors. If a biopsy seems justified during the examination, the doctor will take a small amount of tissue for testing.

Some cystoscopic biopsy reports come back with a diagnosis of "squamous metaplasia," a form of cellular change often seen in the bladder. Physicians do not widely agree that this is an indicator of cancer—many people, disabled and nondisabled, have squamous metaplasia but never develop cancer. Yet some doctors feel this change sometimes is a precursor to bladder cancer.

The strategy for preventing bladder cancer is to limit irritation to the bladder. Prevention measures include:

- Controlling infections and stones by drinking enough fluids (see the discussion of bladder management later in this chapter)
- If you have a suprapubic catheter, keeping the area around its insertion in the abdomen clean and shaved
- Cleaning drainage bags and tubing with chlorine bleach and water
- Reducing or quitting smoking
- Switching sides with your leg and/or bedside drainage bags; this changes where the catheter contacts the bladder, rather than having it always contact the same spot
- Using catheters that are less irritating; for example, hydrophilic catheters are softer than other catheters and are lubricated
- Taking antioxidant vitamins such as E, C, and B6, which are thought to reduce the effects of carcinogens on cells
- Having regular cystoscopic exams, as frequently as every two years if you are a longtime user of an indwelling catheter

Deep Vein Thrombosis

When we do not walk, circulation through the legs is reduced. Contractions of the leg muscles are part of the circulatory system—an important mechanism for how blood is pumped through the body. For people with paralysis in the legs, blood may pool in the lower extremities.

The danger is that blood could begin to clot in a vein, coagulating into a more solid state, known as deep vein thrombosis (DVT). DVT limits circulation further, at the least. At worst, the clot could dislodge and travel through the body into the lungs or brain, causing a stroke or death. This is called a pulmonary embolism. A 1979 study found that 35% of people with DVT who were untreated died of an embolism.[1] A clot in the thigh is the greatest concern, since this location gives a more direct route to the lungs.

DVTs are a greater concern at the acute stage of an SCI, when someone is inactive for an extended period of time during extended bedrest. DVTs have been observed as soon as 72 hours after injury. Researchers suspect that 80% of DVTs occur within two weeks of injury. Studies of people at this stage have found incidence rates from 15% to 47%. Studies have also found slightly higher rates of DVTs for those with complete SCIs compared to incomplete injuries.[2]

During periods of extended inactivity and bedrest, pneumatic compression stockings or wrapping with elastic bandages is often recommended. The drug heparin is sometimes used to reduce blood viscosity, improving flow. Electrical stimulation of calf muscles has also been explored.

Heterotopic Ossification

Heterotopic ossification is a condition in which bone develops outside of the normal system, potentially clogging joints and limiting or freezing movement. It occurs in acute SCI, brain injury, and other neurologic traumas and takes a year or more to develop, making it difficult to diagnose early. Remaining active and keeping up regular range-of-motion exercises play an important preventive role.

Heterotopic ossification only occurs below the level of injury, commonly at the hips. It can lead to scoliosis problems as the nonneutral position of the pelvis puts curvature pressure on the spine. The condition can ultimately require surgical intervention. Some doctors use anti-inflammatory drugs to manage heterotopic ossification. Although studies have reported from 16% to 53% of occurrence of heterotopic ossification in people with SCIs, adequate acute management substantially reduces the need for surgery to free joints or correct scoliosis due to heterotopic ossification.

Osteoporosis

Without the regular loading of weight from walking, bones begin to lose calcium. This leads to osteoporosis, in which bones become more brittle and prone to fracture. The hips are a common site of fracture, as are the legs, spine, and arms.

Osteoporosis commonly occurs with aging, particularly in post-menopausal women. Risk is increased with diabetes, vitamin D deficiencies, or diets low in calcium. Smoking and alcohol abuse exacerbate the condition, as do lack of activity and lack of sunlight. If you are able to stand or walk, it is a good idea to do it as much as you can—with safety being your first priority—to help your bones remain strong. People with traumatic disabilities such as traumatic brain injury, SCI, or amputation tend to spend an extended initial period in bed, which invites osteoporosis to begin.

If you have osteoporosis or are at high risk for developing brittle bones, avoid stresses to your bones. To help prevent breaks, remove your feet from heel loops or restraining straps first when you make transfers to and from your wheels, making sure nothing will prevent your foot and ankle from rotating, and straighten your legs before rolling over in bed to minimize excessive strain to your bones. Just having a toe caught under a footrest when you transfer can be enough to break an ankle.

If you don't have sensation in your lower body, you might incur a fracture and not know it—for example, a hairline fracture that produces only moderate symptoms. Pay attention to changes in spasticity or occurrences of dysreflexia. These could indicate a fracture that might not otherwise be apparent. If you hear a snap or other unusual sound, don't ignore it. A bruise from internal bleeding is another potential sign, which you could mistakenly assume is from an impact you didn't feel during the day.

Spasticity has a mixed impact on osteoporosis. When muscles spasm, they place a load on bones that help maintain their density. But severe spasms can break osteoporitic bones. For people who never stand, managing extreme spasticity is all the more important.

There are also wheelchairs capable of elevating you into a standing position, thus bearing weight on your legs. Such a chair would provide you with more frequent opportunity to stand, so it could contribute more to prevention of osteoporosis.

Standing Frames

Standing frames address both osteoporosis and circulation. The act of walking helps pump blood through the body. Legs that are inactive have less efficient circulation, since their muscles are not helping the process. Always sitting also limits circulation to the legs because of the angles that veins and arteries must pass at the hips and knees. Standing lets gravity help circulation, as blood passes straight down the body without having to turn corners. Circulation is also a matter of hydraulics—the assistance of gravity to bring blood down to your legs also helps it flow upward in the closed pressure system of the body.

The risks of softer leg bones and poorer circulation can be addressed with standing frames, which comprise a growing segment of the medical supply industry. There are three types of standing frames:

- Fixed. The frame remains in one place and does not have a seated position.
- Movable. The frame includes wheels within reach, linked by a chain or belt to smaller wheels at the bottom so you can move within a room. Some frames are motorized and move by means of a joystick control, like a power wheelchair.
- Integrated. Another kind of product is a wheelchair with the capacity to transform into a standing frame. Such a frame is intended for people at work, such as a mechanic who would need to stand beneath an elevated car, or for situations in which an extended reach is needed, such as at a supermarket. There are both manual and power models.

Other benefits of standing frames pointed to by manufacturers are reduction of spasms and muscle shortening, less chance of pressure sores, and improved urinary and bowel function, since the colon and intestines are constrained in the sitting position (although some physicians do not subscribe to this view). If you have shortened muscles from sitting for many years, a standing frame can be a means of getting your body straightened out again. A product that is able to be set at intermediate angles can allow you to therapeutically stretch in the frame and gradually lengthen your tissues out to a normal posture.

Standing frames support you with a surface behind you, which generally contacts the buttocks and might extend as far as down to behind the knees or as far up as the lower back. Although it is true that there is still some pressure on them, it is much less than if you were sitting directly on them. The knees are braced in front, and another support is generally located at the abdomen. All supports are padded for the prevention of pressure sores. Some frames include adjustable footplates. Frames are available with various options, such as a desk platform for writing or reading, storage compartments, and drink holders. Some come in a range of colors.

People with very brittle bones, cardiac disorders, or significant short-ening of hip and knee flexor muscles might need to avoid standing frames but might be able to work their way toward using them with stretching and therapy. You may require a prescription to purchase one, and a consultation with your physical medicine physician and therapist is recommended.

Pain

There are many reasons why a chair user might experience pain—far too many to detail here. The causes may or may not relate to your disability.

Pain is usually thought of as a message telling us something is wrong in our body. The International Association for the Study of Pain defines pain as "an unpleasant sensory and emotional experience associated with actual or potential tissue damage."[3]

But a disability might involve conditions in which pain is a continu-ing feature. When the nervous system is affected by injury or an autoim-mune event like multiple sclerosis (MS) or amyotrophic lateral sclerosis (ALS), nerve messages get mixed up. Impulses fly through the body and can be experienced as pain. In these cases, you manage and adapt to pain, rather than always thinking of it as an indicator of something to be fixed.

> I had a lot of pain the first couple of years after my SCI. I don't know exactly what it was. No one could tell me. It was in my back. I think it was because the bones were fusing. One day a friend said to me, "You haven't complained about your back hurting for days." It was just gone all of a sudden. I thought I would always be in pain because of my injury.

Pain is a very personal experience. What is unbearable to one person might be no big deal to another. Many people with disabilities experience sensations that stem from their disability, but they define those sensations as discomfort rather than pain. Other people experience their pain as more immobilizing than their physical condition.

It is your task to identify your boundaries and manage activities to minimize pain. Some people find that sitting or lying for extended periods exacerbates pain, whereas others experience greater pain when active. Extremes of either will probably increase pain. The body requires variety of movement but has limits to how much it can endure. Even sitting still involves muscular exertion and can become fatiguing. Your attitude affects your experience of pain and your ability to respond. Being overrun by fear of pain will increase it. The ability to stop and breathe can cause your pain to abate.

Stronger measures might be required to interrupt the pain if it interferes with your ability to function. This woman with SCI finds her pain from spasticity disabling:

> More than spasticity, the pain has limited me socially. I had to
> quit a part-time job because I can't sit for eight hours a day
> (the pain is usually worse in the buttocks, aggravated by sit-
> ting). I've often said that the pain is the real disability, not so
> much the paralysis.

As time progresses after an injury or disability, people tend to report less pain. Studies have shown large differences between what people report while in the hospital and what they report later in follow-up meetings with their doctor. In a 1985 study, 60% reported pain while in the hospital, compared with 17% as outpatients.[4] This difference is partly explained by the lesser response of the nervous system as we age but is probably more related to our capacity to adapt. What was once frightening and uncomfortable simply becomes an accustomed sensation we don't even notice unless we put our attention to it. This paraplegic man, 25 years after his SCI, reports:

> I have a strong tingling in my legs and feet that feels like I
> have been shot with a lot of Novocain, like the dentist uses.
> But I'm not even aware of it unless I think of it. I know that
> anybody else feeling what I do in my legs would be very upset
> and scared by it. To me it's just normal.

To the degree that someone experiences greater pain over time, it is often a result of poor health maintenance, which allows urinary, gastrointestinal, skin breakdown, or other health problems to occur.

Of people with SCIs, estimates of people who experience pain range from 33% to 95%. A very small number of these people describe their pain as severe. Dr. Elliot Roth of the Rehabilitation Institute of Chicago estimates that

> Between one third and one half of all people with SCI have
> pain and about 10% to 20% of all patients have severe, dis-
> abling pain. Only about 5% of them or less undergo surgery
> for pain.[4]

Most spinal cord pain develops within the first year. In a 1979 study, two thirds of people with SCIs reported onset within six months. It has been observed that those people injured by gunshot are more likely to experience chronic pain.

If pain appears significantly later after an SCI, your physician can explore the possibility of syringomyelia, the presence of fluid-filled sacs in the spinal cord. This is found in a minority of cases of late-onset pain and in only 5% of all spinal cord cases overall. For quadriplegics of level C4 and higher, syringomyelia needs to be caught early if it occurs. At that level of injury, breathing is a critical matter, possibly already assisted with a mechanical ventilator. Syringomyelia can effectively raise the injury level and further threaten respiratory function.

Syringomyelia often appears early. After an injury, testing with magnetic resonance imaging studies can be complicated if a halo vest is still being worn to stabilize the neck; however, there are halos made of metals that do not interfere with the imaging process.

There has been a correlation made between pain and intelligence—among other factors—as Dr. Roth notes in his study on pain in spinal cord injury:

> Interference with daily activities by the pain tended to occur in patients who were older, of higher intelligence, more depressed, experiencing greater levels of distress, and involved with more negative psychosocial environments.[4]

Difficult to Judge

Pain is hard to diagnose. Doctors do their best, but there are so many possibilities that the task is daunting. Descriptions of pain are subjective, not exact. People variously describe pain as being burning, tingling, stabbing, achy, pins and needles, numb, shooting, throbbing, cramping, freezing, stinging, or crushing. X-rays do not show soft tissue, often the source of pain. Magnetic resonance imaging studies or computerized tomography scans are expensive and sometimes uncomfortable.

The difficulty of diagnosis forces doctors to use a process of elimination. They make an informed guess of the cause and treat accordingly. If the treatment doesn't work, they move on to the next possible theory. They will do this process conservatively, beginning with the least invasive approach. Some doctors might suggest beginning with biofeedback or self-hypnosis. Most doctors will save surgery for the last resort.

Symptoms can overlap or be misdiagnosed. Pain is sometimes referred—experienced in a different part of the body. With tissue pain, trigger points can be activated in the muscles, but the pain is usually experienced in another location. This is known as myofascial trigger point theory, and not all doctors subscribe to its concepts. Yet most doctors do understand that a disorder in one part of the body can express itself elsewhere. For example, gall bladder pain can sometimes appear as pain in the shoulder.

Doctors might not take your pain seriously. If examination and tests reveal nothing physical, they might say it's "all in your head" and leave it for you to deal with. This was the experience of a woman with postpoliomyelitis syndrome. After feeling stable for many years, she began to experience pain:

> *I have been reluctant to talk to my doctor about my muscle pains because every time I go, she insists that it is merely a muscle pull or tendonitis. I have gone to her so much about these "muscle pains" she thinks I am a hypochondriac and refuses to believe that postpolio even exists!*

Tissue Pain

Musculoskeletal or mechanical pain involves muscles, tendons, ligaments, or bony abnormalities. It can result from overuse. This type of pain is increasingly typical of longtime chair riders.

Muscles are generally able to recover with rest, stretching, and appropriate exercise. When tendons or bursae—fluid-filled sacs that help lubricate and cushion movement in joints—are involved, recovery can be more difficult, and chronic recurrence is more likely. There is less blood flowing to these tissues, so the body has more difficulty repairing strained cells.

Shoulder tendonitis is the most common tissue pain in longtime chair users. Chair users, particularly manual chair users, use their arms to replace the work of the legs and place an increased workload on shoulders. For those with quadriplegia, shoulder, arm, and neck pain are also common because those muscles are the only ones available to do the work once shared by muscles in the trunk. In SCI populations, studies have found rates of shoulder tendonitis as high as 31%. Another study equated shoulder pain to years of disability; it found 52% reporting pain after five years, 62% at 10 years, 72% at 15 years, and 100% at 20 years.[4]

Learn optimal transfer techniques to minimize tissue strain, which can produce pain. Transferring to and from your chair from different heights, over a distance, or without brakes (which requires you to grip with more force or throw yourself into the chair) is more likely to cause pain or injury over time.

Carpal tunnel syndrome is common for manual wheelers. When wheeling, the wrist is in a position of extension (bent backwards at the wrist) while applying pressure on the palm. This strains the median nerve, which travels through a narrow opening in the wrist called the carpal tunnel. Symptoms usually include tingling in the fingertips, thumb, or palm. Nerve injuries such as this—including ulnar nerve entrapment at the elbow and wrist or thoracic outlet syndrome in which nerves are compressed in the neck and shoulder—are serious and can become permanent if allowed to become advanced.

When muscles are weakened or unusable, and if a joint is limited or bone fused—as in a spinal fusion of neighboring vertebrae—more stress is placed on nearby tissues and joints. If a muscle is not doing its share, other muscles must pitch in to make up the difference, and so the risk of overuse is increased. In the same way, if a vertebra cannot move, more force is transferred to the neighboring vertebrae. Spinal fusions are common in SCI, as is the installation of metal rods to either manage scoliosis or reduce the time of acute hospitalization prior to rehab. The resulting overuse of neighboring tissues and structure becomes a source of musculoskeletal pain.

These measures will help you minimize mechanical pain:

- Be active. Keep your body flexible and strong.
- Move patiently and with awareness, avoiding unnecessary force, exertion, and strain.
- Design exercises that do not stress tissues.
- Reduce stress in your environment—the spring tension in doors, the weight of objects, an incorrect or poorly maintained wheelchair, etc.
- Adjust the wheelchair for optimal propulsion, keep tires inflated, etc.

Visceral or Abdominal Pain

Visceral (deep) pain is equated with abdominal pain. It can be caused by bladder and kidney infections, bowel constipation and impaction, peptic ulcers, or gall bladder or kidney stones. Sweating, changes in blood pressure, or increased spasticity are often associated with visceral pain and pressure sores.

When control of the abdominal muscles is lost, internal organs have a weakened support structure. The lack of support can stress kidneys, bladder, stomach, etc. Initial sensations, such as spasticity, nausea, or fever, might not be perceived or could be mistaken for something else, such as a UTI. Dr. Roth writes that, "Acute abdominal catastrophes were responsible for up to 10% of deaths in patients with SCI" (in two reviewed studies).[4]

Spasticity in abdominal wall muscles can be very painful and possibly mistaken for problems in internal organs. As with spasticity in general, movement or sensory stimulation might evoke the spasm. Spasms localized to the abdomen could indicate a deeper, systemic problem. Your physician should first attempt to rule out spasticity as the cause of pain before settling on a diagnosis of a deeper organ disorder.

Most visceral pain involves constipation and impaction, which can be experienced as a feeling of fullness or bloatedness. Keeping a regular bowel program helps your doctor diagnose pain. Your doctor can more easily rule out the bowels and determine the source of your pain sooner, avoiding the chance of a problem escalating into a life-threatening emergency.

Neuropathic Pain

Many disabilities affect the nervous system. Pathways that generate and carry messages of pain are functionally impaired; pain signals can result from sensory confusion in the body. Spasticity is an example of how the nervous system gets caught in a loop, with muscle impulses bouncing around in muscles because the brain can't turn them off. Sensory signals are thought to be capable of behaving in a similar way. "Phantom" pain, experienced by people with amputation, is a case in point. The limb is no longer there, but the sensory system still thinks it is and continues to generate sensations, which seem to come from the missing limb. Pain from brain and spinal cord conditions seem to share some of the mechanisms related to phantom pain.

Pain can signal that something is going on in the body that merits attention, just as muscle spasms can signal infection, a full bladder, or other conditions. Pain is your early warning system, and if you ignore the first alarms, they'll get louder.

> I don't experience spasmodic muscle contractions, but, when I have an infection, or a sore, or even the flu or a cold, there is a spot on my right thigh that will spasm with pain. Sometimes it is just like someone plunging a knife into my leg. The spasms only last for seconds at a time, but, if I am really sick, it can happen many times an hour and is really exhausting. I have learned to pay attention very early if I feel the smaller shocks that usually appear at first. Sometimes it just means I've been sitting too long.

The same therapies used to manage muscle spasticity often help with pain, although doctors can't always explain why. The drug 4-aminopyridine is presently in tests as a method of increasing function for people with SCI and MS. It helps amplifying nerve impulses past areas where myelin, the material that insulates nerves, is damaged. Researchers were surprised to find that a drug that increases nerve impulses also helped to temper muscle and sensory spasticity in some people.

Pain Management

Pain management demands a good working relationship with your physician to develop the best strategy. Physicians can't magically identify the exact cause and make it go away. Dr. Roth, writing for other physicians who specialize in the treatment of SCIs, states:

> Successful treatment of pain relies heavily on the patience,
> cooperation, collaboration, and ingenuity of the patient and
> the professional alike. This means that active listening and
> taking complaints seriously are keys to successful diagnosis
> and management.[4]

The least invasive approach to manage pain is always preferred. Start with an active lifestyle—even if it is only performing regular range-of-motion exercises with an assistant or alternating time in and out of your wheels as you're able—and maintain a healthy diet. Avoid factors that cause pain, such as infections, sores, or bladder and bowel disorders. Don't abuse alcohol, drugs, or tobacco. These things might seem like a source of relief from your pain, but, in the long-term, they only exacerbate it.

People are increasingly exploring what are called alternative (or complementary or holistic) measures to manage pain.

Emotions have a great impact on pain and don't have to be treated with drugs. Dr. Roth writes:

> Emotional well-being appears to exert a great positive effect
> on pain relief. Psychological stress, hostility, anxiety, or
> depression may precipitate or exacerbate pain.[4]

Fostering friendships, having satisfying activities, getting out into the world, or watching a funny movie can play important roles in your health. They help keep you out of pain. They help you remain focused on the external rather than dwelling on the internal.

Biofeedback is a method in which electrodes are placed on your head to read brain waves. A readout of brain activity appears on a meter or a computer screen. By relaxing and noticing the effects of your thoughts and breathing on brain-wave activity, you can learn to control stress and muscle tension. Biofeedback training allows you to take these skills into your daily life, using what you learned while using the machine.

In the film *Mask*, a young man has a disfiguring disease that sometimes puts great pressure on his brain and spine, causing great pain. His solution is to visualize a beautiful place and describe it in detail, closing his eyes and breathing deeply. Although this example is fictional, visualization is a valid pain-management technique.

This woman found benefits in acupressure, a form of massage therapy that uses some of the same theories as Chinese acupuncture:

> *I never believed in acupressure. My fiancé took a course in it before I met him. He did the acupressure and it worked. For the first time in 15 years I was pain free. I can't tell you how much massage and getting the blood to flow makes a difference. I can't move at times. I lie down and he does his thing and I am pain free the rest of the day. My problem has been insurance companies and doctors not believing me.*

There has been much interest in electrical stimulation as a means of pain management. TENS—transcutaneous electrical nerve stimulation—stimulates peripheral nerves and has the effect of diminishing pain. A TENS unit can be used at home without skilled assistance, after it has been set up by a therapist or trained professional and explained to you. It is a small unit—the size of a transistor radio—with electrodes that are applied to the surface of the skin. Its effect is temporary, but a 1977 study of seven quadriplegic and 32 paraplegic subjects showed that half of them found complete or nearly complete relief with TENS. Another 41% had moderate relief. TENS was more effective with musculoskeletal pain. Pain rooted closer to the spinal cord or brain did not respond as well.[4]

Strong pain elicits strong emotions, and, at some point, you need a break. If you are disabled by pain, if it interrupts your sleep cycle, if it prevents you from being able to maintain your health with exercise and activity, then it might make sense to cautiously and carefully employ drugs to manage your pain.

Many drugs are used to manage pain. Some of them have significant side effects, such as reducing your sexual impulses. Many pain drugs are also sedatives, which will affect your clarity, cause constipation, or affect your appetite. A pain medication could interact badly with a drug you are taking for another reason. Drugs should be used only when their value outweighs the side effects. Any prescribing physician should know all of the drugs you take.

The body has a way of adapting to drugs. After a while, you might need a larger dose or the drug might not work at all. Some drugs entail a risk of physical or psychological addiction.

The last resort to treating pain is surgery. Dorsal rhizotomy is a procedure to cut nerves to simply turn off the pain impulse. More extreme is surgery to cut the spinal cord below the level of injury. This procedure is known as a cordotomy. Since it obviously can't be reversed, it is performed in only the most severe cases. If injury to the spinal cord was not complete before the surgery, some function or useful sensation could be lost after the surgery.

Success rates are not high with these surgical procedures. Studies have found only half of people who underwent cordotomy experienced permanent relief. The percentage was 65% for people who had dorsal rhizotomy.[4]

Shoulder Strain

For manual chair wheelers, the shoulders are especially prone to overstrain, as they bear the greatest burden of making up for what your legs used to do to carry you through space. Doing your own transfers gives your shoulders extra duty. You can protect your shoulders from chronic pain and eventual shutdown through a combination of being in shape, maintaining your chair, and refining your wheeling style.

The more strength your shoulders have, the more they can weather the demands placed on them by full-time wheeling. Gentle but regular exercise will help maintain optimal strength. You don't need to be "bulked up" in order for your shoulders to be up to the task at hand. In fact, too much bulk can begin to limit the range of motion of your arms at the shoulders, ironically making muscles work even harder. An exercise approach based on bulking up also means working with heavier free weights or higher settings on machines, which forces you to exert greater force with your hands and wrists, putting them at risk as well. Go easy on the weight, and you'll still get and stay strong with a regular exercise routine and active lifestyle.

Muscle strength is directly related to how far your muscles can shorten during a contraction. Our muscles tighten with overuse, so stretching to help them maintain this elasticity is another important component of proactive safety for your shoulders. See the section below on yoga and stretching.

Having your chair in good shape helps keep you in good shape. As the tires go soft, if the frame gets loose, if your joystick is in a poor location, or if your wheel rims are in the wrong relationship to your hands and arms, then you will be unnecessarily straining your shoulders. The right chair properly maintained and adjusted (see Chapter 4, Wheelchair Selection) will put the least demand on your shoulders.

Even the perfect chair doesn't get you all the way to shoulder safety if you don't learn how to use it well. Coast whenever you get the chance, go easy on the speed, and let somebody who knows what they're doing give you a push on the major slopes rather than push yourself to your limits.

Pressure Sores

Perhaps the greatest scourge of full-time wheelchair users is developing pressure sores from sitting for long periods of time or from being in bed. Sores—or decubitus ulcers—can take months to heal or may require surgery or hospitalization, though typically only if they are not treated early. If the sores are allowed to advance far enough, you are likely to find yourself spending a lot of time in bed—or worse, in a nursing facility.

Pressure sores form when oxygen and blood are restricted in skin tissue by the weight of the body pressed continuously on a small area of skin. For people unable to use the gluteus maximus muscles of the buttocks, pressure is increased as those muscles atrophy (thin from disuse). The skin comes in closer contact with the bone, limiting circulation further. Two bony areas are of particular concern: the ischial bones of the pelvis upon which we directly sit, which are somewhat pointed and apply direct pressure to a small area, and the sacrum at the base of the spine.

Pressure sores can be serious enough to kill, if not cared for properly. Large sores become infected more easily, with so much tissue exposed, often at deep levels below the skin. Small sores ignored will inevitably become large if left untreated. There are three stages of pressure-sore development:

- Stage One: Redness of the skin. This stage might last for a short time, as circulation is restored to the area. The longer it lasts, the higher the risk of skin breakdown and the greater the need for caution. The area will be warm to the touch if it is approaching skin breakdown.
- Stage Two: An open area or blister appears. The skin might darken to a blackish color. This indicates cell death, at which point an open sore is inevitable. Remove all contact from the area to minimize any further cell death and to prevent the resulting sore from becoming any deeper.
- Stage Three: Open wound into deeper layers of the skin. Risk of infection is very high, particularly for sores close to the anal opening, where there is a great deal of infectious bacteria.

At its worst, a severe sore can progress into tendon, muscle, and even bone tissues. Such sores are likely to require surgery, either to stitch them closed (not always possible) or to perform a "flap," in which a thin layer of skin is taken from another part of the body and grafted onto the sore. A long nursing facility stay will be necessary to allow the skin to integrate itself into the new location and for the wound where the flap was taken to heal. Flaps do not always take, so all this time can be spent for naught. The need to limit your activity and stay in bed can produce additional sores in the process, trapping you in a downward spiral of skin breakdown. Be very serious about pressure sores. They are not worth the risk of these horrible possibilities.

Caring for a Sore

Keep the sore clean so it can heal. Dead tissue or bacteria will slow the healing process and increase the chance of infection. Dead tissue and dried blood must be removed for healing to proceed effectively. You may be able to remove this yourself—for example, with wet-to-dry dressings. This process should not be painful. If it is, see your doctor. A doctor might need to remove the tissue with a process called debridement.

The sore should be cleaned every time bandages are changed. Your doctor might recommend a cleaning solution, such as saline solution, to irrigate the sore. Saline solution can be purchased at the drugstore, or you can make it yourself by dissolving eight teaspoons of table salt in one gallon of distilled water. Make sure that the salt is completely dissolved and that you use clean utensils for measuring and stirring. Antiseptics such as hydrogen peroxide or iodine—although known for killing bacteria—are not recommended, as they can damage sensitive tissue. It is also important to keep the skin moist. Sufficient cell hydration is crucial to the healing process.

Your doctor might recommend any of several measures to help the sore heal:

- Wet-to-dry dressings. Dead tissue adheres to this special dressing as it dries and comes off when the bandage is removed.
- Hydrocolloid dressings. These dressings retain oxygen and moisture. Sometimes they are left on for days at a time.
- Enzyme medications. These medications dissolve only dead tissues.
- Gauze. Often gauze is soaked with saline solution. It must be kept moist, or it could pull off new tissue when it is removed.
- Hydroactive dressings. Dressings such as DuoDerm® are left on for days and allow the body's own enzymes to dissolve dead tissue.
- Electrotherapy. Application of a very small current to the tissue to stimulate healing.

When there is infection present, dressings must be changed often, so hydrocolloid and hydroactive dressings are not used. Infection can spread to tissues or bone, so do not delay reporting any redness or swelling to your physician.

Diet for Healing Pressure Sores

Diet plays a very important role in the healing of a pressure sore. The body is trying to rebuild a part of itself and needs proteins and nutrients as building materials.

When a sore occurs, a great deal of protein can be lost from the sore itself, depending on its size. Protein should be included in a healing diet. Good-quality protein for healing comes from eating whole grains—brown rice, quinoa, bulgar wheat, and rye—and beans—lentils, peas, chickpeas, kidney, pinto, and lima. Vegetable and grain proteins are more effectively metabolized by the body than is meat, and don't include other elements that place a load on the body, such as fats or remnants of drugs used to fatten livestock. Use animal foods judiciously rather than relying on them as a primary protein source. Processed sugar—hidden in most commercially produced foods—uses up other nutrients when it is digested, robbing the areas that need them. White, processed flour has a similar effect.

Stress also disrupts the process of healing, causing nutrients to be excreted from the body. B vitamins and vitamin C can be easily supplemented in your diet to make up for loss from stress, but it is best to control stress. Although it is upsetting to have a sore—with the possibility of having to limit yourself for weeks or more—giving in to fears hinders the process of healing. Do what you can to avoid falling into the trap of constant emotional—and therefore physical—stress, which only interferes with your recovery. Don't expect yourself to be upbeat all the time—it's natural to be upset about a sore. But it need not be a continual state that will only interfere with healing.

Prevention with Skin Care

The risk of pressure sores is higher when a person is new to managing his condition, before good skin care becomes habitual. You can prevent pressure sores with vigilant skin care every day:

- Avoid unnecessary areas of pressure, noting contact at the knees, hips, buttocks, and sacral bone, ensuring proper fit and contact with braces, catheters, and clothing.
- Regularly inspect areas that receive pressure.
- Use the appropriate wheelchair cushion, and maintain it well.
- Do push-ups often in your wheelchair for pressure relief.
- Shift your position and weight in your wheelchair if you are unable to use your arms to fully lift your body.

■   Use a tilt or recline system with your wheelchair if you are completely unable to accomplish posture shifts.

■   Do not wear rough or irritating undergarments.

■   Do not wear loose undergarments—wrinkles can cause increased pressure in small areas.

■   Keep your buttocks clean, particularly after your bowel program.

■   If your skin is dry, use moisturizers in area of regular contact.

■   If your skin is wet, bacteria and fungi can grow. "Moist" is different from "wet."

■   Eat a balanced diet rich in nutrients needed for skin health—protein; vitamins C, A, and B complex; and zinc. Drink plenty of water to keep tissues moist and flexible.

Inspecting the Skin

You or a personal assistant should observe your skin daily for any indications of pressure sore development. Take Stage One indications just as seriously as an open sore. Use a mirror to check areas where contact normally occurs—the ischium, the sacrum at the bottom of the spine, hips, elbows, heels, insides of the knees, and so on. Inspection mirrors are available that include a strap for use by people with limited grip.

Skin breakdown can also occur from infection. The ischial area where you sit is at high risk because of its regular exposure to bacteria from your stool during bowel movements or from urine from incontinence or catheter accidents. It is possible for a microscopic invasion of the skin to occur and for infection to develop beneath the surface, resulting in significant skin breakdown. Prevention is simple. Keep the area very clean with good habits in your bowel program. Also pay attention to fevers, increases in spasticity, or episodes of hyperreflexia, which can be indicators of infection.

> I got a sore in the emergency room when I was injured. They didn't turn me since they were afraid of doing damage. It needed surgery. I spent two months going side to side because the sore was on my back, so I couldn't lie back. It was on my sacrum. It was very rough. And it delayed my ability to start rehab.

Users of mechanical ventilators run some risk of developing skin breakdown at the tracheal opening in the neck. The tracheal opening is already an open wound and so can attract bacteria. When using a cuffed tracheostomy tube to create a more effective vacuum for air flow, the covered area should be inspected daily. It is usually the goal to wean such a user from the cuff, since it also interferes with the ability to speak.

Rashes

You'll also want to look in those narrow places where the sun doesn't shine, as they say. Locations such as in the groin on either side of your genitals are places that easily become moist. They don't get much opportunity to breathe because you're sitting down most, if not all, of the time. After bathing or showering, you want to make a special point of drying these areas well, even using a hair dryer on cool setting if needed.

The presence of moisture invites the growth of fungus and bacteria that can cause a rash. This is essentially the same as athlete's foot, so the spaces between your toes—easily ignored because they seem so far away and may not be easy for you to reach—also need your special attention.

Use of baby powder is a good preventive strategy, helping to absorb moisture from the surface of the skin. If a rash develops, an over-the-counter treatment such as Tinactin® spray can help manage it. If the condition persists, see your doctor. And be careful not to mistake the redness of a pending skin breakdown for a rash. If this occurs in an area where you have no sensation, you will not be able to judge the difference, since a rash tends to itch in a way that a pressure sore does not.

Cushions

The design of wheelchair cushions to minimize sores has become very advanced. It is critical for people who sit for long periods of time or who have reduced ischial muscle mass to sit on an appropriate surface that properly spreads and reduces pressure and to practice good pressure-relief habits. The basic types of cushions are air flotation, gel, foam, urethane, and alternating pressure. Cushions are described in more detail in Chapter 4, Wheelchair Selection.

For people less mobile in their chair, cushioning is also important for wheelchair backs. Continuous contact with the back of the chair can lead to scapular sores in the shoulder area. There are wheelchair back options with scapular cutouts to prevent this from happening.

Your bed is another important place to ensure even pressure distribution as a way to prevent sores. Spending more time in bed than in your chair—for example, after surgery or during an extended illness—is a high-risk period when you need to be extra vigilant. "Eggcrate" pads for the bed are commonly used in hospitals and are moderately priced for home use; the foam surface spreads and reduces pressure by means of peaks and valleys.

Some sophisticated bed-cushioning products include an air or water pump that maintains pressure throughout the pad, or alters it gradually, alternating pressure changes across the body to provide relief to one part while the other is more supported.

> *Even though my mattress is extra soft, it still needs something to help spread the pressure more evenly. An egg-crate pad has worked perfectly. I rotate it every so often and, at some point, have to get a new one because it gets sort of compressed. I also like it because it's comfortable for my wife, too, and, as it's under the sheet, it doesn't make our bed seem like a hospital bed.*

Sheepskins are also popular bed cushioning. The wool is trimmed and the sheepskins are laid under the bottom sheet. They are soft and comfortable and minimize pressure points, particularly on the hips, elbows, and knee joints, which tend to get the most contact while lying down. Some sheepskins cannot be laundered; the skin becomes hard and brittle.

Scoliosis

Excessive curvature of the spine is a serious problem. The spine supports you and allows you to bend and twist. The spine is meant to work in cooperation with the muscles of your trunk, the job of which is to balance and move us and to maintain the intended, optimal functional shape of the spine.

The spine's gently curving shape is part of its flexibility. Because the curves are gentle, the spine's structural capacity remains strong. When the curves become severe—or when the spine curves to the side, out of its natural symmetry—the spine's ability to do its job of structural support is compromised. Muscles must start to do more of the work of carrying us, leading to fatigue, back pain, and continuing degradation of the spine. The further curvature and degradation progresses, the faster the damage happens.

Some people with disabilities have limited use of trunk muscles, particularly with high-level quadriplegia from SCI and those with CP, progressive stages of certain muscular dystrophies, MS, and ALS. Such people are at greater risk of spinal curvature because muscles are too weak or paralyzed to help keep the spine in alignment.

Prevention

The spine—and the body in general—learns from how it is used. If you spend enough time in slumped and twisted postures, your body learns this state. Muscles, ligaments, and bones will begin to adapt, changing shape and adopting the curvature as normal. Your sitting habits—in or out of the wheelchair—and sleeping positions can either support the proper shape of the spine or teach it to go out of line.

Many chair users hook an arm behind them on a push handle to support the upper body while they reach with the other hand. If you have limited upper-body balance, you are at risk of falling over unless you anchor yourself somehow. There is a tendency to reach with your dominant hand and always twist in the same direction, thus teaching the spine to adopt a curve in that direction.

For some people without sufficient upper-body strength and balance, pushing a manual wheelchair puts deforming strains on the spine. This man with spinal cord quadriplegia in his early 30s found that using a manual wheelchair was not really appropriate for him:

> I used a manual chair for 10 years. For me it was an ego thing. I really felt that people looked at me differently in a power chair than in a manual chair. The biomechanics of a quadriplegic or a paraplegic operating a manual chair are like the difference between night and day. I have a severe scoliosis from using a manual chair and also from hooking my arm around the back.

The proper specification of wheelchair and positioning systems—backs, cushions, stabilization accessories, and so on—along with vigilant posture management are crucial to preventing spinal curvature. Therapists often do not teach people enough about posture during the rehabilitation process. In the attempt to get comfortable, you might establish poor habits that can contribute to scoliosis. If spinal curvature has not progressed too far, it can be corrected by changing those habits. This man changed habits when he began to see a chiropractor:

> I used to sit in all kinds of curvy, slumping postures. Sitting in a wheelchair most of the day gets uncomfortable, so I was just trying to get some variety. No one ever talked to me about these issues. Then I went to see a chiropractor who took x-rays that showed my spine was very curvy. He taught me better posture, got me using a back cushion, and did regular adjustments to free up my spine to realign itself. After six months, the difference in the x-rays was amazing, and now people comment on my good posture. Best of all, it's my natural posture now, even though at first it was an effort to sit straight. Now it's comfortable.

Wheelchair riders need a variety of postures because the body needs movement and comfort. Good posture is a matter of being conscious of how you hold your body, spending more time comfortably supported upright, and spending brief amounts of time in nonneutral postures. When you slouch to the right, next time do it to the left.

To the degree that you still have sufficient upper-body balance and control, the risk of spinal curvature can be prevented by having the right equipment and knowing how you use your body. Being active, maintaining range of motion, having properly-specified, well-maintained equipment, and being aware of your posture are key to maintaining the health of your spine and avoiding the daunting impact of scoliosis.

What Goes Wrong?

A number of undesirable things happen when the spine goes out of shape. The muscles and ligaments around the spine get stretched out of shape, compromising their ability to support the spine and causing discomfort and pain. In the long term, it becomes difficult to sit for more than brief periods of time.

When the spine deforms, the rib cage also deforms; the lungs are compressed, compromising the ability to breathe fully and provide the oxygen your muscles and metabolism require.

As the spine deforms, the discs between the vertebrae get squeezed. Discs are gelatinous cushions, key to the flexibility of the spine. When the discs get compressed, they change their shape, get pushed out of position, and begin to lose some of their gelatinous fluid. It is very difficult for the discs to regain their shape, and, once fluid is lost, it cannot be replaced. Damage is permanent.

Discs also help maintain the space where nerves extend from the spinal cord to the rest of the body. When the space between vertebrae gets smaller, nerves are pressed, causing damage and pain. This compression might cost you the ability to use parts of the body previously unaffected by your disability. Ultimately, neighboring vertebrae come into contact and begin to fuse. The flexibility of that "joint" in the spine is lost. If the curvature is severe enough, the spinal cord itself can be at risk of a compression injury.

Surgery

When scoliosis is allowed to progress, surgery becomes necessary. The typical approach is the installation of Harrington rods, steel bars attached to the straightened spine. Harrington rods maintain the shape of the spine without relying on muscles of the back. The surgery is very involved, and the rods limit the freedom of the spine to move, imposing a rigid upright posture on the person. In rare instances, there is a risk of injury to the spinal cord from the surgery.

When scoliosis has become progressive, the surgery can be lifesaving. Many people feel a great relief to have an upright, symmetrical posture again, despite the rigidity. For people born with CP, certain muscular dystrophies, or other childhood disabilities that affect the back, this surgery is often necessary early in life and can make a significant difference in their quality of life.

Spasticity

Spasticity is an issue for people with spastic CP, SCIs in the thoracic and cervical regions, MS, ALS, and other conditions involving the spinal cord and brain. Spasticity can be a daily event—painful and significant enough to interfere with daily activities. How seriously spasms affect someone's life varies widely. They can be extremely painful and severely limit your ability to function. Or they can be an aggravating, occasional event, as this woman with an SCI reports:

> Generally spasms aren't terribly painful, just terribly both-
> ersome. They make it hard to transfer and keep me awake
> sometimes at night. I have had a decrease in spasms since
> my release from rehab in 1996. I attribute the decrease to
> better medications. One kind of spasm has never changed:
> every time I lie down flat on my back, I get terrific extensor
> spasms (my legs become stiff as boards and my feet and
> toes curl outward). This usually subsides within a few
> seconds. But sometimes when I try to get up, it happens
> all over again.

Contracting a muscle is not a simple, one-way communication, where the brain sends a message and the muscle contracts. Instead, the communication between brain and muscle is two way and more complex. The brain is getting immediate feedback from the muscle, about how much it has contracted, whether it is fatigued, and if there is pain, for instance. The communication is a loop of nerve impulses going back and forth.

Not all impulses to a muscle originate in the brain. Direct stimulation of the muscle causes a reflex response. This is what happens when a doctor taps you on the elbow with that little rubber hammer. The muscle responds with a contraction. With a central nervous system disruption, this loop of communication between brain and muscle can get interrupted. Reflexes run amuck, resulting in spasms; the brain is unable to sense the muscle contracting and then send the appropriate messages to the muscle to calm the reflex. Spasms could be a brief episode in which parts of your body suddenly move, sometimes in a repetitive, vibrating manner.

Spasticity can also be chronic, pulling the body into positions, which can lead to scoliosis, digestive problems, or limited range of motion.

Not All Bad News

Spasticity is not always a bad thing. Spasms exercise your muscles, since they are contracting and maintaining some degree of muscle bulk; the only other way to exercise paralyzed muscles is with direct electrical stimulation. By maintaining muscle tone, you can be protected from pressure sores that are more likely to develop with atrophied muscles. With quadriplegia, this muscle tone can help maintain postural integrity—the increased muscle bulk provides better trunk support. Many people find they are able to wear shorts, being less self-conscious of their legs, which remain muscular. Some who are counting on the future results of spinal cord cure research feel that keeping muscle tone improves their chances of being able to benefit from possible advances.

Increases in spasticity can serve as an early warning system for other changes in health, such as infections, an over-full bladder, a pressure sore, the presence of an injury you cannot feel, or more serious conditions such as the development of a spinal cyst (known as syringomyelia), spinal tumors, transverse myelitis, or Guillain-Barré syndrome, for example. Any changes in the general pattern of your spasticity should not be ignored—it might be an important sign.

Some people take advantage of spasticity to help them make transfers to and from their wheels or to assist in emptying their bladder. However, spasms can also interfere with transfers, when they are more likely to occur. Spasms can force you constantly out of position in your chair, adding to the challenge of anyone assisting you who must manage your posture throughout the day.

There are three approaches to spasticity, depending on how it affects you: managing it on your own, pharmaceutical, and surgical. Doctors will often not treat spasticity unless it is disrupting the ability to make transfers or the ability to sleep or is a substantial source of pain. Other times, you might be treated by a doctor who considers spasticity something to always prevent.

> I use spasticity. I work out my legs by inducing spasms. I just
> know how to do it. It was another irony of rehab that they put
> me on baclofen to get rid of my spasms. When my leg extends
> in a spasm, I can feel it and it feels good. They wanted to get
> rid of that. To the extent where spasticity gets in the way of

*function, I would say yes, that needs to be controlled. I've
known people who've had spasms where they almost fall out
of their chair. But they didn't really assess me well enough to
gauge that.*

Managing It on Your Own

Some people manage their moderate spasticity on their own, learning how
to avoid stimulations that cause spasms and knowing how to respond to
calm the response if it occurs. For others, the spasticity is too strong a
response and needs more significant measures to manage.

Stress increases spasticity, so relaxation methods are valuable. Simple
breathing exercises and self-hypnosis can help moderate spasms. If you
sense spasms coming and they are painful for you, you are more likely to
become tense and upset, which actually promotes the spasms. Learning how
to relax in response to the onset of spasms is a useful skill.

This woman with SCI has found a gentle approach to managing her
spasticity:

*Warm water and massage are definitely helpful. I'm fortu-
nate that one of my former rehab nurses has a massage certificate and comes to my home twice a month for massage
sessions. She also does range-of-motion [exercises] and I can
ask her questions about SCI-related topics. She is a gem!
Massage is so beneficial, not only with spasticity and pain
management, but it gives such a feeling of well-being and
relaxation.*

Certain postures are known to promote or inhibit specific reflex patterns. Lying in the prone position, face down, tends to inhibit flexion, in
which the body would close toward the fetal position. Standing also inhibits
flexion, which would interfere with walking. Sitting promotes flexion. Lying
on your side or face up (supine) tends to inhibit extension in which the
arms, legs, and hips open up.

Spasticity promotes contracture—in which muscles are trained into
chronically shortened positions. It is important to counteract spastic muscles with stretching and range-of-motion exercises in the opposite direction
to prevent the body from becoming restricted in its ability to move and
achieve comfortable postures.

Stimulants like coffee and caffeinated tea generate more nervous system activity and so can increase spasms. Relaxing drinks like chamomile
tea have a calming effect. Kava kava is an herb that some people have found
helps them manage symptoms.

> *I read about kava kava online. I use it at night when my*
> *spasms are worse. They would keep me up at night. Using*
> *kava kava, I have been getting the best night sleep in years. I*
> *have tried both baclofen and Robaxin®, and the kava kava*
> *works better than either for me.*

Your general health has an impact on spasticity. Being overweight and eating a poor diet—especially with too much sugar, which is a stimulant—adds stress to your nervous system.

Pharmaceutical Management

The most well-known drug for managing spasticity is baclofen, known commercially as Lioresal®. Baclofen is similar in chemical structure to GABA, a neurotransmitter deficient in people with spasticity. In some cases, baclofen has also been found to improve bladder control. In rare instances, reversible coma has occurred from toxic levels of baclofen.

Baclofen is available as an oral medication, but, if taken orally, little of the drug actually reaches the spinal fluid where it must do its work. The oral form only lasts in the bloodstream for eight hours.

Baclofen is more commonly used with an intrathecal pump, which supplies a continuous stream of the drug directly to the spinal fluid. With this method of distribution, only 1/100th of the typical oral dose need be taken. The baclofen pump is surgically implanted underneath the skin and needs to be replaced every four to five years. The pump must be refilled every month or two by means of an injection.

The next most common medication is diazepam, which may also be sold as Valium®. Diazepam is a muscle relaxant and sedative. It is absorbed quickly by the body and stays in the system longer than baclofen when taken orally. Still, diazepam needs to be taken two to three times per day. Diazepam works on the brain, causes drowsiness, and can lead to dependence.

The medication dantrolene—sold as Dantrium®—weakens the muscles themselves, so is less likely to cause drowsiness or other central nervous system side effects that are common with the use of sedatives. Dantrolene is more preferred for cerebral forms of spasticity. It is considered helpful for spasticity in MS, which is predominately spinal. In a small percentage of users, the drug has caused slight liver damage. There is some concern that it could exacerbate seizures in people with CP.

Several other drugs are also used for spasticity, including tizanidine (Zanaflex®) and vigabatrin (Sabril®). As with all medications, be sure to ask your doctor specifically how the drugs function in your body, why she recommends it in your case, the effects on libido, and what possible side effects could occur. For example, the medications might affect memory, emotional state, concentration, and energy level.

Drugs can also be injected directly into muscles, selectively impeding the spastic response. Alcohol and phenol have commonly been used for this purpose over the last 20 years, but are painful to people with sensation. Botulinum toxin (Botox® or Myobloc©) is a purified form of the toxin that causes botulism or food poisoning. It is safely injected into muscle and is now frequently used, particularly with children with CP. Botulinum toxin injections are also found useful for abnormal facial contractions in MS. Botulinum toxin usually takes two to three days to take effect and can last for as long as two to four months.

> We tried Valium during rehab and I cried for three days—
> not a good choice. Baclofen definitely helps (I take 100
> mg/day). Another beneficial drug is Dantrium. I have had
> good luck with it, but unfortunately it is extremely expensive
> and sort of hard on your liver. I'm trying to decrease it (from
> 300 mg/day to 200 mg/day). I have a quadriplegic friend
> who had a baclofen pump installed and he said it changed
> his life.

Surgical Treatment

The baclofen pump has also supplanted surgical measures, which were once used widely. Aside from the aforementioned cutting of tendons—known as a tenotomy—the most typical surgery was the dorsal rhizotomy, which is still an option in some cases. In a dorsal rhizotomy, the surgeon operates on the nerves in the spinal canal, which branch out to the areas where a person experiences spasms. Under general anesthesia, he will literally test each nerve branch for abnormal responses to stimulation and then cut, burn, or chemically injure those peripheral nerves to interrupt the spastic response.

For people who are functionally impaired by spasticity, experience considerable pain, and have no expectation of recovering use of the muscles fed by those nerves, a dorsal rhizotomy might remain a valid option that could make a great difference in quality of life. It is generally reserved for severe cases.

Tendon transfer is another option a surgeon might consider. This procedure moves the tendon attached to a spastic muscle to another connection where its force can be used. For example, it could use a spastic response to aid in the movement of a hand or elbow or the ability to lift a foot while walking, a common issue for stroke survivors. This operation is very complex and requires a surgeon to identify very specifically what muscles are impaired and which ones have a controllable spastic response in order to determine if a transfer could be of rehabilitative value.

Spasticity and Aging

Getting older might itself lessen the effects of spasticity. Nerve conduction slows as we age, and muscle mass and blood flow to the spinal cord become reduced. At the same time, as you age, your body also gets more sensitive and your ability to be patient with spasms or pain might be reduced. If you experience overuse injuries with age, this also might cause spasms to be painful, which in the past could be better endured.

Stress

The human body's stress reaction is referred to as the "fight or flight" response. To help you fight with your arms or run away from danger, the body increases its heart rate and sends blood to the extremities. When you are experiencing stress reaction, blood is taken away from your digestive tract. While you are under stress, you are not absorbing nutrients effectively; they are instead excreted through your bodily wastes. Vitamin C is lost in large amounts to the stress response.

Under stress, there is a tendency to limit your breathing and the amount of fresh oxygen you take into your body. Shallow breathing also involves holding muscles of the trunk, abdomen, and often the shoulders and neck in constant, low-level exertion. For people with pulmonary limitations as a factor of their disability, stress only decreases their respiratory efficiency.

There are a number of unique stresses you might experience as a wheelchair user:

- Pushing a wheelchair to overexertion raises your body's metabolic processes in ways that mimic a continual stress response.
- Awkwardness in handling your body while wheeling, transferring, or performing daily tasks such as work or cooking is stressful and fatiguing over the course of a day.
- Some daily tasks such as dressing or using the bathroom could be strenuous for you.
- Worrying how others see you, particularly at stages of disability when you are adapting to your new identity as a chair rider, can by psychologically stressful.
- You might experience discrimination, such as being denied access to jobs or transportation.

■   Stresses with bureaucracies such as Social Security, Vocational Rehabil-
      itation, Medicaid, Medicare, or other systems that you must rely on
      for support.

The simple act of breathing is an extremely valuable stress manager.
When you take a couple of deep breaths and close your eyes, you can discover where you are holding physical tension in your muscles. Breathing
allows you to notice that your belly is tight or your shoulders are slightly
raised or that you are holding your head in a limited range. If you don't have
the use of your trunk muscles, keeping the area around the lungs relaxed is
all the more important.

You already know how to breathe, of course, but you might be in the
habit of breathing only in your chest. Even if your disability precludes the
use of your abdominal muscles, you can imagine your breath starting from
that part of your body. Imagine that the air you are breathing first goes all
the way down to the very bottom of your lungs and out to the farthest small
branches of the bronchial "trees" that make up your lungs. As you practice
this method, you will find that you are able to comfortably take in more air.
This ability to breathe deeply will help you counteract the stress response.

Another important technique for stress management is your own
thinking. When there are parts of your life that are upsetting, staying focused
on those problems increases the negative impact of the resulting stress. In
time, you lose perspective and the ability to think objectively. Certainly it is
healthy to experience emotions about events and challenges in your life,
but it is not healthy to be continually overwhelmed by them. You can minimize the effect of stress by doing your best to relax, giving your attention
to other activities and allowing your mind to have a rest from what is troubling you. When you come back to thinking about a problem, you will likely
have a fresh perspective, and your body will not suffer so much from the tension, loss of nutrients, and other detrimental effects of excessive stress.

Meditation might sound like something that only Buddhist monks or
Californians do, but it is a simple and powerful tool available to anyone,
anywhere. Meditation is not about going into a trance, nor is it about super-
human concentration. To meditate, all you do is sit comfortably and pay
attention to your breathing. That's all. Your thoughts will continue but, each
time you notice getting caught up in a certain thought, just put your attention back to your breathing. Decide that for the 15 minutes you will spend
in meditation—or longer, if you choose—that any thought that comes
to you will still be around later, and you don't have to stop and explore
it. The simple act of observing your breathing will allow you to gain a fresh

perspective and help to moderate physical tension and emotions. Try it once a day for a week, without judgment, and see what happens.

Bowel and Bladder Issues

Urinary Tract Infections

Urinary tract infections or bladder infections are a constant risk for those with a neurogenic bladder. If not cared for promptly, a UTI can make you severely ill with high fever, spread to the kidneys, and ultimately kill you. However, the only reason an infection would reach these proportions is if you don't take care of yourself.

Multiple sclerosis is often treated with immunosuppressive drugs that increase the risk of infection. Urinary complications are common with MS. Women more frequently have neurogenic bladders with MS than do men, and so they have more UTIs. When men with MS get infections, however, they tend to be more severe.

Some people with disabilities experience low-grade bladder infections two or three times a year without the infections being a major problem. Many other people find they constantly struggle with more severe UTIs. They find it difficult to hold a job or make social commitments because of the frequency of occurrence.

Despite a good bladder program, some people continue to struggle with UTIs. It has been a chronic problem for this 35-year-old woman with L5 paraplegia from an SCI:

> *I've been plagued by UTIs. I've been getting them every month. They've been associated with my period. It's been like clock-work, when my period's ending. I've tried almost everything. Drinking a lot. Cranberry juice and pills. I've tried herbal remedies. Anticholinergics. Vitamin C. Irrigation. The only thing I haven't tried is prophylactic antibiotics.*

The most common contributors to UTI are:

- Failing to drink enough and empty the bladder often
- Excessive intake of dehydrating drinks—caffeine or alcohol—and salty foods
- Picking up infection from a sexual partner
- Bacteria carried into the bladder on a catheter

The answer to the first is obvious—drink enough appropriate liquids and commit to a regular bladder program appropriate to your needs and minimize dehydrating foods. The third is solved by using condoms, urinating after sex, and paying attention to signs of infection, which indicate that you should employ sexual options other than intercourse until the condition clears. People who use catheters have a harder time preventing infections completely because they are regularly inserting a foreign object into their body. No matter how well you clean the catheter, some bacteria are going to get in. Nonetheless, practice the cleanest habits you can. Signs of a urinary infection include:

■   Fever
■   Sweating and chills
■   Nausea and vomiting
■   Increased spasticity
■   Difficulty urinating
■   Pain during urination
■   Cloudy or foul smelling urine
■   Bloody urine (pink, red, or rusty in color)
■   Change in volume of urine—either more or less
■   Sudden onset of leaking between catheterizations

When you have a UTI, you need to drink two to three additional glasses of water each day to help flush out the bacteria and prevent the bacteria from multiplying and the infection from spreading. Visit your urologist, who will culture your urine to determine an appropriate antibiotic, if necessary. People with chronic infections need to be careful; overuse allows the body to build a resistance to antibiotics, rendering them ineffective for treating future infections.

Stones are another risk with a neurogenic bladder. Excessive calcium can collect in the bladder, kidney, or ureters, which are the tubes that connect the kidneys and bladder. The formation of stones is encouraged by residual urine, chronic infections, incorrect catheterization, lack of fluids, or lack of physical activity. The ureters can become blocked by stones, increasing backup of urine into the kidneys. Symptoms include sweating, severe pain, blood in the urine, increased spasticity, or pain in the lower back or abdomen. Stones are usually removed surgically, though there are new techniques being developed such as using sound waves to crush the stones.

As a diagnostic test, a urologist might perform:

■   A renal scan or ultrasound, in which a dye is injected into the body and then is flushed through the kidneys. An x-ray is then able to reveal the condition of the urinary tract.

■   A cystoscopy, which is a visual examination inside the urinary tract
     with a cystoscope, inserted by catheter through the urethra, to inspect
     for stones.

Many physiatrists recommend that bladder diagnostics be routinely
performed every two years for people with neurogenic bladders as a preventive management measure.

Bowel and Bladder Management

The ability to evacuate your bowels and bladder depends on your particular disability. For example, the ability depends on the level of a condition
that otherwise affects your nervous system, such as a brain injury, MS, or
ALS, the level of a spinal cord disability, or the strength of surrounding muscles of the bladder, such as the urinary sphincter.

Normal, reflexive emptying happens when the bowels or bladder
become full and send a message to a particular area of the spinal cord. The
message then goes to the brain, which can send back the instruction to relax
the sphincter muscle or to hold on until later.

Injury or disease can interfere with this communication process. For
example, in an SCI, if the spinal cord is damaged above T12, the message
will reach the reflex arc, but not the brain. This is known as a reflex or spastic bladder or bowel; you will not be able to control when your bowel and
bladder will empty. If the cord obstruction is below L2, the message will not
reach the cord at all, and your body does not know it is time to respond. This
is known as a nonreflex or flaccid condition, sometimes referred to as a
frozen bladder.

Management of these neurogenic conditions is central to the degree
of independence possible in your life. Tremendous amounts of time can be
spent dealing with your bowels and bladder—but this depends considerably on how consistent and well-designed your bowel and bladder programs are. A poor bladder program can invite nearly constant infections.
Surgeries could become necessary, such as installation of a suprapubic
catheter through the abdomen or cutting the sphincter muscle to allow
urine to flow.

A poor bowel program can allow constipation, making evacuation
very difficult. You might spend hours dealing with evoking a bowel movement, inserting suppositories, stimulating the area, manually cleaning out
the stool with a gloved hand, or relying on a personal assistant to do so.
For some, bowel management unavoidably takes some time, but you have
some control over how much time it takes, depending on your habits and
discipline.

Soft Stool and Constipation

A good bowel program starts with maintaining a good consistency in your stool. When your feces becomes too dry and firm, not only will you have more difficulty in emptying your bowels, but you are allowing bacteria to remain in your body for a longer period of time. Bacteria can multiply and become the cause of infections and other problems.

Firm stool is irritating to the colon and can cause hemorrhoids. It might also require you to apply more aggressive manual stimulation in your bowel program, which can further irritate those delicate tissues. Diarrhea can be an indication of constipation, since the runny stool can be from the water lost from the fecal matter farther up the intestines. The more severe the diarrhea becomes, the more likely you are to become impacted. You need to drink more water to replace the fluids lost with diarrhea.

Avoid becoming reliant on laxatives, which dull the nerves of the bowel and compromise whatever reflex activity you might have retained. If you continue to have chronic constipation, there might be another medical issue involved, and you should see your doctor. Enemas are also a poor standard method. They stretch the colon and compromise its tone. Your body can develop a dependency on these measures if they are overused.

Start with Food

Diet plays an important role in managing stool softness. Before relying on drugs such as stool softeners to manage your bowels, start with food. Foods that prevent or cure constipation include fluids, wheat bran, rice bran, vegetables, and fruits—especially prunes, figs, and dates.

The advice you have heard for years is true: include fiber and bulk in your diet. Fibrous food absorbs and retains water, keeping your stool at an appropriate softness. Fiber remains in the intestines because it is not digested. Humans are not equipped with the enzymes capable of breaking down cellulose and absorbing it into the body (only termites have that ability!). Fiber helps stimulate the nerve reflexes in the colon wall that trigger bowel movement. Fiber also reduces your chances of developing hemorrhoids, varicose veins, or diverticulitis, which results from the formation of small pockets in the intestines where stool becomes trapped, allowing bacteria to grow.

Fiber can be overdone. Add fiber gradually, making note of how it affects your stool, and work your way up to a consistent level, allowing your body to adapt. Because fiber absorbs water, you must increase fluid intake as you increase bulk in your diet. Too much fiber without enough fluid can cause hard stools—and eventually impaction. Diuretic medicines, designed to remove fluid from the body, will also affect the amount of fiber you can accommodate, as do the diuretic effects of coffee and alcohol.

The modern, highly processed diet in general is much lower in fiber than in the past. To add fiber to your diet, choose whole grain or coarse breads or use a bread machine to make high-fiber breads. Miller's bran and rice bran are available in powdered form to sprinkle on cereals, salads, and other creative alternatives. Whole fresh fruits and vegetables provide bulk and fiber.

The age-old belief in prunes is true. Prunes are high in fiber and vitamin A, have no cholesterol or fat, and have a laxative effect. A glass of prune juice each day can help manage your bowels. Or keep a supply of pitted prunes around so you can pop one in your mouth now and then during the day.

Don't use coffee as a tool to manage your bowels or health. For some people, a cup of coffee has a laxative effect, but not because of the caffeine, which can be a cause of constipation. If you have chronic problems, either with constipation or diarrhea, look at your coffee habits. Too much coffee also amplifies stress.

Dairy foods, by virtue of their calcium content, contribute to constipation. Milk should not be too large a part of your diet.

Medications influence your diet and how you process foods. Ask your physician how drugs she prescribes for you will affect your stool consistency and bowel program.

Have a Program

Most of you will have received guidance in a rehabilitation program or been advised by your physician on what bowel and bladder management program will work best for you. However, sometimes a doctor or program will simply apply a given model that doesn't take individual abilities and needs into account. Your own personal experience will show what your individual capabilities are and guide you in determining the best management program. Many brain or spinal cord traumas—whether from injury, infection, birth defect, or disease—are not complete, so some messages from the nerves might be getting through, giving you access to some degree of use of your bladder or bowel sphincter muscles. Your ability to tighten or relax these muscles can determine whether the process requires manual support or how much of your day you must devote to elimination. Although you might be diagnosed as having no control or sensation, you might retain some manual control of the sphincter muscles or have some capacity to sense when your bowel or bladder is full.

> *Rehab had me use a leg bag attached to a condom to continu-*
> *ously collect drips from my weak bladder. I found that I had*
> *enough control to only need to put a cap in the condom,*
> *assuming I used the bathroom before my bladder would fill.*
> *That is when I experience involuntary urination. This contin-*
> *ues to surprise doctors, given my level of SCI.*

The Bladder Program

A neurogenic bladder has a difficult time emptying itself completely. Urine left behind in the bladder—known as "residual"—will stagnate and allow growth of bacteria, which causes infection. A very full bladder can eventually back up into the kidneys, disrupting the important filtration task they perform and leading to infection and disease.

You must drink plenty of water, as much as three quarts per day or a glass every hour. All of this fresh fluid keeps flushing you out and reduces the risk of bacteria remaining in place long enough to cause trouble. But chair users face a contradiction in drinking extra fluids. For many chair riders, using the bathroom is time consuming and involves a lot of mechanical or physical effort or the time involved in cleaning an intermittent catheter. You must find a balance for yourself, putting a priority on your safety and health while reducing inconvenience.

> *I was avoiding going to the bathroom because I didn't want*
> *to have to do all the work of getting my pants off and back*
> *on. I have some control, but it is not a reflex. That means I*
> *have to push continuously to urinate, and it can be tiring.*
> *But I discovered that I wasn't drinking enough and so got*
> *infections more often. Or else I would delay going, and my*
> *external catheter would slip and get me all wet. Now I know*
> *I have to drink enough. I do my best to stay calm in the*
> *bathroom and do the whole routine with the least possible*
> *strain. It turns out I didn't have to push as hard to urinate*
> *after all.*

With a flaccid bladder, some ability to know when it is time to empty is lost. There is already a disruption in the automated system of your brain getting the signal that it is time to empty and sending back the message for the sphincter muscle to release. The bladder cannot develop enough pressure to overcome the resistance of the sphincter muscle, so urine is held in. If the bladder fills too much, it begins to stretch, known as "overdistention," and urine begins to back into the kidneys. Remaining muscle tone will be damaged, and what bladder function you have can be lost. Since your body is not giving you the sensations to know when these events are happening, you must practice a regular bladder program and be very conscious of how much fluid you take into your body and how your body determines when you need to void.

It might be possible to empty a flaccid bladder if you use the Credé technique—pressing against your bladder with your fist to overcome the resistance of the sphincter. Discuss this method with your doctor to ensure that it is safe for you. This technique is likely to leave behind residual urine, but, depending on your fluid intake, this could be a manageable approach. It might be necessary on occasion to catheterize yourself.

A spastic bladder might try to empty itself at any time; the amount can be small, leaving behind residual urine. The reflex is most likely to occur when the bladder is full, but it can also be triggered by contractions from muscle spasticity in your legs, if that is an issue for you. Spasms in the bladder will increase with the presence of an infection or stones. The spastic bladder can be triggered by massaging the abdomen, by leaning forward or doing pushups from the sitting position, or by stimulating the rectum with a gloved finger. Once the reflex begins, it will continue, so you need either to be sitting on a toilet or commode or have an appropriate collection system in place. Women rely on medication, urine-absorbing pads or, as a last resort, bladder augmentation surgery.

With either a flaccid or spastic bladder, you will want to limit your fluid intake in the evening to reduce your need for emptying during the night.

Catheterization

A catheter is a narrow tube inserted through the urethra, beyond the sphincter muscle, and into the bladder, allowing it to drain. There are two kinds of catheterization, indwelling and intermittent. Which kind you use depends on the bladder condition you have and other considerations such as convenience, lifestyle, and cost. An indwelling catheter remains in the bladder for up to several days and is usually attached to a drainage bag that straps onto the leg and collects urine. With intermittent catheterization, urine is emptied into a plastic urinal or container or directly into a standard urinal.

A flaccid bladder typically must be emptied with an indwelling catheter, since the sphincter muscle is frozen and cannot be consciously relaxed. A spastic bladder might not be capable of emptying itself completely, so occasional use of a catheter might be necessary to remove residual urine. Males with spastic bladders or some control of the urinary sphincter can often manage well with male urinary condoms.

This woman who uses intermittent catheterization describes her routine:

> *I prefer to cath in bed because it's easier for me to pull my*
> *pants up and down. I do clean cath, I don't do sterile. I don't*
> *use gloves or Betadine. I boil my catheters to clean them. I use*
> *a mirror, which makes it easier for me to find the spot. I don't*
> *want to be poking around because I'm so prone to UTIs, and I*
> *don't want to chance causing irritation.*

Catheters come in various sizes, identified in French units, which indicate the outside circumference—16 and 18 Fr. are common sizes. The overall size does not indicate the size of the inside channel, so it is important to learn more about the design of the product you choose. You might want to cut open a used catheter to become familiar with its design. The size of the inside channel will determine how quickly the catheter might become clogged. A larger catheter is not always a good solution, as it can still plug up and cause complications in the urethra.

Catheters are made of latex or silicone. Some latex catheters are coated with Teflon to ease their passage. However, latex catheters will generally be smaller inside because of the extra surface layer. Some people develop latex sensitivity and so must use the more costly silicone type.

Either intermittent or indwelling catheters entail a risk of chronic infection because you are necessarily introducing a foreign object into your urinary tract. Again, religiously keeping the catheter clean, using a fresh one as often as possible, and drinking plenty of water will go a long way toward protecting you from infection.

Indwelling or Foley Catheters

An indwelling or Foley catheter remains in place for days at a time, allowing the bladder to empty continuously into a leg or bedside drainage bag. Indwelling catheters include a small balloon at the internal end that is filled with water to keep the catheter from pulling out. The "Foley kit" used for sterile insertion includes the water-filled syringe for this purpose. An indwelling catheter is also the solution for quadriplegics who cannot perform intermittent catheterization for lack of hand dexterity.

A suprapubic catheter is a type of indwelling catheter inserted surgically through the abdomen into the bladder because of conditions that prevent entry through the urethra. Some people experience leakage around the opening where the catheter enters. There is a chance of having to relocate a suprapubic catheter after some years; the previous opening could take a while to close, requiring you to deal with leaking from the opening until it heals.

With indwelling and suprapubic catheters, there is an increased risk of infection from the continuous presence of a foreign object in the body. Catheters can become clogged in time if the urine contains sediment or is cloudy from a persistent infection. It is very important to pay attention to whether you are voiding as much fluid as you are taking in.

Indwelling and suprapubic catheters empty the bladder continuously. As a result, the bladder shrinks and loses muscle tone. Eventually, bladder walls can become firm. Carefully consider whether to go ahead with either of these two options, since they can result in a change to your bladder that might not be reversible. Consult with your physician on the reasons to use them. Despite these permanent changes, one of these options might be the right thing for you to do. In particular, those without the hand dexterity for self-catheterization benefit from continuous drainage. The logistics of getting assistance or the difficulty of trying to do it alone when it challenges your ability might not be worth the effort to avoid the possible complications. If you will continue to use an indwelling approach, a smaller bladder might not matter to you.

Spasms can cause leakage around a catheter, since the strength of the muscle contraction may force more urine into the tube than it can accommodate. The excess will flow around the tube instead. Some spasms can be powerful enough to force out an indwelling catheter even with its balloon inflated, which can stretch the bladder and cause damage to the urethra. This is more of an issue for women, whose urethras are shorter than men's. There are two commonly recommended anticholinergic medications for this problem, Probanthine and Ditropan, which relax the bladder to minimize spasms.

If you are having to change your catheter more often than usual, take time to find out why. Not drinking enough fluid is the most common reason for a catheter to become prematurely clogged. Water is the best fluid to drink. Tea, lemonade, and fruit juices are also good. Cranberry juice has long been thought to be healthy for the bladder and even part of a treatment program for infections, although there is no hard research to support it. Do not choose products that rely heavily on sugar, corn syrup, or artificial flavors and sweeteners.

A clogged catheter might also be an indication that you are developing stones. Stones do not develop when your urine, rather than becoming too alkaline, maintains a sufficient acid level. Carbonated drinks and certain foods make the urine more alkaline, noticeable by a stronger odor. The best way to get your urine back to an acid level is simply to drink more water. You can test this yourself with pH paper found at any pharmacy. A good pH level is from 5 to 6.5.

Intermittent Catheterization

With intermittent catheterization, you insert a catheter when it is time to empty the bladder, performing the process several times per day. A nurse or therapist trains you in the proper techniques for self-catheterization. In the hospital, a fresh catheter is used each time. After discharge, the same catheter can be reused, assuming you practice very clean habits. If you use intermittent catheters, you would carry catheters and supplies for cleaning; these can be carried in a pack on the back of your wheelchair.

Historically, bladder catheterization programs have been based on a time model. Such a program encouraged you to empty your bladder every four to six hours. At times, there would be a small amount of urine, meaning that the invasion of a catheter was an unnecessary act. In that interval between catheterizations, the bladder might also have become very full and distended, an even more undesirable state. Without sensation, there was no way to know how full the bladder was.

There are new catheterization products being developed. For example, Diagnostic Ultrasound Corporation has released a product based on volume-dependent catheterization. The BladderManager™ PCI 5000 is an ultrasound device that can be worn continuously and can warn you when your bladder reaches a selected percentage of fullness. The company's research found that 67% of timed intermittent catheterizations were performed prematurely and 16% were performed too late. The BladderManager is promoted as a means to limit infections, upper urinary tract damage, and costs for healthcare and supplies.

The O'Neil catheter is designed to limit UTIs. It is a catheter already placed inside a sterile collection bag. The special tip is first inserted into the opening of the urethra. The manufacturer claims that its opening goes beyond the area where bacteria are most likely to invade. The sterile catheter is then extended from inside the drainage bag and enters the urethra beyond the entry tip, supposedly bypassing the place where it could pick up bacteria from the urethral opening and carry it into the bladder. O'Neil catheters are portable, and the integrated drainage bag is convenient. The company claims that it considerably reduces the incidence of UTIs. O'Neil catheters are a single-use product and cost more per unit. The cost of such catheters might be covered by your private insurance carrier, Medicare, or Medicaid.

Intermittent catheterization can be more costly than an indwelling catheter if you rely on additional personal assistance services to change them. Dr. Alex Barchuk of the Kentfield Rehabilitation Hospital in California observes:

The difference in cost for a high quadriplegic on intermittent catheterization versus having an indwelling catheter is unbelievable. It's almost triple the cost of an indwelling catheter because someone who can't catheterize himself has to have either an attendant or a nurse. You have to have someone around every four to six hours to do it, which costs a lot of money. If you don't have the attendant—or if the attendant doesn't show up, which happens a lot—you have to go through an agency. An agency costs $35 an hour for a nurse to come out and do the catheterization. The cost difference is astronomical.

For someone with sufficient hand dexterity to do the intermittent procedure themselves, the cost might not be a concern, particularly with good insurance coverage.

Male Condoms or External Catheters

Many men with spastic bladders or a degree of manual control of the urinary sphincter can manage well with a male urinary condom, also known as an external catheter. Men using condoms will need to catheterize only occasionally, if at all, to remove residual urine. The condom is changed or reapplied at least once a day to provide the skin a chance to breathe and be inspected for irritation. It is a good general practice to swab the penis for hygienic reasons. There are three types of male urinary condoms:

■   The Texas catheter is held in place with an external strap, either made of sticky foam or with a Velcro tab at the end. The strap must be applied carefully. If it is too loose, the catheter will leak. If it is too tight, the skin of the penis can become irritated or break into a sore.
■   Another design uses a two-sided sticky foam strap that is first applied to the penis and then adheres to the condom as it is rolled over the strap.
■   The third type is self-adhesive and adheres as it is rolled onto the penis.

Some urinary condoms are supplied with a small pad of skin protector. The skin protector is also available as a separate product you can order from a medical supply store or catalog.

Condoms are typically made of latex. Some men develop latex sensitivity, in which the skin of the penis becomes dry, red, and irritated. Some men experience a temporary allergy and are able to return to the use of latex. Silicone catheters are available in the self-adhesive type only. Latex, as with balloons, is capable of stretching. Silicone has very little elasticity.

My latex sensitivity appeared twenty years after my injury. At
first I thought the condoms I used were defective, but instead I
needed to switch to the silicone condom. Then, after a few
years, suddenly the sensitivity ceased and I could go back to
latex, which I preferred.

Urinary condoms come out of the package rolled up, just as with con-doms for sexual use, although they include a tubed end for drainage of urine. The tube might be an extension of the material of the condom or a separate plastic tube attached at the end of a latex catheter. Urinary con-doms come in several sizes, and the latex types are flexible enough to accom-modate the changes in size that some men experience throughout the day.

When a man has severe ongoing problems with bladder infections and other complications, a urologist might recommend a sphincterotomy. Sur-geons cut the bladder sphincter muscle and release its capacity to keep the bladder closed. The bladder empties continuously, and a condom and leg bag system collect the urine. This very invasive procedure should be considered a last resort. Take care not to allow your physician to overly influence you. Consider him a provider of information. Take time to understand the full implications of such a measure, talking to others who have been through it. A sphincterotomy is not reversible.

Keep Things Clean

Bacteria grow like crazy on the appliances used for bladder management. Indwelling and external catheters and leg or bedside drainage bags are environments in which the *E. coli* that cause infection grow. Cleanliness must be a high priority to protect yourself from chronic UTIs—and the increased risk of developing bladder cancer that is associated with having chronic UTIs.

Use new internal catheters as often as you can, employing the best clean practices you can in the meantime. Always wash your hands before and after you insert a new catheter, and store the catheter in an antibacter-ial solution such as Betadine®. Know that indwelling catheters harbor bac-teria after only days, so the catheters need to be replaced often. External condom catheters should be replaced daily—some urine inevitably remains on the inner surface, breeds bacteria, and can migrate back up the urethra.

Each time you remove a catheter from a collection bag, clean the end of the catheter and the collection bag with alcohol before replacing them. Keep a bottle of alcohol and cotton balls in your bathroom, and carry indi-vidual alcohol wipes with you everywhere you go. This commitment to the cleanest practices—along with drinking sufficient amounts of water and ensuring that you are efficiently emptying your bladder—will help ensure your greatest protection from immobilizing and ultimately life-threatening UTIs.

The Bowel Program

If you don't have a bowel movement every day, you don't necessarily have constipation. It can be normal to have a bowel movement every two to three days. What counts is that you have a routine and that you manage your stool consistency. You need to establish a pattern in a managed bowel program that depends on what kind of neurogenic bowel you have. Evacuate your bowels often enough to ensure that you do not become impacted, yet not so often that you unnecessarily disrupt your schedule or risk the health of the tissues of the rectum and colon, especially if your bowel program regularly involves manual removal. Without an effective bowel program, some people can eventually require a colostomy—whereby the bowels must empty into an external bag—after falling into patterns of constipation and impaction.

The less your nervous system allows you control of the sphincter muscles, the more you need to train it to prepare for defecation at a time when you can control and induce it by the use of one or more following techniques:

- Digital stimulation. Gentle massage of the area around the anal sphincter muscle encourages it to relax.
- Manual removal. Wearing a latex glove, you or your PA gently scoops out stool with a finger.
- Suppositories. There are two types: bisacodyl (Dulcolax®) suppositories, which work by stimulating the nerve endings in the rectum, causing the bowel to contract, and glycerin suppositories, which draw water into the stool to stimulate evacuation. Overuse of suppositories or laxatives can cause deterioration of the tissue in the colon.
- Mini-enema. Softens, lubricates, and draws water into the stool.

A program that relies on the aid of suppositories or enemas can take from 30 to 60 minutes to complete. In a 1997 study of 100 people with SCIs, 23% of them took more than 45 minutes with their bowel program.[5] Some of that time might be spent lying down waiting for the treatments to have their effect. You will develop a sense of when you would need to be on the toilet, though a protective bed pad is always a good precaution.

If you have sufficient balance to sit on a toilet or commode chair, gravity can help you along. Many people with high quadriplegia are unable to be stable sitting on a toilet or commode for a bowel program, so it must be performed by an assistant while you are lying down.

If you can contract your anal sphincter on your own, that is certainly more attractive than having to put on a glove and dig, or sit waiting for a suppository to act. If you have some manual control of the anal sphincter, beware of the inclination to push continuously to force the feces out. It seems reasonable to think that, since the muscle is weakened, you have to make up for it with more effort, but such a strategy is exhausting and stressful. The rectum actually works somewhat on its own. If you can make a contraction, you will achieve more effect by alternately pushing down and relaxing. Alternately pushing and relaxing allows the natural reflex of these muscles to work with you, and you will find that stool will evacuate more easily.

Take care not to irritate the delicate lining of the rectum, which can cause bleeding or development of hemorrhoids. Emphasize this with any PA who aids you with your program.

> While I was in rehab, I remember a nurse's aide who seemed to be pretty rough doing my bowel program before I had been taught to do it myself. And then I noticed blood on her glove. I bled almost every time I moved my bowels for years, until I finally had hemorrhoid surgery to correct it.

Being Healthy

Now that we've reviewed the risks specifically associated with being a wheelchair user, and certain disabilities, now let's discuss the best ways to avoid these potential pitfalls—by being as healthy as possible. Health and disability are not mutually exclusive concepts. "Impairment" is not the same as "illness." You can be very healthy in the context of your disability. The place to start is by keeping in shape.

Exercise

If you use your body, you will live longer and more happily. It is especially important for chair riders to exercise to the degree possible. An inactive, sedentary lifestyle is an invitation to a variety of undesirable results:

- Weak muscles
- Cardiovascular loss
- Osteoporosis
- Weight gain

Our overall health relies on blood being able to flow efficiently, carrying the vital nutrients and metabolic components we need throughout the body. The pumping of the heart does not do this job alone, but relies on the movement and contraction of our muscles to assist in moving blood through the miles of arteries and veins in our bodies.

This is especially true in the legs, where veins that return blood to the heart employ a system of valves to prevent blood from flowing back down toward our feet. It is the contraction of our leg muscles that assists the hydraulic flow of blood up against gravity and back to the heart. If we are not using our legs, then our heart is working harder, so we need our heart to be healthy. Any physical activity that is available to us contributes to the health of our circulation.

Strength-Building Exercise

You don't have to be a bodybuilder to maintain strength. Muscle strength is as much a matter of softness and elasticity as it is of bulk. Flexible muscles can travel further when they contract, which translates to additional strength.

Whatever muscles you have voluntary control of can be exercised and kept at an optimal level of mass and elasticity. You can do this without an extreme amount of exertion. It is a myth that, to exercise a muscle, you have to strain it to exhaustion. A regular routine of gentle and slow repetitions with little weight will maintain muscle tone, at least, and gradually build strength, at best. Exercising moderately two or three times a week will take you a long way toward attaining the strength, stamina, and general health you desire.

> *I find that a very simple routine of exercising—doing push-ups in my wheelchair, using moderate free weights, and other resistance types of workout—really makes a big difference. Once after an extended illness I lost some of that tone and really noticed the change in strength.*

For people with limited hand strength and ability to grasp, a quad cuff, such as the one shown in Figure 2-1 from Preston Sammons (www.prestonsammons.com), will allow you to use exercise machines and free weights.

Aerobic Exercise

Aerobic exercise has a number of important benefits:

- It makes the heart stronger and improves circulatory efficiency. The heart is, after all, a muscle, too.

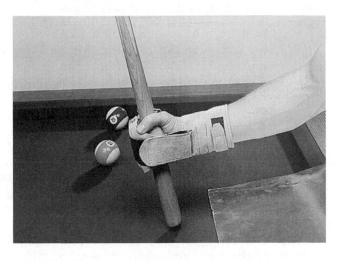

Figure 2-1 A quad cuff, for use by people with limited grip.

- It helps reduce blood pressure and heart rate.
- It helps control your weight.
- It increases endurance for physical activity by helping more blood and oxygen to reach muscles.

Only some manual chair riders are active enough that pushing the chair alone is adequate aerobic exercise to benefit the heart and general fitness. Most manual wheelers do not push enough in the course of an average day to provide for optimal health, nor do they work up a sweat or maintain an increased heart rate for long enough in the process, indicators of productive aerobic exercise.

Exercise Programs

Unfortunately, medical schools do not teach much about exercise physiology or the preventive values of exercise. Your doctor will encourage you to be active to the degree you are able and might refer you to physical therapy, but usually for practical purposes like activities of daily living. You should directly ask your doctor and therapists to develop an exercise program specific to your needs. Exercise needs to be a continuing program—not just short-term therapy.

Keeping to an exercise program might seem like an unwanted burden on top of everything else required of you by your disability. But even small amounts of regular exercise make a remarkable difference in a short period of time and more than compensate for whatever inconvenience the exercise entails.

After extensive exercise and training in rehab, this person noticed a decrease in physical abilities as he exercised less:

> *I became very busy with my new business out of an office at home. This meant that I was not wheeling around the place where I used to work, not commuting back and forth, and not traveling or going to meetings as I used to. I think all of that physical activity helped keep me in shape. I especially noticed that it was becoming more difficult to transfer into and out of my chair. Suddenly I seemed to be throwing my body more than lifting it. So I started doing simple upper body exercises a few times each week for about fifteen or twenty minutes and was amazed by how quickly I started to feel the difference. Now my exercise routine is important to me because I know it really works.*

The type and duration of exercise appropriate for you is a matter of experimentation and building endurance. You will need to design a program for yourself working with the best qualified doctor and therapist you can find. Any professional who develops an exercise plan for you must clearly understand the physiology of your disability as well as your personal experience. For example, people with MS are sensitive to being overheated and must not let body temperature rise much. People with paraplegia need to take care not to overstrain their shoulders. For people with postpolio syndrome, certain types of exercise can be exactly the wrong thing to do.

> *For a long time I pushed and forced myself to exercise, to use a stationary bike, etc., to help my respiratory system and to get myself "fit" after my daughter was born. I didn't know it then, but that was the worst thing that I could have done. Yes, I did need exercise, but I was modeling my exercise program on one that healthy people use. I overtaxed my respiratory system. I made the muscles that had taken over for those that were atrophied work even harder.*

Even if you have high quadriplegia or experience fatigue easily, you can be physically active in ways that benefit your general fitness. Aerobic exercise is very good for the heart, but just being outside enjoying even modest activity and getting some sun is worthwhile. It helps you maintain a more positive attitude and higher spirits.

An exercise program doesn't have to mean lifting weights, pulling on rubber straps, or using some exercise machine. There is a tremendous array of athletic options available. Almost anyone can participate in some form of sport. Many can swim or exercise in water. Bowling, shooting, or archery can be performed even with high quadriplegia with the use of newly developed adaptive devices. Those with higher degrees of function can participate in sports like wheelchair basketball or quad rugby. Accessible sports are discussed in Chapter 8, Getting Out There.

Health Clubs

Of the vast number of health facilities, few are well equipped for wheelchair access, and staff is rarely trained in issues that relate to disability. Most weight trainers come from a bodybuilding point of view. They are interested in building muscle mass to give your body a bulkier, sculpted look. Building to a "bulked up" degree of muscle mass—which can limit your range of motion—is generally not appropriate for a wheelchair user, although those wheelchair users involved in weight lifting or certain other wheelchair sports can benefit from this approach.

Ask whether your physical therapist can visit the health facility with you. She can review the various exercise machines, discuss whether swimming would be an option and how you would actually do it, and help you prepare a program. Asking for such consultation is not an unreasonable request on your part. Therapists are often given approval to make such visits. It is especially important that your program is balanced among the various muscle groups you are able to control.

As a wheelchair user going to a health club, you might find yourself uncomfortably conspicuous at first:

> I'd really like to go someplace where I can swim and use the
> exercise equipment, but it's important to me to have a place to
> dress and shower in private. I'd rather not be in public with
> my skinny legs or revealing my catheter. A few newer places
> are starting to include private dressing rooms with showers,
> but nothing close enough to where I live at the moment.

Health clubs are highly unlikely to have any of the equipment that has been designed for doing exercise from your wheelchair. Examples of such equipment include offerings from Apex Designs (www.apexeq.com), RTM Fitness (www.grouprmt.com), or the Quadriciser (www.quadriciser.com).

Brooks Rehabilitation Hospital in Jacksonville, Florida, has built a substantial health center that is available to any users with a disability, equipped with all the appropriate equipment as well as a full gym and pool, whirlpools, and sauna. It is open to the public, yet includes disability-specific services such as the postrehabilitation fitness program (www. brooks rehab.org/healthandfitness).

Quad Belly

For those with little or no muscle tone in the abdominal area, development of a "quad belly" is very common, but not entirely inevitable. The muscles in your abdomen can no longer work to keep your internal organs in place. Your stomach, intestines, pancreas, and liver are all contained snugly in that space, held there as well by ligaments and the peritoneum—a membrane that encloses the area. As the muscles atrophy, the organs literally slide down and out causing the quad belly.

Some people regularly wear an abdominal binder, which wraps around the body and can be adjusted for a firm fit—somewhat like a girdle. Although this will not prevent the atrophy of abdominal muscles, it will limit the stretching of the peritoneum—the membrane that contains this abdominal region—simply by preventing gravity from pulling your organs down and out.

Abdominal muscle tone can be maintained using electrical stimulation, but you have to really keep it up.

> *If you use electric stimulation religiously you can begin to gain back abdominal tone. You want to ramp up the power gradually; don't go full power when first beginning. You will injure muscles if you proceed too aggressively. Don't get discouraged when you don't see instant results. You have to do it daily for a long time, but you will begin to notice a difference. Find a muscle chart on the Internet and target the muscles you want to stimulate.*

Diet

The human organism is a biochemical machine. The body relies on water, vitamins, proteins, carbohydrates, fats, and minerals from a balanced diet of pure and healthy foods. The fact of being a chair user, or particular features of your disability, raises specific issues about diet.

Manual and power chair users have some different dietary considerations. A manual chair rider burns more calories in the act of pushing the chair, whereas a power chair user does not exert himself in the same way while using a joystick. Manual riders need more usable calories, whereas power chair riders should take extra care not to gain unnecessary weight.

People with high quadriplegia are particularly at risk of weight gain because their ability to perform aerobic activity is very limited and because any muscles that have atrophied require fewer calories. They are well advised to work closely with a dietitian to develop a dietary plan that includes foods they enjoy but defines appropriate amounts for the sake of weight management.

All chair users need to take extra care of their skin, already at risk from the pressure of sitting for long periods. Power chair users have a more difficult time shifting their position if they have limited arm strength, so added weight gain only increases the potential for more pressure where they sit. Healthy skin can be promoted by a balanced diet with a complete range of nutrients.

> *In the early years after my injury, I had a lot of problems with pressure sores. Looking back, I'm convinced that part of the problem was the meat and potatoes diet I grew up with, not to mention my sugar addiction! A few years after my accident, I switched to whole foods, no red meat, and a lot less sugar, and now I don't get pressure sores. Of course I also take better care of my skin, do my pressure-relief pushups religiously, and make sure I'm properly supported and cushioned in my chair, but the diet was definitely a big part of getting it under control.*

Some Important Nutrients

A variety of whole foods with minimal processing is the best source of nutrients needed by the body. A few examples are included here.

- Vitamin A helps in the growth and repair of body tissues and maintenance of healthy skin. It is derived by the body from carotene, which is abundant in carrots, green leafy vegetables, and broccoli.
- Vitamin B complex is a group of B vitamins that work together to produce energy by helping the body to convert carbohydrates to glucose, the source of your body's energy. They are also crucial to the nervous system. They are found in whole grains, liver, and brewer's yeast. Some antibiotics limit the ability of the body to produce B vitamins in the intestines.
- Vitamin C, or ascorbic acid, plays a role in the healing of wounds by maintaining collagen, the protein that forms connective tissue in the body. It also helps fight bacterial infections. It is found in fresh fruits and vegetables.
- Calcium is the most abundant mineral in the body. It must be accompanied by vitamins A, C, and D, as well as magnesium and phosphorus. It is crucial to bones and teeth, as well as the proper function of muscles, which cannot contract and release without calcium. The best known source is in dairy products, but calcium is also found in

many fruits, vegetables, and grains, particularly in figs, greens, and soy products.

■ Iron exists in every living cell. It works with protein and copper to carry oxygen from the lungs to the tissues of the body. It is found in liver, oysters, lean meats, molasses, and green leafy vegetables.

■ Potassium is involved in maintaining the water balance of cells, which is necessary for cell growth and to stimulate nerve impulses to muscles. It also stimulates the kidneys to eliminate toxins from the body. Potassium is found in all vegetables, oranges, whole grains, sunflower seeds, potatoes, and bananas.

■ Zinc is a crucial nutrient for chair users because of its importance to blood formation and the skin, particularly the healing of wounds.

The behaviors of nutrients in the body are a complex set of interactions. Certain vitamins, proteins, or minerals do not work on their own but, instead, rely on interactions with others to accomplish their task. Supplements are poorly absorbed unless accompanied by a balanced diet; they are not food and should not be relied upon to provide the basic needs of your body. However, a good vitamin-mineral supplement is a worthwhile addition to support a balanced, whole-foods diet.

Alternative Health Practices

More and more people are exploring so-called alternative healthcare options to maintain their health. Many have been in use for a very long time. Chinese acupuncture is thousands of years old. Herbal medicines are even more ancient. One man, a polio survivor, reports:

> I've been on total disability since 1991 and the only thing that
> helps me stay fairly mobile is my chiropractic/acupuncture/
> massage treatments. Depending on how I feel, I may get
> one or all of the above treatments. Treatment is painless and
> very relaxing.

Using these health practices does not mean that modern medicine has no place or that you should eschew the use of drugs altogether. Modern medicine continues to uncover amazing discoveries and therapies that reduce suffering and promote quality of life. Those who use alternative health practices typically try to find a balance—partaking of more natural and less invasive (and costly) measures where they make sense, while relying on modern, technical medicine for the things it does best. Following is a brief description of some widely used alternative health practices you might be interested in exploring.

Yoga/Stretching

Yoga may be one of the best activities for a person with a disability. The stretches that a physical therapist teaches you have essentially the same effect. Even if stretches are performed passively with assistance to improve and maintain your range of motion, the body benefits in much the same way.

When muscles are not used—whether paralyzed or due to a sedentary lifestyle—they shorten and get tight. This shortening of muscles is the reason that you feel stiff when you wake up in the morning and want to stretch—which shows us that the process can happen pretty quickly. As muscles get short, they become weaker and begin to restrict movement and eventually define and limit posture. Scoliosis, for example, sometimes results from muscles adapting into shorter lengths, pulling the spine into curvature.

The fact of sitting for most of the day gives the muscle-shortening process even more opportunity to advance and is all the more reason that a regular habit of stretching and range of motion is important to offset this effect. Specific muscles at risk of chronic shortening include the psoas muscle—which connects from your pelvis to the lower part of your spine—and the hamstrings—a group of three muscles that connect just above and below the knee. A surefire way to judge if contracture is taking hold is if your knees do not lay flat when you lie down on your back.

Alex Barchuk, physiatrist at the Kentfield Rehabilitation Hospital in northern California, feels that yoga and stretching are some of the best habits a person with a disability can develop:

> Strong, active wheelchair users are already getting aerobic exercise from how they get around. Stretching helps prevent trigger points from forming, which are painful and can limit muscle strength. Keeping muscles elastic is all the more important as you age.

Most yoga exercises involve the whole body, but you can adapt them to your capabilities. If you can, get a consultation with your physical therapist to develop a set of yoga stretches that work for you. The therapist will advise you on how often to do the stretches and will guide you in subtle issues of how to move and where the stretches are having their effect. Yoga has made a difference for this woman with an L5 SCI:

> I was watching TV at five A.M. one day and saw this incredible woman doing yoga. They announced a video for people sitting down, and I ordered it sight unseen. It has two fifteen-minute

*stretching routines, and I love it. I have to be so limited in
how I use my body, so the yoga helps me use muscles that I
don't always use. It's like nirvana for me. It's sensual. It's a
great feeling.*

Acupuncture/Acupressure

Chinese medicine—which has developed over the last 5000 years—believes
the body has a great capacity to heal itself and uses the body's own forces to
accomplish healing. The basic life force is called Qi (pronounced "chee").
Pathways throughout the body—specifically mapped—relate to all systems
of health and life. A practitioner working in this mode will activate points
on these pathways to free up blockages and promote the movement of Qi to
allow the body to regain its natural state of health. An acupuncturist acti-
vates these points by use of needles; acupressure involves pressing on the
points with the fingertips.

If you have never tried acupuncture, you might fear that it is painful—
the same as getting an injection with a syringe. This is not the case.
Acupuncture needles are very thin and do not go in very deep; a skilled
acupuncturist knows how to apply them in a way that is not noticed or that
feels like a very small sting. There are some points on the body that are sensitive, so an acupuncture needle is sometimes briefly painful.

Acupuncture and acupressure have been found helpful for pain management, to promote healing, to level intense emotions, and to aid recovery
from illness. Acupuncture has gained much in popularity. Increasingly,
scientific study is bearing out the positive effects of this approach.

Feldenkrais/Alexander

Although the Feldenkrais and Alexander methods are two distinct disciplines, they have similarities. Each method involves an awareness of the
body. Instruction/treatment in each discipline guides you to become attuned
to your movements. Practitioners are certified in training programs that last
for years and are often trained in other health fields as well.

Both methods are based on the observation that people use their bodies in an unconscious fashion, not fully aware of how they are moving, what
muscles are involved or their relationship to the environment, and missing
the chance to use energy efficiently. Both methods seek to increase your
awareness of subtlety. You are shown how to use small movements to renew
your brain's awareness of its connection to your whole body. Large movements are not the goal. The act of thought is powerful; almost the exact
same impulses are sent out through your nervous system when you imagine a movement as when you actually perform it. You can enhance the qual-

ity of how you use your body by employing small, subtle movements and by using your mind.

Frederick Matthias Alexander was an actor in the late 19th century who developed chronic laryngitis. Rather than give up his craft, he devised this method of body awareness to regain his voice. The Alexander Technique, as it is called, is commonly taught to actors today. You are taught to be aware of the spine, to imagine lengthening and opening it as you sit. You are taught to allow the rib cage to open and close with the breath, freeing the lungs to expand and receive more oxygen. By being aware of the forces at play in your movement, you increase the ability to move fluidly and naturally.

Moshe Feldenkrais was a scientist who saw that people suffered poor health because they were not integrated and because their life experience created "sensory motor amnesia," in which the brain is not fully in contact with the body. A person slumped over in pain, he saw, was suffering from chronic muscle tightness that could be relieved by teaching him to renew contact with the muscles so as to release them and regain control:

> I learned that the arms are not just limbs that pivot at the shoulder joint, but involve one half of the entire trunk. Muscles in the chest and the back are very much involved with our arms. For those, like me, who have control of abdominal and pelvic muscles, there is tremendous power when those muscles are used integrally with the arms. When I open a door, rather than simply pulling from the shoulder, I employ my back muscles and turn my trunk as I pull. It is remarkable how much more power I can draw on this way, and how much less strain there is to my shoulders.
>
> The same thing is true for wheeling technique. Friends independently observed how my wheeling style changed after the Feldenkrais work. It was visibly evident that I was involving my entire body in a new way.

Chiropractic and Osteopathy

Chiropractors are fully trained in anatomy and physiology. The central skill they are taught is to make adjustments in your skeleton, usually the spine:

> When I went through rehab in 1973, no one ever taught me anything about posture, and I found that I was comfortable in some pretty twisted looking positions! In 1986, someone recommended I see a chiropractor, who took x-rays that showed my spine was getting very curved. So they taught me about

> *posture, gave me a lumbar cushion, and I went for adjust-*
> *ments a couple of times each week. After six months, they*
> *took another set of pictures and my spine was incredibly dif-*
> *ferent, back into its proper alignment and natural curvature.*
> *Now a proper, upright posture is what's most comfortable for*
> *me. It was amazing to see how my body could adjust back to*
> *the right shape.*

Osteopathic physicians are fully trained medical doctors, but they take an extra level of study in what they call osteopathic manipulative treatment. Both osteopathic and chiropractic practitioners are focused on the spine and overall skeleton and tend to be holistic in their approaches. Osteopathic manipulation is gentle compared to the high-velocity method used by some chiropractors. Osteopathic physicians focus more on soft tissues than chiropractors. Each works well in conjunction with massage therapy and exercise to keep muscles well conditioned.

You will also find differences within each field. Osteopathic manipulation is actually practiced by a minority of osteopaths these days, whose practices are closer to traditional—or allopathic—medical doctors. Although there are chiropractors who perform spinal adjustment as their entire practice, many have begun to incorporate other disciplines. In both cases, you will often find practitioners who have studied for and become certified in subspecialties such as orthopedics, nutrition, or various holistic practices such as herbal medicine.

Osteopathic doctors are conscious of the movement of cerebrospinal fluid around the brain and down the spinal column. They are attuned to the four diaphragms in the body—the pelvis, the abdomen, the chest, and the brain. They are concerned with the freedom of movement of the ribs and practice a mode called craniosacral work, which senses the relative movement of the sections of the skull.

Massage Therapy

People's bodies absorb toxins from the environment and foods. These elements become held in our tissues and can weaken the body or immune system. Metabolic waste from the contraction of muscles gets trapped between the muscle fibers, leading to stiffness and soreness and limiting the full strength of those muscles.

The goal of massage therapists—no matter what style they employ—is to rub the muscles to release toxins and allow the bloodstream to carry them out. Massage therapists study anatomy, so they know what muscles they are working on, how they are connected to the skeleton, and how they should feel under their hands when they are normal and healthy. They will generally work toward the heart, to help the blood carry toxins into the kidneys and out in the urine. It is a good idea to drink plenty of water after a massage to help this process of elimination.

There are many types of massage. Some are very gentle. It is quite wonderful to be rubbed gently, in a peaceful, trusting setting. Touch is itself healing, as even traditional physicians increasingly recognize.

Other types of massage can be deep and intense. Many massage therapists will say that it is important to work deep, even if it is a bit painful, in order to release the locked tissues and clear the toxins. For example, "Rolfing" is a style of very deep massage therapy called Structural Integration, developed by Dr. Ida Rolf. Good Rolfers are able to start gently and work down deeper.

Homeopathy

Homeopathic doctors see illness as a message trying to tell you something about your life. Homeopathic doctors want to determine what your body is telling you. They believe the symptoms exist for a reason, and conventional treatment might not work if the root issues are not addressed. Even an injury can raise important questions about what led you to that moment.

At the initial visit, homeopathic doctors will do an extensive interview about your life. Practitioners treat with granules—very small doses of certain substances, usually herbal, but processed commercially. These granules are microdoses of the disease you are suffering. According to the homeopathic view, homeopathic medications attempt to stimulate the body's own reaction to the illness, much in the same way that a vaccine works by putting a small amount of a disease into you.

Steve and Aviva Waldstein, homeopaths in the Denver area, write:

> These natural remedies are made from plants, minerals, and other natural substances. They are prepared by a process of step-by-step repeated dilution and shaking, which makes them capable of stimulating the body's own defense system. Homeopaths recognize the importance of intervening as little as possible. They know the body is intelligent and produces symptoms for a reason. Rather than giving a medicine that ignores the intelligence of the body, homeopaths choose the one homeopathic remedy that can strengthen the body and allow it to heal itself.[6]

Homeopathic medications are now widely found in health food markets and are extremely popular in Europe. Homeopathy is the primary approach to health in some countries.

What Happens when You Age?

Life itself is a degenerative process. But you still have considerable control over the quality of life as you age. When you understand the innate changes in your body over time, you are better able to craft a lifestyle to maintain optimal health and reduce the chances of catastrophic problems.

It is common to lose muscle mass, although this is largely the result of less activity. Range of motion becomes limited as muscles shorten and tendons and ligaments become less elastic. Some degree of arthritis might affect the joints. Muscles remain responsive to exercise and stretching but require regular use to prevent significant, functional weakening.

The skin becomes less elastic and thinner, bringing with it increased risk of bruising, cuts, and skin breakdown from pressure.

Bones become more brittle. Osteoporosis is common in elderly people, particularly women. You are at higher risk for breaking bones as you age is because your bones have lost calcium and therefore break more easily.

As you age, your senses lose sensitivity, reflexes slow down, and coordination is reduced. Ultimately your short-term memory becomes less acute, although longer-term memories typically remain intact. Recent research indicates that mental acuity when aging is maintained by regular mental activity, including playing games or writing a journal. Energy levels get lower, and you need less sleep.

These facts of life are not inevitably limiting. For nondisabled people, quality of life can be maintained by keeping active.

Aging is a mix of psychological losses and gains. There can be sadness over the loss of youthful health, fear of approaching death, regret over certain life choices or missed opportunities, the loss of friends and loved ones, and increasing dependency on others. Aging also can bring increased maturity, wisdom, perspective, certainty of one's identity, joy in reaching a point of completion, and peace. Psychological benefits can help offset physical decline.

Increased Risks with Disability

The lost muscle mass that normally occurs with age becomes a greater issue when muscles are already weakened by paralysis or a genetic disorder, such as a muscular dystrophy. As you age, you need to continue to exercise moderately to maintain relative strength as muscle mass declines so that you can function as independently as possible. The ability to transfer to and from your wheelchair is probably the greatest concern. Loss of this ability is a key reason why a previously independent chair user might require the use of attendant services.

Chair riders are already at increased risk of skin breakdown from sitting because their skin becomes thinner and more brittle with age and increases this risk. As you age, you will need to take extra care with keeping your skin clean, doing pressure-relief push-ups and changes of position, possibly changing your cushioning strategy, and being vigilant about maintenance of your wheelchair and cushion to ensure proper pressure distribution and support. Since aging increases susceptibility to other heath problems such as pneumonia and flu, you might find yourself spending more time in bed. If so, change positions often and consider using a different mattress or cushion.

As a chair rider, you must rely on the remaining parts of your body that you are able to control. The arms and shoulders take on a lot of the work once performed by the legs, whether pushing your chair, transferring yourself in and out of it, or adjusting yourself in bed or in a favorite recliner in the living room. The shoulders are forced to do much more than they were designed to do. After enough years of extra work, there is a high risk of chronic pain or joint overstrain. A young chair rider able to push long distances over sloped or rough terrain might discover in his 50s that he overused his shoulders and has to switch to a power wheelchair.

For a person with a disability, it is vitally important to manage the aging process. Drs. Gale Whiteneck, PhD, and Robert Menter, MD, write:

> *Most of the changes and declines associated with aging might*
> *be prevented through awareness, vigilance, active health*
> *maintenance, and wellness strategies.*[7]

How Old and How Long

Most aging studies look at both the age of onset of the disability and the length of time one has a disability. People who acquire disability when they are older tend to recover and adapt less effectively than do younger chair riders. When older people are injured, they are already dealing with some results of the aging process, which make adjustments to disability more difficult. The length of time you have a disability is another factor that affects the degree of change you might encounter as you age.

These two factors sometimes have opposite effects. Pressure sores, for example, are found to increase with the age of the person but decrease with the length of disability. The skin is frailer when people get older, but a more experienced chair user will have better skin-care habits and skills.

Other conditions more closely related to an older age at onset are heart problems, pneumonia, respiratory infections, kidney stones, fainting, and headaches. A longer period of time after the injury is more associated with

musculoskeletal overuse strain, tendon and joint pain and stiffness, hemorrhoids, and urinary problems among men.

In general, signs of aging occur earlier in the disability population than
in able-bodied people.

Using Personal Assistance Services

Your ability to stay healthy and have a full life might rely on being assisted
with certain tasks. The kind of support you might require could be as simple as some light cooking or running a few errands or as significant as help
with your bowel program, getting dressed, and getting into and out of your
wheels. A PA might also administer an injection or perform simple physical
therapy tasks such as range-of-motion and stretching exercises. Certain tasks
might need to be performed by a registered nurse; some states require this
for catheterization, for instance.

The basic questions to ask include the following:

- How much support do you need?
- Who will do it?
- How do you find these people?
- Will it be a family member or friend?
- If necessary, how will they be paid?
- How do you ensure the quality of services?

It might already be clear that you are limited in the performance of
various personal functions. A person with high quadriplegia doesn't have
to wonder if some personal assistance is necessary. A person with lower
quadriplegia or someone with MS experiencing a significant exacerbation
could do many things for himself but might quickly fatigue if he does. There
is a point where personal assistance makes sense in order to preserve your
energy for the rest of the day. No one likes to surrender independence, so
people in this gray area will face more difficult decisions. For example,
deciding to allow someone else to perform a very personal task like a bowel
program can be a difficult line to cross.

> In fact, when you come right down to the nitty-gritty, PAS
> (personal assistant services) is an interruption of the flow of
> my life. I'd really rather do it myself.

A good goal is to find a balance that optimizes your energy so you can
do what you want with each day. That could mean assistance from someone

every morning and evening or perhaps just an hour or two every other day. Some people perform their bowel programs on alternate days but are able to dress and perform basic household tasks. To the degree possible, continue to do what you can to optimize your capacity and independence, keeping an eye out for undiscovered strategies or new products that allow you to do more for yourself.

The Assistant's Role

Ideally, PAs are the means to gain control over your own life. Personal assistance is a tool you can use to adapt to your disability. Assistance allows you to make your own choices and pursue the level of activity you prefer, according to your ability, on your terms.

The relationship between you and an assistant is a human relationship, with feelings on both sides. Many people avoid receiving assistance from someone they know and prefer to hire someone or work through various agencies that provide these services. That way, the assistant is an employee, and his role is easier to define. Personal relationships can become complicated by this mixture of roles.

Many people develop a detailed job description for an assistant, with a list of specific tasks. The job description does not have to be cast in stone, preventing you from asking for other kinds of assistance. A job description lists what is needed and helps define what the relationship will be like, including:

- Clearly defined tasks, such as dressing, administering medication, bowel and bladder programs, or cooking
- Hours to be worked
- Your requirements for notice of late arrival or nonarrival
- Provisions for vacation coverage or illness
- Payment

While working out the description of what a PA will be doing, you can discuss such tasks as running errands, house cleaning, or anything else with which you feel you need help. Some of these things might not be acceptable to an assistant or might be precluded by the overseeing agency. This does not mean such requests are impossible—assistants might be willing to do things on their own time or make exceptions to policies in order to provide what you need.

Assistants are not there to be slaves, any more than they are there to tell you what to do. You must respect them and understand that they will be conscious of a boundary they should not cross, such as when you ask for something that would injure you. One PA describes this dilemma:

> *The only time this is a problem is if a person may want or is doing something I know is not necessarily good for their own physical or mental health. For example, my employer asked me to stop and get him some beer. He is diabetic, a stroke victim, and has heart problems. I had to take a deep breath and decide that he knew the risks, and that it's his life. So I got him the beer. But only a six-pack, not a case. I don't know if this was right or wrong, probably wrong according to an agency.*

Some tasks have to be done at a certain time, such as catheterization or getting dressed. Other tasks, like house cleaning, can be scheduled more flexibly. These things get worked out over time in a relaxed, collaborative relationship. Doing a description up front gets this process off to the best possible start.

A working relationship can develop into a friendship, although still with clear boundaries. Hopefully you will work with compassionate people, who will inevitably come to care about you as a person, as any friend would. Two personal assistants talk about their jobs:

> *Sometimes all I did was have coffee with him and share the day's news from the paper, or come sit while he played online, especially when he was depressed. Or he would call at night, his wife not having come home, needing to be put to bed or just have someone with him. This was done on my own time because of the limitations the agencies have on hours. Certainly both parties need to know what the PA is comfortable with doing, especially regarding personal care. But the rest comes from getting to know each other and honesty on both sides.*

> *The majority of the people I have assisted require some personal care—hygiene, meal prep and feeding, transferring, etc. They also need help with day-to-day activities like walking the dog, changing kitty litter, rearranging furniture, shopping, gardening, etc. Yes, every person's situation is different. The only way I have managed to stay in this field that I love for seven years is to be flexible.*

How to Find a Personal Assistant

Start by checking with your medical funder, be it insurance or government healthcare. Medicare provides funds for home health but has some restrictions on how much you can be out of the home to remain eligible. Many local centers for independent living (CILs) run PA services programs. The center might be limited to offering you classes on using a PA or be an actual provider of services with a database of assistants. Some CILs have contracts with their respective state to run a program using government funds.

Your CIL is not the only possible administrator of PA programs. The city of San Francisco, for instance, offers services with city money, and the state of California runs the IHSS (In Home Supportive Services) program.

One type of program is not necessarily better than another. Do your own research on what programs are well administered, provide the best range of services, and screen their workers well. The following man had a mixed experience with his agency:

> I'm a thirty-four-year-old quad. I've been getting PA services through an agency for fourteen years. I've always thought it would be nice to hire my own PAs, but never followed up on it because the service I received from the agency has been good. However, the agency has been screwing up big time lately; PAs not showing up at all, no one calling to tell me so, two PAs showing up at the same time, etc.

You are, of course, free to hire people on your own. Many people advertise in local papers or list themselves at the local CILs looking for people to work. Other places you might advertise include the unemployment office, community agencies such as Catholic Community Services, grocery stores, senior centers, social service agencies, colleges, or hospitals. Also spread the word to friends, acquaintances, and neighbors.

Don't rush the hiring process. You might feel you have an urgent need to hire someone, possibly because a personal relationship is being strained. But this is an important choice. Like any employer, you have to take the necessary time to find the right person whom you will be comfortable with and can trust. Otherwise, you'll end up doing it all over again. Or worse, although by far the exception, you could find yourself taken advantage of or even injured.

Family Member or Friend?

Many people who use PAs report that allowing someone already close to them to play this role can be fraught with problems. That doesn't mean that a parent, child, or spouse taking the job guarantees problems, but it will almost necessarily influence the relationship. This is a complex relationship that requires patience and communication. There is a tendency to get caught up in power issues or just plain get tired of too much contact. Sometimes the relationship changes for the better—deeper intimacy and trust and increasing friendship and mutual appreciation.

Even more complex are the dynamics with a spouse. The desire to be equal partners is a strong part of the marital relationship, and the person being assisted can struggle greatly with feelings of not carrying his share. When it comes to sexuality, it can be difficult to get in the mood when you have just shared the process of a bowel program.

But having an intimate partner play this role does not have to ruin the sexual relationship. If you can talk openly about how the roles are affecting you and find ways to plan time so that personal tasks don't interfere with sensual times, you can make it work. Some people have even found ways to make something like catheterization a form of foreplay. Others have experimented with someone else performing assistant tasks specifically to help them prepare for sex, and even address the topic in the initial employment interview.

It's a Bureaucracy

If you are getting help through a medical funder or center for independent living (CIL) program, there will be a process to evaluate your needs. Most programs have a formal requirement. The program balances making sure your needs are met and confirming that services are being used appropriately, all within the boundaries of their available budget and mandate under law.

Some people with disabilities are concerned when the evaluation is performed by the funding source. They are afraid that the need to control a budget will override the priority of optimal assistance.

You are really the expert on what you need. Your needs are not limited to clinical services but include being supported in any way that allows you to have enough energy to function in the world, rather than being exhausted by everything you can do alone but that would fatigue you. Defining needs is tricky. Sometimes the process can leave you unsure you deserve assistance.

> I've lived with postpolio residual all my life and now get the extra kickers postpolio syndrome throws my way. Suffice it to say that after four months of "doing it myself," my arms were giving me severe pain, and fatigue was robbing me of productive hours. The muscles that were barely allowing me to live without a personal assistant were weaker and their endurance had dropped to almost zilch.

We're constantly guilt tripped for needing assistance in order to live independently. I say, from wiping my butt to preparing the food for a dinner party to which I have invited friends, I deserve all the assistance I need, and only I can decide what I need.

When you are working with government coverage or local programs—depending on how they are structured—there will be some amount of paperwork. You have to confirm time sheets for payment or might be asked to evaluate PAs work. Despite a clear ongoing disability, some people are made to repeatedly establish their need for support.

I have to continue to prove need even though it is very evident that my condition, cerebral palsy, will not improve and I will need the service for the rest of my life. This results in mounds of paperwork and requires calls and visits to see if I have indeed found the right snake oil and can walk again! My case manager has to come over and fill out extensive forms every two months. This takes at least three hours of our time. Sometimes this wall of paper blocks me from getting to work on time.

Who Chooses to be a Personal Assistant?

Workers include students doing part-time work while in school, nurses and aides who work for home health agencies, and good-hearted people who don't really need the money but are interested in helping.

There is a wide range of possible motives for someone to choose this work. When you are interviewing, ask questions to gauge the interviewee's reasons for seeking this work. And ask specifically about their feelings about disability. You will be screening for a caretaker of a needy person—or anything along the lines of pity and charity. You are looking for someone to be your partner in expanding your independence, someone who will work with you in a mode of respect.

You will also want to take great care that the person is trustworthy. Follow up on references and do a background check; plenty of services are available via the Internet for a reasonable price. There are, sadly, all too many examples of people who have been taken advantage of.

When I made the transition to an intelligent, resourceful, and experienced caregiver, my life began to change. Sadly, this came at a great price. After two almost perfect years, she was caught embezzling money from me. She is now in prison.[8]

Not everyone has some ulterior or misguided motivation. Some PAs find great meaning in helping people who need support to continue living at home rather than in an institutional setting.

I learned what a joy and how rewarding it is to be able to help a person live at home, where they want to be, and, in most cases, can be. Whether permanently or temporarily handicapped or dying, it makes no sense to put a person in an institution that costs so much more than home-based services, and takes away dignity, self-worth, and freedom, not to mention loved ones and familiar surroundings.

Checking Up on Potential Assistants

It is important to interview people carefully, to have others around if possible during the early stage of the working relationship, and even to do criminal background checks. Careful screening is standard procedure for some agencies and programs, and you should ask whether that is the case. You should request it. Even if it is refused, it is possible to hire a detective agency at nominal cost to do a simple background check.

Some people are simply desperate for work or unfortunately interested in taking advantage of someone who is vulnerable. Desperation might lead people to prey on you. There are reported instances of physical and other abuse.

> My friend caught her PA with her hand in her purse—stealing not money but her prescription pain medications. Turns out meds were missing at a couple of the other homes too. The PA had a back injury a few years ago; she is addicted to pain meds and her own doctor won't prescribe as much as she wants.

This employer of personal assistants found college students more reliable and advertised in the college newspaper:

> I hire college students almost exclusively. I find that only about one out of fifteen are no-shows for the interview. On the other hand, when I advertise in the local newspaper, no-shows are more than 50%.

Payment

What does a job as a PA pay? Not much. One of the great challenges of filling the needs of the disability population is the limited supply of people who are able—or willing—to work for minimum wage.

> *Here in California, our IHSS system only allows us to pay*
> *minimum wage, presently $8.00. Most people are able to*
> *pad their hours a little bit, so they can pay a little more.*
> *That is to say, some people are able to be allocated a few*
> *more hours than they really need, allowing them more flexi-*
> *bility in what they pay their PAs. People like myself who*
> *need more hours than the state pays for—283 hours per*
> *month—are put at a significant disadvantage because we*
> *don't have a "pad."*

Your program might pay for your PA, or may simply be a service to provide referrals and training to help you find and use such services. Funding could come from sources such as Vocational Rehabilitation or the Veterans Administration.

Payment is usually provided by means of vouchers authorized for a specific number of hours. You typically fill out forms reporting hours, submit them properly signed for payment, and hope they go through. Payment is not always an efficient process, as a PA describes:

> *I would receive a voucher to take to my employer who would*
> *have to fill it out. Both of us sign. I mail it in. If I was lucky I*
> *would get my check in two weeks. Usually it took at least a*
> *month—sometimes many phone calls and a couple of*
> *months. I soon learned not to include my paycheck in the*
> *monthly budget.*

Restrictions

A Medicare regulation regarding payment for assistance in the home only pays when your absences from home are "infrequent and for periods of relatively short duration," which "require a considerable and taxing effort." Otherwise they will not cover visiting aides and certainly not at a place of work. This is known as the "In-Home Rule."

An article in the September 1997 issue of *New Mobility* magazine describes the experience of two people, needing assistance in the morning and evening to get into and out of their wheels, who found themselves cut off from coverage when it was discovered that one of them was volunteering at the local school and the other was driving a modified van once his elderly parents were unable to do so.[9] A worker provided by an agency blew the whistle because the agency is forced to protect its status as a provider of Medicare-covered services. The choice of these two people was to either stay at home or to surrender coverage.

The article explains that CMS, the Federal agency that runs Medicare and Medicaid, is aware of the problem. CMS explained that when home health coverage was established, it was meant as a short-term solution. It was progressive coverage at the time. There are legislative attempts underway to correct the problem. The restrictions on home care have become obsolete as the ability to function outside of the home with basic levels of support is more possible—and more demanded by people with disabilities.

The Americans with Disabilities Act addresses your rights in the workplace and requires employers to provide "reasonable accommodation" that allows you to meet the requirements of the job. Personal assistance does not qualify as a reasonable accommodation. It is not something that an employer is obligated to provide, so you would need to make your own arrangements if you need support in the workplace, such as help with emptying your bladder.

An agency you work with who provides and funds a PA might have a variety of specific restrictions, often based on the criteria of "medical necessity." Many times, such services are designed for people thought to be sick or bedridden, not as support services to allow someone to be active.

> *Is it medically necessary for me to go with my personal care worker to a conference on health promotion and safe sex? My agency says no. Are short vacations medically necessary with your personal care worker? "No!" my agency exclaims. Can my personal care worker take me to visit the chiropractor three times a week, regardless of medical outcome? My agency says yes. These are deemed medically necessary. My case manager cannot come to my work environment and do her paperwork because I am supposed to be sick in bed or something. I'm a square peg that doesn't fit into the round hole.*

Keeping Them Happy

Al DeGraff, in *Home Health Aides: How to Manage the People Who Help You*,[10] lists 10 reasons personal assistants quit their jobs:

1.   Their initial job description was incomplete or keeps changing.
2.   The method and order in which they must perform their duties are illogical, inefficient, and waste time.
3.   Their working environment is messy, unpleasant, disorganized, etc.
4.   They're not paid enough, don't get appropriate raises, or don't feel their work is appreciated.

5.   The employer (you) is either too passive or too aggressive in his/her style of interaction.
6.   They feel another personal assistant is favored over them.
7.   The employer is dishonest about the hours worked or the salary owed or has inappropriate expectations, such as monetary loans or sexual favors.
8.   There are unreasonable duties—those the employer is reasonably able to perform alone, those that cannot be performed in the allotted time, or those that are too tightly supervised.
9.   The employer is intolerant of honest mistakes, the need for sick time, etc.
10. The employer doesn't respect the personal assistant's personal life and expects that his or her needs should take priority over all else in the personal assistant's life.

Service Animals

You might be able to get some help from service animals, using programs that train animals and place them. A dog can learn a surprising number of tasks, such as to pick something up from the floor for you or to open a door, turn on a light, answer the phone, push elevator buttons, or pull you over a curb in your chair. In the bargain, you also get a loyal companion.

There is cost involved. The training is expensive, and animals do have to be fed regularly. Some programs will also cover veterinary costs. Programs that train and provide service dogs do their best to raise money to help cover the costs to make them available to more people.

You could even train your own service animal. It's a substantial commitment, but it is achievable if you commit to learning how. It starts with identifying the breed and specific dog that has the right temperament and personality and that connects with you personally and then fully committing to a process of training and conditioning so that the dog will happily respond to your cues and commands. This is a process that can easily take a couple of years. There are a lot of dog-training resources and programs, including classes offered by your local humane society. The books *Teamwork* and *Teamwork II* by Stewart Nordensson and Lydia Kelley specifically guide you in training your own service dog.

Boston-based Helping Hands provides capuchin monkeys, the type usually depicted with an organ grinder, to clients with quadriplegia. They are raised in foster homes and placed at the age of four years. A key requirement, says program director, Jody Zazula, when she brings a monkey to meet someone for the first time, is that "they fall in love with each other."

Your Choice

Whatever your disability, whether stable or progressive, you have a tremendous amount of control over the quality of your health and life. There is an optimal level of health that is possible for you—and a much lower level if you neglect yourself and elect not to practice at least some of the concepts discussed in this chapter.

You may well struggle with depression, disappointment, frustration with cultural attitudes, financial limitations, or many other difficulties that people face in the disability experience. But none of that needs to stop you from eating well, doing simple exercises, getting into the sun from time to time, and following basic medical principles to protect yourself from skin breakdown, infections, and other risks inherent in being a wheelchair user. There is always something new to try, and there are many people out there who are true healers who work in many different therapeutic modes with their skills—and hearts—to offer, not to mention a vast offering of information on the Internet.

On the other hand, if you are really out there, working, traveling, playing, raising a family, engaged in a fully active life, then you must be conscious of your limits—as everyone must be, disability or no. Your lifestyle is simply more strenuous, so you must take more care with your health.

Trying to make too many changes at once is a recipe for failure. Take one change at a time. Wait until the change becomes integrated into your daily life before adding another. Maybe you start with a little stretching, add a new food to your diet—like eating a couple of prunes every day—or cut back on the ice cream. The benefits in improved health and energy will be so precious that you will come to enjoy and value health-management habits that might have seemed unappealing at first glance.

Taking care of yourself is a lifelong process. Good health habits are crucial for your life on wheels.

References

1. The 2004 National Organization on Disability /Harris Survey of Americans with Disabilities. New York: National Organization on Disability; 2004.
2. Paralyzed Veterans of America/Consortium for Spinal Cord Medicine. Prevention of thromboembolism in spinal cord injury. Washington: Paralyzed Veterans of America; 1999. Available at: www.pva.org/site/ DocServer/DVT.pdf?docID=644. Accessed on: March 3, 2008.
3. The International Association for the Study of Pain. IASP Pain Terminology. Available at: http://www.iasp-pain.org/AM/Template.cfm?Section=

General_Resource_Links&Template=/CM/HTMLDisplay.cfm&ContentID
=3058#Pain. Assessed on: March 3, 2008.

4. Roth EJ. Pain management strategies. In: Yarkony GM, ed. *Spinal Cord Injury: Medical Management and Rehabilitation.* Gaithersburg: Aspen Publishers; 1994.

5. Kirshblum SC, Gulati M, O'Connor KC, Voorman SJ. Bowel care practices in chronic spinal cord injury patients. *Arch Phys Med Rehab* 1998:79(1):20.

6. Learn More About Homeopathy. Available at: www.homeopathy-cures.com/html/about_homeopathy.html. Accessed on: March 3, 2008.

7. Whiteneck G, Menter RR. Where do we go from here? In: Whiteneck G, ed. *Aging with Spinal Cord Injury.* New York: Demos Medical Publishing; 1993.

8. Moran A. *From There to Here: Stories of Adjustment to Spinal Cord Injury.* Horsham, PA: No Limits Communications; 2004:108.

9. Braunstein M. Homeward bound and wishing they weren't: Medicare's homebound regulation is an idea whose time has gone. *New Mobility*; 1997. Available at: www.newmobility.com/articleViewIE.cfm?id=44. Accessed on: March 3, 2008.

10. DeGraff AH. *Home Health Aides: How to Manage the People Who Help You.* Clifton Park, NY: Saratoga Access Publications; 1989.

Chapter 3

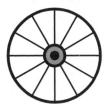

The Experience of Disability

Each of us experiences disability in our own way. No one can tell you how disability is supposed to feel or how you are going to respond to yours. There are, however, some common patterns in the emotions and beliefs experienced by people with disabilities.

Change of Identity

Acquiring a disability often challenges your very notion of who you are and, so, requires adjusting your sense of identity. According to disability psychologist Carol Gill, a polio survivor, reconciling your identity as a disabled person with previously held notions about what being disabled means is a common hurdle:

> *When you become a member of the group that you have previously felt fear or pity for, you can't help but turn those feelings on yourself.*

A traumatic injury or diagnosis of disease that suddenly makes you a member of "the disabled" community is often a shock to your sense of self. Whatever image you had of disability will be the image you first apply to yourself. Before the onset of your disability, what were your reactions to people you saw or heard about who had a disability? How did you react when you saw a person using a wheelchair? Did you feel pity? Did the notion of it happening to you fill you with dread? What was your image of what their lives must be like? Could you imagine them with careers and families, being creative or athletic, having sex? Or was the only image you could conjure one of sadness, dependency, pain, and loss?

Even if you know someone who has lived an active life with a disability, you might doubt you could do it. Despite the increasing public visibility of active chair riders, US culture still tends to promote negative beliefs about the experience of disability—including the idea that only rare, special people live well with disability.

In his book *Missing Pieces*, the late sociologist and disability researcher Irving Zola—himself a polio survivor—wrote:

> *The very vocabulary we use to describe ourselves is borrowed from that society. We are de-formed, dis-eased, dis-abled, dis-ordered, ab-normal, and, most telling of all, called an in-valid.*[1]

For most people, the onset of disability heralds an intensive self-evaluation, the beginning of a process that never actually reaches conclusion. You are now a member of a minority foreign to most nondisabled people you will meet. You will remember your previous identity and always retain a sense of it. In the case of a traumatic disability, a part of you—for some initial period of time—will understandably resist accepting membership in the society of chair riders.

Most chair users eventually accept the internal contradiction between their disabled and nondisabled identities. But this adaptation takes time. The early years are marked by a series of adjustments that are deep and sometimes troubling. But your life after these significant initial adjustments can be meaningful and rich—if you let it. Notes Carol Gill:

> *We all differ in the degree of "equipment" we have to even look at such things as our values. But the people who can do that end up with different values. They redefine important aspects of living. They redefine roles, for example. Mothers and fathers redefine what being mothers and fathers means. What being lovers means. What being productive and contributing members of society means. This is how they adapt.*

If you think your self-esteem relies on whether or not you can walk, you limit yourself. Your self-esteem is more truly related to your compassion, generosity, and doing your best in any situation. You don't have to be able to walk to take pride in yourself or to be recognized and appreciated by the people you care about and who care about you.

You Are Still Yourself

In the ways that really matter, disability does not change you. Rather, disability threatens concepts you have held about who you are. You bring to your disability whatever mix of attitudes, beliefs, fears, talents, charisma, or social skills you have—or have the capacity to develop. Who you are in the essential ways that really matter will inform your adjustment to disability. Notes a man who has been on wheels for years:

> *The most common question I've been asked by people who know someone with a recent disability is, "What can I do to help?" My answer has always been, "First, understand that they are the same person they were before their disability. Don't treat them any differently, don't expect them to be any stronger or weaker than before, but don't be surprised if they discover new qualities in themselves that never came to the surface before."*

A disability forces the issue of "finding yourself." Some people take pride in what they learn about themselves through their disability experience and appreciate the way in which it helps define their values—and their sense of their true identity.

Many psychological adjustments have little to do with your disability and more to do with issues common to all of us. For example, you might be frustrated by the difficulty of finding a mate and think that your disability is the central cause of your loneliness. But this issue is part of many people's lives—disabled or not. Don't make your disability a scapegoat for issues that may well have come up in your life anyway. A disability in and of itself does not preclude finding a mate, as many people have proven.

For most people, disabilities do not define them but are something to deal with when necessary.

> *My name is not cerebral palsy. There's a lot more to me than my disability and the problems surrounding it. That's what I call the disability trap. This country has a telethon mentality toward disability that thinks disabled people are not supposed to talk about anything but their disabilities.*

> *I had a girlfriend back in the '60s. One day we discussed the idea that the whole human race is disabled because we can't live in peace with each other. This was always so and it will continue that way in the future. So who is "normal?"*

Sexual Identity

You might believe that you are not entitled to a sexual identity, that no one could possibly see you as a sexual being, or that you don't have sexual "performance" options. These conclusions are not true. Exploring your sexual identity can be a valuable part of your adjustment, whether you acquired your disability later in life or are making adjustments in teen or adult years with a disability since birth or childhood.

Irving Zola wrote:

> While I agree that sex involves many skills, it seems to me limited and foolish to focus on one organ, one ability, one sensation, to the neglect and exclusion of all others. The loss of bodily sensation and function associated with many disorders, and its replacement with a physical as well as psychological numbness, has made sexuality a natural place to begin the process of reclaiming some of one's selfhood.[1]

Chapter 5, Intimacy, Sex, and Babies, discusses sexuality in detail.

Lawsuits

If you were injured in a way that has led to a personal injury lawsuit, you face another complication in adjusting to your self-image with a disability. Typically, attorneys will urge you not to work during the case because working reduces the apparent impact of your disability on your life and, so, reduces the amount of money you are likely to be awarded.

Deborah Kaplan is an attorney and consultant, the former director of the World Institute on Disability in Oakland, California, and a wheelchair rider. She is concerned about the message people get during the extended process of the lawsuit:

> The legal system and the personal injury system—and I think the lawyers aid and abet it—are premised on the same notion: that disability equals inability to work. One of my concerns is the impact on somebody who has just gone through a huge shift in their life, a huge shift in their self-respect and self-image. They sit through a trial where all they hear, over and over and over, even from their own advocates, is how worthless their lives are. I think it's difficult for someone who's had all that negativity instilled in them to then go out with self-respect, get an education, get a job, and be productive.

Passing

In US culture—so imbued with fear of disability—it's probably fair to say that anyone with a recent disability will, to some degree, resist fully adopting the identity of disability. One of the most common ways to deny disability identity is to try as hard as possible to function in the culture as if your disability did not exist. This is known in the disability community as "passing."

What's the problem with passing? After all, the disability movement is working hard for full inclusion in society and for removing barriers to the ability to function as independently and fully as possible. However, passing is not about interacting in the world, being involved with able-bodied people, having a non-disability–related career, or dancing at your cousin's wedding. If you can be an auto mechanic or a dance instructor because you found a way to adapt to the task and you have some real expertise to offer, what could be wrong with that?

Passing is crossing some line where the acting as if you are not disabled causes a problem. For example, perhaps you resist using an adaptive device necessary for your safety. Perhaps you are quadriplegic with use of your arms, but you exhaust yourself using a manual chair because you resist the image of being a person using a power wheelchair. There is a borderline between challenging yourself within reasonable boundaries and risking your health and safety because you don't want to define yourself as a person with a disability.

Passing is effectively denying the truth of who you are and the real possibilities in your life. Psychologist Carol Gill describes passing in this way:

> I think passing is trying to convince society that we're more like nondisabled people. We just happen to have this disability. I think a lot of people want to be assimilated into the mainstream and try to act the part of what they think people in the mainstream are like. "Passing" to me implies some dishonesty.

Trying to pass as something you're not is always bad, unless you can carry it off so well and you have an emotional makeup that doesn't require honesty and authenticity. It's true! Some people can be happy playing a role all their lives. They'd be playing one role or another even if they weren't disabled—rather than looking inside and being at peace with who they really are.

The cultural pressure to pass is great, as this deaf woman observes:

> *When I was growing up, adults made it very clear that bring-*
> *ing up my deafness would signify that I was slacking—if I*
> *"tried hard enough" I could get by. The message was clear:*
> *Shut up about it, and look like you're doing okay. I think that*
> *as long as "overcoming" disability is such a cherished cultural*
> *myth, social pressure to engage in passing behavior will be*
> *part of the disability experience.*

If you can be free from having to prove yourself, your choices will not be tainted by this skewed motivation. If you are able to look at yourself honestly and with acceptance, you can see this motivation and not allow it to affect your choice.

Passing doesn't have to be only about how you are viewed by the broader culture. It can be an attempt to make up for your losses: being athletic, seductive, capable of robust physical work, and so on. People with disabilities are driven to substitute. Irving Zola wrote:

> *An uncomfortable assessment of my last twenty years was*
> *that they represented a continuing effort to reclaim what I*
> *had lost.*[1]

Thinking about where your motivations are coming from and what you're trying to prove can be complicated.

> *I have felt some satisfaction in having my disability disappear*
> *in the eyes of colleagues and friends, but does that mean I was*
> *necessarily passing? Or was my desire to minimize the social*
> *impact of my disability a motivating force that helped me*
> *accomplish what I have with my life?*

The boundary between making the most of your abilities and trying to pass as not disabled is a fine line. Only you can know what drives you as you integrate your disability into your life in a balanced way. A man with a spinal cord injury recalls:

> *A man I used to work for, impressed with my level of activity*
> *and work, once said to me, "You're not really disabled!" He*
> *thought he was complimenting me. He didn't realize he was*
> *exposing his belief that it was a bad thing to be disabled.*

> *I remember mixed feelings. On one hand, I took some pride in*
> *having participated fully in my career and being accepted as*
> *an equal. On the other hand, his comment was upsetting*
> *because it denied an essential part of who I am—a person*
> *with a disability. I wish he could have said, "Through know-*

*ing you, I now understand that a physical disability is not
necessarily the limiting, tragic experience I had believed it
to be."*

A woman who got polio at the age of five observes:

*For those of us who grew up with disability, that is a very
common crossroads we face—the moment where we discover
we were trying to pass and it just is not worth the effort.
"Wait a minute! This is costing us too much!" It's much more
fun to be a person with a disability if we just relax into it.
Then we'll save ourselves a lot of energy.*

The dividing lines take time to sort out. Figuring out the subtleties
might not be a priority for you following a recently acquired disability.
Many of them will become clear to you in their own time anyway. Whatever choices you make are basically driven by a desire for comfort and security. If you're at peace with yourself, no one can fairly accuse you of trying
to pass.

Recently Acquired Disability

Most able-bodied people imagine disability to be a far more negative and
difficult experience than it is—or needs to be. At first, you have no conception of how someone functions using a wheelchair full-time, so it appears
to be a life of complete dependency and endless difficulty.

When you've suddenly acquired a disability by injury or a disease, you
bring your previous notions of disability to it. It is no surprise that many
people find themselves experiencing depression, anger, anxiety, fear, and a
very deep sense of loss in the early stages of the disability experience.
Regardless of how well-adjusted, mature, or emotionally strong you are, this
is a catastrophic event that can shake your basic beliefs about life. It also asks
you to draw upon coping skills you might never have needed before.

Strong emotions are a natural response to this shock. A woman who
has made her own adjustment to disability counsels someone raw from the
experience struggling with dark, angry feelings:

*You have every right to those feelings that threaten to drown
you, but you will learn that they will not drown you, and
that things will get easier, and that there are things that
make life worth living. But you don't want to hear that now,
so just keep howling at the moon and, most important of all,
keep breathing.*

You will have many questions floating around in your mind about your life with a disability. Will I be able to work? How will my friends and family feel about me? Can I be loved? Can I make love? How will I get around? Can I travel? Where will I live? Why did this happen?

Your future can seem so uncertain, with no way to grasp an image of where your life can go from here. According to Jeri Morris, PhD, of Northwestern University Medical School in Chicago, this uncertainty of the future can be so extensive that you "feel virtually without a lifestyle."[2]

There is a wide range of disability and experience. You might have low-level spinal cord paraplegia and be highly capable of independence. Or, at the other extreme, you might have sustained a traumatic brain injury or broken neck that has paralyzed you almost completely. Each situation entails its own set of adjustments, some admittedly more challenging than others. Yet, what all such people have in common is the challenge of separating their misconceptions from reality, discovering over time what adjustments can be made, and learning that even the most significant disability need not preclude a meaningful life.

Being a person who uses a wheelchair is not an easy experience. But it can be an opportunity. Psychologist Carol Gill contracted polio at the age of five. She has worked directly with people as a counselor and has performed research. She knows from her own experience how large a challenge a disability is. However, Gill notes:

> When you go through any crisis, any experience that tests you, in which you feel you may fail but you triumph instead and come out on the other side, I think that deepens you. I think it gives you a lot of perspective on life.

Gill carries an image in her mind of

> ... a piece of pottery going through a kiln. The temperature is very hot. If it's too hot, the piece can melt down and break, but, if it's just right, the piece comes out stronger with lots of color, a beautiful piece of art. I think that's what happens with most people with a disability.

Just the fact of getting through the rehabilitation process is the first proof for people of what might be possible, as this quadriplegic woman says:

> I remember toward the end of my rehab, thinking, well I broke my neck and I got through it, I can do anything.

While your experience might be marked by negative emotions, fatigue, confusion, or a sense of powerlessness, you also have the chance to experience hope and confidence as you witness your ability to deal with such a challenging situation. The fact is that most people who acquire a disability make the adjustment in ways they never dreamed possible. Plenty of people before you had similar feelings and could not imagine how they would adjust.

Notes Carol Gill:

> The overwhelming majority of people can and will adjust, given proper social support, meaning not just family and friends, but society at large. I worked in rehab for many years, and it's just amazing how people can take this in stride, given adequate social support. People I never would have predicted would have the inner resources to deal with a disability, just do!

Emotional Responses

Regardless of how well-adjusted, mature, or emotionally strong you are, powerful emotions are a natural reaction to a crisis and part of the recovery and adaptive process. Emotions are neither positive nor negative (although you sometimes experience them that way—most people would rather feel happy than angry). They are a natural part of your being human.

It's important to recognize that the emotions related to your disability experience will rise and fall, come and go. Keep in mind—especially when you are feeling emotionally overwhelmed—that these reactions are not lasting. Most of all, when you are troubled, remember it is because of what happened to you, not because there is anything wrong with your mind.

Following are common emotional responses experienced by those with a disability. Whether you experience some or all of them, and to what degree, depends on a number of factors, including your individual situation and temperament.

Sense of Tragedy

Whether or not you think of having a disability as a tragedy depends on how you believe it will affect your life. Society ascribes images of dependency, pain, isolation, and fear to disability. These qualities are not true of the experience for many people with a disability or may not be present to the degree you might imagine. Your sense of tragedy may be amplified by these assumptions. Such exaggerated beliefs about disability are a source of unnecessary suffering.

Says this man with paraplegia, 33 years following his spinal cord injury:

> When I was 18, I had a tragic experience, but I am not a
> tragic person because of it.

That is not to say that you should be expected to just "get over it." Carol Gill says:

> As a therapist I would select a tone with people who are deal-
> ing with a new disability, which says, "Yeah, this is a crisis
> that is catastrophic for you." I would not try to minimize that.
> After all, who wants to become disabled?

In *Sexual Adjustment*, Martha Gregory writes:

> For healthy persons, the thought of spending the future
> [with a disability] may be so completely endowed with
> tragic overtones that they assume no one could be stable
> and happy.[3]

If you consistently project only the negative aspects of the experience of your disability to your family, friends, and the public, they are more likely to reflect negativity back to you. The way you feel about yourself and your disability affects others' reactions to you. You might also feel negative messages about your disability from others. It goes both ways. Self-confidence is no guarantee that some others won't see you in tragic terms, but revealing your positive side will often overcome the initial discomfort some people might have with your disability.

Your sense of tragedy about the experience of disability is important to face. Are you willing to consider that it's not as horrible as you always imagined? Michael Yapko, PhD, in his book *Breaking the Patterns of Depression* writes:

> Do you focus on problems, or do you focus on solutions? Do
> you constantly spin around the same negative thoughts and
> feelings about how terrible things are, or do you actively
> search for and identify new things to do that will help? Focus-
> ing on solutions means knowing that your circumstances are,
> at some level, changeable.[4]

Once you can discover that the impact on your life options is less than you feared, the sense of tragedy is reduced. Tragedy is really the beginning of the process. As a man who has spent years on wheels observes:

Those of us with a disability who have made our significant adjustments do not think of ourselves as tragic. Nor do we want to, having gone beyond it to get on with our lives. The tragic part is history—old news.

New people you meet who find out what led to your using a wheelchair will experience your story as tragic and respond with sympathy. This is natural on first contact. They need to feel the tragedy of it themselves and make their own adjustment, especially if they are people with whom you will have a continuing relationship. Just as you adapted beyond the initial sense of tragedy, so, too, will the significant people in your life.

Denial

When reality is too hard to bear all at once, the mind protects itself by using defense mechanisms, one of which is denial. In the short term, denial can help you get through difficult situations. Denial buys you time to gradually come to terms with what has happened. It gives you some control over the pace of psychological adjustment. A new disability is so powerful an experience that people just can't take it all in right away. Denial is one of our miraculous, self-adjusting "design features."

Lying on the ground, having fallen 25 feet, unable to move my legs, I remember very clearly thinking that they would take me to the hospital and I would be home that afternoon. Walking and fine.

There are a number of ways in which denial can manifest itself. A person might:

- Forget what the doctor has said about his condition
- Discount the facts of her medical status
- Suppress grieving emotions, keeping up a happy countenance, despite his true feelings
- Grant the facts about her condition but resist the idea that her life will need to change

According to psychologist Ann Marie Fleming:

Some people will say, "Well, I'm the same me I've always been, so I should be able to do all the same things I used to— let me at it." They want to go back to their normal life, regardless of what kind or degree of disability. But once they get through their hospitalization and rehab and get back

home, once they get out there and try everything, at some
point they're going to hit a wall and say, "Ouch. Omigod, this
is hard!" It is a big shock, but that's when the real adjustment
begins.

Denial gets to be a problem when it continues well past the initial
shock of a crisis and is so pervasive it keeps you from acting in your own
best interest. For instance, someone in denial:

- Might not take recommended medication or participate fully in a treat-
  ment or rehab program
- Might not arrange for needed support at home, thereby risking injury
- Might not make necessary home-access adjustments, risking injury
- Might not speak honestly to family and friends so that they can know
  what support is needed
- Might be careless about health maintenance, for example, not respond-
  ing to early signs of a pressure sore or infection

Staying stuck in denial about your condition can also drive you to
overachieve, unnecessarily trying to prove that you aren't disabled. That can
be a great waste of energy and put your health at risk. As a result, denying
the needs of your disability costs you freedom and independence. The more
you realistically meet the needs of your disability, the more your options
actually increase.

It's so strange that for most of my life after polio, all I could
think about was to keep going as fast as I could. Never did I
want to think about polio. I would also ignore my physical
discomfort and limitations completely—unless, of course,
they had me flat on my back or hospitalized. Even then, as
soon as I was back on my feet, I'd be back on that treadmill.
Now after all these years, I realize the need to heal all of the
wounds inside.[4]

If others—medical professionals, family, friends—tell you that you're
in denial, it's worth asking yourself if they might be right and to what degree
it might be limiting you. But no one else can know what you are experiencing, and you have to find your way the best you can. Psychologist Carol Gill
has respect for the help denial can offer individuals:

If a person stays in denial but it insulates them from pain,
who are we to decide it is a bad adjustment? I've met people
who've used denial all their lives and, although I might get
frustrated, if it gets them through, who am I to judge?

Blame

There are many, many ways one can place blame for having a disability—whether on themselves or on others. Perhaps you were injured because of a poor decision on your part—be it climbing up a tree or driving when you were tired or under the influence. Or maybe another person was driving the car or was unnecessarily rough as an opponent in a football game. Maybe you blame God. Clearly this paragraph could go on for a very long time, which means that you face a compelling temptation to place blame.

Blaming implies a sense of injustice, and, often, what comes along with that is anger, or even a desire for revenge. This is a common feature of people with a violently acquired injury, particularly those who come from a culture that involves guns or knives and the imperative to defend yourself and those to whom you consider yourself devoted.

For those with a childhood disability, the blame could be directed at a parent simply for being the carrier of a gene or for having been irresponsible during the pregnancy. A pregnant woman who drinks or takes drugs indeed puts the fetus at risk.

Blame is also easily directed at one's self, for having damaged your own body—and life—in which case punishment is an equally possible option. You don't have to go far to injure the blamed party when it's you.

Or it might simply be that you blame the circumstances that led to your disability. Ultimately it comes down to a question of whether you were in control of the events surrounding your disability. Now the question is whether you are in control of your response to it. Clinical psychologist Michael Yapko writes:

> ... if you recognize that negative things are not always the result of your personal shortcomings, that lousy circumstances can and will change, and you limit your conclusions to the specific situation at hand, then you are far less likely to experience a negative perspective.

Grief

Some people say that, at the moment of their disability, they died. The person they were was gone. The natural response to loss is grief. You grieve for the loss of your former self—lost plans, lost capacities, lost relationships. Whether or not these fears come true, the feelings are real and merit attention.

Ann Marie Fleming, a rehabilitation psychologist, observes:

> When you become disabled, you lose some part of yourself that you knew and cherished. Everybody goes through

multiple, major adjustments that affect their career, marriage, and relationships.

There are a number of stages following a recent disability that can elicit more feelings of loss and grief. After dealing with the injury itself, you might face disappointment about how much recovery you accomplish in the initial months. When you are released from hospital care or rehabilitation, you will face certain limitations in the outside world, such as not being able to easily go wherever you want. Relationships will change. Until you move through these milestones and face these losses and changes, it will be more difficult to redefine yourself and replace those lost parts of your life with new activities, interests, and relationships.

Grief is part of the healing process and diminishes over time. With a new disability, you might well experience a deep, immobilizing grief over being injured or discovering you have a progressive condition of some kind. But it will pass, if you allow yourself to mourn. In time you might continue to feel a sense of loss about your disability, but says Carol Gill:

> *People are complex. We're capable of feeling loss and remembering a sense of grief, but also of pursuing our lives and feeling real joy about other facets of our lives.*

There is great social pressure not to grieve, or at least not openly or not for long. Social norms do not encourage vulnerability, particularly for men. You may already be feeling dependent on family or friends because of your disability, so to also need emotional support can feel like you are demanding even more. Because you care about how your disability has affected loved ones, you naturally want to be strong for them, to not cause them further pain by having to watch you suffer more. Seeing you cry can raise great fear—that you are not adjusting well or that you will continue to be dependent, maybe increasingly so. But if you need to cry, do. Your loved ones may have just as much a need to cry with you. Irving Zola wrote about people's fear of crying:

> *[They believe] once started, it, like self-pity, will never stop. My own observation is that those people with an oversupply of tears are ones who have been unable to mourn their losses fully, especially when they first occurred. As a result they "leak" and mourn a little bit at a time.[1]*

Anger

Some features of early disability and rehab can understandably lead to angry feelings. The future can seem ruined, you have to submit to the care of strangers, who often must perform invasive , undignified medical or personal care procedures—sometimes with a cavalier attitude. This often feels like a loss of control and dignity. These feelings need not necessarily occur, but you might have thoughts, such as:

- This isn't fair.
- Why did this happen to me?
- It was my fault. How could I have been so stupid to let this happen?
- It was their fault, and I will hate them forever for what they did to me—or didn't do to protect me.
- I will never have the life I wanted, so nothing can be okay now.

You have the power to decide how to express the anger, and how to face the source of it so that you can move on with your life. It's exhausting to go through life angry.

> I'm a C4-5 quadriplegic. It takes way too much energy to get through the typical day living with my disability to be spending the bulk of that energy on hostility, denial, and rebellion.

You will also find yourself in situations that will likely arouse anger. There will be people who will speak to your companions on your behalf rather than directly addressing you. You might be left waiting for the wheelchair you need because your insurance is refusing to pay. You might be trying to find an apartment to rent and discover how few meet your access needs. The list goes on.

If you use a wheelchair, your anger—no matter what its source—is often seen as bitterness about your disability. Carol Gill explains:

> I think anger is one of those emotions that gets interpreted by outsiders in the context of what they think about us in general. It's been said that when a man is aggressive in his profession he's considered a go-getter, but when a woman is aggressive she's a bitch. I think those same contextual interpretations exist for people with disabilities. If a nondisabled person was told, "You can't get into this store, we're not going to move this box so you can get down this aisle," they would become angry and leave the store in a huff. That would be considered justified. But if a disabled person got equally angry about not having access to that store, he would be viewed as having a chip on his shoulder.

Even if you never see people from these encounters again, they might interpret your behavior as bitter—the "angry cripple"—another widely held social stereotype. Learning to manage anger will not only save you a lot of trouble, it will help foster an accurate perception of people with disabilities in the broader community. Managing anger does not mean keeping quiet. It means recognizing you are angry before your anger gets out of control and knowing that you have a choice about how to express it.

When you are angry—for whatever reason—you might feel like screaming, throwing things, or hurting yourself or others, actions most people associate with anger. Since these expressions are not socially acceptable, many people will instead suffer in silence, repressing their emotions. But anger that is held in has a way of finding its way out, often in subtle ways you may not notice. You might begin to be more cynical or sarcastic, or more of a tease—which can be a disguised form of attack. You might begin to drive more aggressively or start hitting the keys of your computer keyboard harder. Many people with disabilities throw their legs—such as while getting into or out of bed—or fail to be as gentle as necessary in bowel and bladder management. These subtle ways of venting pent-up anger can be harmful to you.

Fortunately, there are healthful ways of expressing anger, although they may take practice. For instance, you can talk about your anger with people you trust, making it clear that your anger is your experience and not about them—that you need to vent. This paraplegic man in his 20s, now a social worker in a major rehab center, describes learning that lesson the hard way:

> I was really into being a tough guy at the time I was injured, so I felt that I couldn't let people run my life once I broke my back. I really put my family through a lot of hell, but then I realized I was just stuck in a trap. One day I got on the phone and called a lot of people and apologized. They let me know that it sure wasn't fun to be treated badly when I was rude to them, but they tried their best to understand. It helped clear the air, and we're all the closer now for having talked about it.

When you're feeling explosive—and not in the mood for a heart-to-heart chat with anyone—you can channel your anger into some physical activity. If you're able to exercise, that can release a lot of angry tension. Other ways to physically release anger are to throw darts or blow up balloons and then pop them, all the while reciting the reasons for your wrath. Sometimes your only outlet is your voice. If it helps you feel better, go ahead and yell, but make sure anyone in hearing range knows that you're not in danger—nor is anyone else. Or you can sing. As strange as it sounds, singing when you're angry not only releases energy, but makes you feel better. You can even make up your own angry words to popular melodies. Use creativity as an outlet for anger that works for you.

Anger doesn't have to be full blown. Living with a disability can make your life harder at times, and being frustrated is a logical reaction.

> *If I'm having problems transferring [to and from my chair] and I'm exhausted and it's hard for me, it means I'm having a bad day like anyone can. People with disabilities have those day-to-day frustrations, too.*

> *When I feel angry and most frustrated about being disabled, it is almost invariably when I'm trying to be too nondisabled. Say I'm putting on a dinner party, which is pretty difficult for a quadriplegic to do. If something goes wrong, I get pretty frustrated. Now, someone might say that it means I really hate being disabled, but I say, "What was I trying to do!?" It's frustrating when you get caught up in the expectations of what you think you're supposed to be able to do. When I'm having a bad day, it's not because I hate having a disability.*

It's not always enough to express anger. If you are being treated poorly or unjustly, you can use your anger as redirected energy to try to resolve the problem. For example, if your insurer won't pay for something you need and you believe you have a right to it, hitting pillows isn't going to change things. You need to do some research, write letters, and make phone calls to make a difference. Righteous anger has moved many a mountain, especially if you take the time to find out the best methods to make your case and enlist the help of the right people.

Feelings of resentment and rage toward society's misconceptions of the disability experience drive many people to become involved in disability activism. Anger played a part in the motivation of trailblazers like Judy Heumann, Justin Dart, Ed Roberts, Bob Kafka, Evan Kemp, John Kemp, and Mary Lou Breslin—among many others—to get out and work for the kinds of changes that have already been accomplished. Despite the passage of the Rehabilitation Act of 1973, the Americans with Disabilities Act, and other victories, there is a great deal to be done. Anger will, and should, stoke that fire.

Depression

There are basically two kinds of depression: the kind almost everyone experiences from time to time, often called "the blues," and chronic, clinical depression. There is a distinct difference in the effects of each kind, how long the depression lasts, and how it is treated.

Common Depression

Few people get through life without ever feeling down. Common depression always has a reason that triggers it. The trigger can be something significant—like dealing with a disability—or more mundane, like a week of rainy weather. During a common depression, brain chemistry is altered, which is why you don't feel like your normal self. The chemical alteration usually rights itself after a few days when the trigger has either dissipated or you have had enough time to begin to cope with it.

It's normal to feel sad and disappointed, maybe even a little hopeless, just following a recent disability. You may wonder, "Will I feel like this forever? How much worse will my life get? Who could ever love me with this disability? Is it my fault that I'm disabled?" These are normal things to worry about, and they can foster feelings of depression.

When you are depressed, it is hard to separate issues associated with your disability from those troubling issues you would have anyway. Be careful not to allow your disability to become a scapegoat for things that have little or nothing to do with it. Blaming everything on your disability means missing the chance to review other aspects of your life that merit attention, and it means defining your disability as an unendurable state that you can never rise above. That can be a lifelong sentence for unnecessary unhappiness.

Common depression can last from a few hours to a couple of weeks. You might feel unmotivated, sluggish, or distracted as well as sad. You might be tempted to retreat into yourself, spend more time sleeping, and be as passive as possible, maybe watching television a lot more than you usually do. However, you will still be able to attend to necessary daily activities, and you will be able to acknowledge that there can be solutions to your problems, even though you might not yet be able to imagine what the solutions are. Although you may not laugh as readily as when you're not depressed, you'll still have a sense of humor. Most important, you will retain a sense of being in control of your life. You just won't feel like working very hard at it.

Clinical Depression

When mental health professionals speak of depression, they are usually referring to a condition much more severe than common depression. Clinical depression affects about one in 20 people in the United States each year. Whereas common depression is a temporary emotional downswing, clinical depression is an illness that can last as long as three years and can be completely debilitating—although this is a worst-case scenario. Unlike common depression, clinical depression doesn't necessarily have a trigger. Even if there is a reason, the depression lasts long beyond the time it normally takes to cope with a trigger event. Clinical depression is more about the alteration of brain chemistry that doesn't right itself than it is about logical reasons for feeling blue.

Although modern research is learning much about brain chemistry and depression, it remains a chicken-and-egg question. It is not clear whether the chemical change is a cause or a symptom of depression. This means that one must be careful of simply taking antidepressant drugs to curtail depression when, at the same time, it might be important to engage in the deep personal and spiritual work of self-evaluation such feelings often elicit.

A person ill with clinical depression requires medical intervention. You should tell your doctor if you have any of the following symptoms and they last more than a couple of weeks:

- Persistent sadness, hopelessness, or pessimism
- Feelings of guilt or worthlessness
- Lack of emotion; a feeling of emptiness
- A sense of helplessness
- Lack of interest in activities you would normally enjoy; inability to find pleasure or humor in anything
- Marked change in sleeping or eating patterns
- Chronic fatigue; exhaustion
- Restlessness or irritability
- Cognitive difficulties: remembering, concentrating, making even simple decisions
- Preoccupation with death or suicide

In the darkest moments of clinical depression, there can seem to be no options remaining for happiness or meaning in one's life. Feeling like nothing can ever be better is part of the insidious nature of the illness. Some people might tell you to "snap out of it!" They might as well tell you to snap out of pneumonia.

If you suspect you are clinically depressed, remember it is not your fault. It is not a sign of weakness.

Take Action

You can help yourself feel better sooner, though, and possibly ward off a more serious depression by taking some small steps, even if you have to push a bit to get started.

One of the most common pieces of advice is to simply do something. The simplest activity can give your mind another perspective and provide the opportunity to become engaged and interested in something other than what is troubling. It's also important to maintain human contact, since loneliness tends to amplify depression, but try to include other topics of conversation besides your woes. Finally, take especially good care of yourself. The following ideas can help lift you out of a common depression:

- Listen to your favorite music. Music has a way of bringing feelings to the surface so you can explore them rather than just being miserable.
- Play with or read to a child. It will help you get out of your world and see things from a simpler perspective.
- Work—or just spend some time—in the garden.
- Straighten up a room or a table, or bring in some flowers.
- Try to distinguish between what you really are unable to do and what you just don't feel like doing. For the latter, try to apply yourself, if only for a couple of minutes. You might discover you are able to do what you thought you couldn't.
- Divide big jobs into small ones. They add up quickly that way and will give you a sense of accomplishment—and feel less overwhelming.
- If you can, exercise. Physical activity is stimulating and can change the chemistry of your brain to lift your spirits.
- Play a game—athletic or otherwise. It will help you focus on the moment. You might even have fun.
- Go out with a friend, perhaps to a funny movie.
- Hug someone or let someone hug you.
- Do something unexpectedly nice for someone.
- Do something unexpectedly nice for yourself.
- Remember to eat as healthfully as possible. Keeping your body well nourished will speed your return to your happier self.
- Observe good hygiene and grooming. You're less likely to feel depressed when you feel clean and look your best.

Part of your goal in breaking out of your depression is to break out of patterns—of thought and of behavior. So, while taking action is beneficial, you also will want to make changes in what you do and how you think. Writes Michael Yapko, in *Breaking the Patterns of Depression*:

> *We are taught, "If at first you don't succeed, try, try again."*
> *I would add "... and when you try, try again, do something*
> *different." For you to break the patterns of depression, your*
> *expectations must be positive and realistic. Change is possi-*

*ble, and you can make good things happen in your life if you
approach each situation intelligently and with some flexibility.
Otherwise, you may keep doing over and over again what
doesn't work.*[4]

Depression is Treatable

Eighty to ninety percent of people with clinical depression can be treated
effectively. Almost everyone benefits to some extent from treatment, which
usually involves a combination of drug therapy and psychotherapy—exploring your feelings and life events with a trained therapist.

Many depressed people fail to seek treatment, despite the fact, as Yapko
writes:

> *... good treatment works. Typically, the depression sufferer
> feels hopeless—perhaps about ever feeling good again, per-
> haps about whatever seems at the base of the depression.
> When you feel hopeless, you usually don't want to spend the
> time and energy it takes to shop for, find, and then build a
> whole new relationship with a therapist. It may seem far too
> big a project, especially when your underlying hopelessness
> has you say, in essence, "Why bother? No one can help
> me anyway."*[4]

Suicide

Having a disability—regardless of the physical severity—sometimes leads
people to the point where they feel their situation is unchangeable and hopeless. They see themselves as having no options, no place to move, no
resources for change, and no one to turn to who could make a difference.
Perhaps the thought of adapting to a life with disability seems unaccept-
able—too far out of line with their notion of what it means to have a full,
rich life. In a moment of utter despair and darkness, a person may consider
that he would be better off ending his life.

The serious consideration of suicide should not be kept secret. If you
find yourself thinking that death is the best solution for you, tell someone
right away. Many cities have a 24-hour hotline (look in the yellow pages
under "crisis intervention"—if there is no agency specific to your need, any
of the listed numbers should be able to help you). No matter how hopeless
or ruined you believe your life to be, one phone call can save it.

If you are worried that someone you love might be thinking about suicide, don't be afraid to say, "I'm concerned you are thinking about taking
your life." It can be a great relief for the person to know someone is willing

to listen. Encourage him or her to get immediate professional counseling. The following are warning signs to watch for:

- Withdrawing from friends and family
- Changes in appetite, weight, behavior, level of activity, or sleep patterns
- Making self-deprecating comments
- Talking, writing, or hinting about suicide
- Purposefully putting personal affairs in order, such as tending to a will or life insurance
- Giving away possessions
- Sudden change from extreme depression to being "at peace" (may indicate a decision to attempt suicide)

There is ample evidence that people with even the most significant disabilities—including those who are mostly paralyzed and ventilator-dependent—consider the value of their lives to be very high. Most medical professionals know this, but you could find yourself influenced by people who do not believe quality of life is possible with a disability. They are wrong. Make sure whoever is helping you is committed to uncovering every conceivable possibility to enrich your life and make it worth living for you.

In *No Pity*, Joseph Shapiro describes Larry McAfee, a 34-year-old engineering student who became quadriplegic from a motorcycle accident and was in an intensive care unit for three months. McAfee was the subject of a high-profile assisted-suicide case. He asked to have a switch installed on his ventilator so that he could turn it off; a court granted permission. After a dizzying series of bureaucratic battles regarding where he could live and being provided access to computer equipment, McAfee's outlook changed. Thanks to the efforts of his family, other individuals, and disability advocacy groups, Larry McAfee finally returned to the community in a group home. According to Shapiro:

> *His mood bounced up and down, but on the whole, he pronounced himself happy to be alive, living a "good" life that had given him "hope."*[5]

Assisted suicide is a controversial topic in the disability community. Some people consider it their innate right to choose their time and method of passage. Yet others feel passionately that people with disabilities are denied the support and counseling that would be afforded anyone else with a wish for suicide, reflecting society's belief that a life lived with a disability is not worth living. Especially in the early stages of a recent disability, this is not a choice that can be reasonably made, and the first order of business should be to aggressively advocate for rehabilitation and equipment and other services that will provide for the optimal living that so many with disabilities of all kinds have proven is possible.

Religion

Each of us has our own particular take on God, the divine, and the realm of spirituality, including the atheist's view that there is no mystical component to our lives. Your beliefs and faith can be an extremely rich source of support, with lessons learned from the teachings of your spiritual tradition, community, or leaders. Most religious traditions tell us that the challenges in our lives have meaning and that we have a capacity to survive them and move through them as a process of learning and deepening of our very sense of self.

The atheist, the reincarnationist, and the humanist equally operate from a philosophy that affirms the good in humanity, and that our purpose in the world is to bring that to bear. This is how it should be: ultimate truths being about the ultimate good and the best of what it is to be human in this lifetime. If you are going to seek guidance from your religious or philosophical community and teachings, then pursue this perspective. It is the one that points you to your capacity to continue in the face of tremendous change and pain.

Unfortunately, some people become overwhelmed by their propensity to self-doubt, which can become translated into the fear—if not belief—that God (or karma, if you choose) has punished you, that you deserve to be in the situation you find yourself in, and it is just further evidence that you are unworthy. "How could God let this happen to me?"

Such a point of view is self-fulfilling. It drains your energy away; it prevents you from being able to see any potential path to renewed life, to see your real possibilities in the world with your disability being a feature of who you are: namely, a person just as capable of living in the world with meaning, giving and receiving among the people you love.

Take care to not allow matters of religion and faith to add to the emotional demands of adapting to your disability. If those thoughts are trying to assert themselves in your mind—and heart—then make the choice to challenge them, reaching out to whomever you trust as a guide to reassert and renew the positive nature that all true religions and philosophies teach is our true essence.

You Really Don't Know

In the early stages of an acquired disability, you are in a state of being overwhelmed. Your brain is limited by its very physiology—it just can't absorb and integrate that much change and emotion at one time. It is actually necessary to exist with a narrow perspective, as a way of protecting you from having a severe emotional breakdown. Then you can begin to put your attention on the decisions and actions needed to renew your sense of balance, gaining a measured understanding of what your life is about in this new and strange context of disability, and what's possible with it.

Postponing decisions does not mean you surrender faith in yourself. It means you have the good sense to know you'll make better decisions when you can think more objectively—when your emotions are in better balance. This day will arrive soon.

Hope

Hope is powerful, giving you strength to overcome grief, denial, and depression. Even a small ray of hope can help keep you moving forward. Sometimes, hope may be all you have. It is only natural to hope for a significant recovery after a disabling injury or diagnosis of a chronic or progressive condition.

After a person is injured or receives a life-changing diagnosis, medical professionals are cautious about encouraging what they fear could be false hope. Every one of them has seen people suffer heartbreak when their hopes didn't come true. Yet doctors, nurses, and others don't want to rob you of a positive outlook or make themselves your adversary. It is a difficult balance for them to achieve. They want to foster your motivation as much as possible while at the same time protecting you from the potential for psychological trauma.

How you discuss your hopes with the medical professionals who care for you makes a difference in how you are perceived and responded to. If they perceive you as being stuck on expecting a complete recovery or cure, to the exclusion of all other possibilities, they might not want to encourage your hopes. On the other hand, if you are asking questions about possible outcomes and what active measures you can take to bring about the best possible result, they'll be more comfortable supporting your hope for a degree of improvement even if they personally doubt you might achieve it.

At its best, hope will spur you to do whatever is necessary to make life as good as possible for you, including participation in the rehabilitation process. Embracing rehabilitation or other adaptations doesn't mean you surrender hope of recovery. It means you recognize that it is the best you can do right now. Should the hoped-for recovery be on its way, full participation in therapy will ensure that you are in optimal health and in the best position to take advantage of it.

Real hope isn't limited to the hope for a full recovery. You might hope you will still be able to pursue the career you want, hope you'll still be able to participate in some of the activities you love, hope you'll find a really great personal attendant, or hope you can learn to pop wheelies as well as some experienced riders you've seen. Your hopes can help bring into focus what is truly important to you and, therefore, help you make it happen. The ancient Roman poet Ovid had the right idea: "My hopes are not always realized, but I always hope."

Acceptance

There will be people who will try to get you to "accept" your disability, as if it is just a simple decision that you make and then are done with it. It is not just an intellectual choice; it is a process. Not only is there a complex set of inner forces at play, but acceptance is supposed to take time. What you learn along the way is worthwhile.

Well-trained medical staff know that people need to be allowed their natural emotional responses and will try to help family members understand this as well. That response might include a refusal to initially accept a new disability.

Attitudes do change. You can reach a balance appropriate for you, as happened for this spinal cord-injured man:

> More than 17 years ago, I remember saying I would not accept my disability. But by investing my life in positive activities, my attitude slowly changed to one of tolerance. Don't believe I have fully accepted it—or want to—because, for me, that would diminish hope. You don't need to accept this situation, but you must learn to deal with it. You have a life you might as well live.

Acceptance doesn't have to mean you're happy about having a disability. It means you accommodate its needs so it won't compromise the quality of your life any more than necessary, if at all. Resisting acceptance implies there is some preferred state, other than the one you are in, or some way to resolve your situation. Buddhist nun Pema Chodron describes seeking resolution this way:

> We don't deserve resolution; we deserve something better than that. We deserve our birthright, which is the middle way, an open state of mind that can relax with paradox and ambiguity. To the degree that we've been avoiding uncertainty, we're naturally going to have withdrawal symptoms—withdrawal

from always thinking that there's a problem and that someone,
somewhere needs to fix it.[6]

Acceptance includes the willingness to let go of always having answers and wanting things to be "solved." It is possible to recognize that things are out of control and still find a way to relax in the face of chaos. The ultimate message: given the hard reality of your loss, why multiply the loss by denying yourself what remains possible?

Humor

You might be surprised at having the ability to laugh about your disability experience. Having a disability does not erase your sense of humor. If anything, it enhances your sense of irony that is the root of much humor. Even tentative humor in the initial stages of adapting can reassure you that things are going to get better. Laughter is healing.

> *We had a lot of fun at the therapy gym where I went for*
> *rehab. It added to the spirit of the hard work, increasing my*
> *motivation.*

Joking about disability makes some people uncomfortable. They are so used to thinking of disability as tragic that to joke about it seems cruel. You will undoubtedly feel more at ease with such humor than the nondisabled people around you. For instance, John Callahan is quadriplegic from a spinal cord injury and is well known for his sometimes-skewed humor about disability. He has drawn many published cartoons, now collected in several books, and has also written a book on his own disability experience, *Don't Worry, He Won't Get Far on Foot*. Another rider collects disability one-liners to use in various situations:

> *I have built a repertoire of lines over the years of using a*
> *wheelchair. When the opportunity presents itself, I can joke*
> *with someone that "I'll never set wheel in here again!" or that*
> *I need to "take a sit" on a certain issue.*

You can find plenty of examples of humor in daily life:

> *There was the man in a movie theater who thought that the*
> *Americans with Disabilities Act entitled me to go ahead of*
> *him in the popcorn line. Or the time I took a spill after trying*
> *to show off a bit too much with wheelies.*

Reynolds Price is a writer who faced an extended experience fighting cancer, which included paralysis. In his book *A Whole New Life*, he writes:

*Best of all, with the help of friends, I managed to laugh a few
times most days. Sometimes the rusty sound of my out-of-
practice chuckle reminded me of how a gift as big as the tendency to laugh in the face of disaster is a literally biological
endowment.*[7]

Your disability need not be off limits to humor. Your friends can
become comfortable with where the boundaries are on joking about your
disability. Spend time with friends you enjoy, and let them know they don't
need to restrain themselves on your behalf.

*I consider it a proof of intimacy and real acceptance when
friends demonstrate they know I won't break down and
cry if something truly funny comes up around being a
chair user.*

Emotional Support

The need for medical treatment and therapy for a person with a new disability is obvious. Your inner self is equally deserving of support, helping see
you through the initial emotional trauma of injury or diagnosis and helping
you gain increasingly deeper insight as you live with disability. Common
sources of emotional support include family and friends, colleagues and
peers from work, support groups, and psychological counseling.

The emotional support of family and friends not only is a tremendous
comfort, but helps get you through the initial process of grieving and adjustment. If you are lucky enough to have strong support from the people closest to you, don't be reluctant to let them help. Because they know you so
well, you can get to the heart of what you are feeling without having to
explain a lot of background about who you are. Trust is already there, so
you don't have to feel as cautious about exposing your deepest emotions.
You also get reinforcement for the ways in which you are still the same person now in the context of your disability. You learn that your disability is not
who you are but is one of many things that makes up your identity. Many
people come to recognize that the disability is not only one of loss, but also
includes unique lessons they might not have otherwise gained in their life.
The quality of your relationships and the emotional support they provide
has much to do with this process. This man with C5 quadriplegia recalls:

*All my friends were super supportive. I remember going out to
dinner when I was still wearing my halo! We were sitting in a
crowded restaurant on a Friday night where all the beautiful*

*people come out. Here I am wearing a halo, so for them to do
that for me, and take me to bars—we were all learning things
together. My family and friends is the single most important
thing. I can give myself credit, but they totally changed how
it went.*

Unfortunately, not all family members and friends will be able to offer
ideal emotional support, especially not at first. They might be having their
own difficulty coping with what has happened to you and may need emotional support, too. It's important that you don't feel responsible for their
emotional needs. That can be a temptation—and a drain. In rare cases, family or friends will have to take time away from you in order to make their
own emotional adjustments.

*I had some friends who just didn't know how to deal with my
injury. They couldn't come to the hospital. It was too much.
Some were honest enough to say they needed time and were
sorry they couldn't be there for me. One of my best friends just
cut off all contact. I found out later that he was overwhelmed
and didn't know how to even approach me. It took a few
years, but, once I was back out in the world, we were able to
resume our friendship, which was very deep. Now he is like
family to me. I could have been angry and chosen not to for-
give him, but I realize how painful the whole thing was for
him and would rather not sacrifice what he means to me now.*

Another source of emotional support is a support group where people
share the experience of disability. Group members can honestly say, "We
know how you feel." It is a chance to meet with people who share your experience. Whether you need someone to understand and relieve your fears
about the future, recommend a helpful product, or share ideas for dealing
with insensitive strangers, group support can be a wonderful resource. You
can find support groups in your city or on the Internet. Many rehab hospitals have support programs that include peer volunteers.

Professional counseling is another option for emotional support.
Going to a psychologist does not mean something is seriously wrong with
your head or that you aren't smart or strong enough to get through rough
times on your own. A professional counselor can save you unnecessary dis-
tress by helping you understand yourself better and see a disability as a part
of your life that offers opportunity as well as challenge. (You may have to
shop around a bit to find someone with whom you feel comfortable. Don't
be discouraged if the first counselor you visit doesn't seem right for you—
it's worth it to keep looking.) Counseling is absolutely confidential, provid-

ing a safe "container" for you to explore your thoughts and feelings. So well recognized is the importance of adequate emotional support immediately after onset of the disability that psychotherapists are now commonly included as part of the rehab team.

There are circumstances when it is extremely important to seek out the services of a psychology professional. If you are suffering from chronic depression or having thoughts of suicide, the sooner you talk to a professional counselor, the better. In these situations, human beings are too emotionally distraught to be of much help to themselves, and nonprofessionals don't have the necessary training. Being depressed or suicidal is nothing to be ashamed of—although it will probably feel that way. Don't hesitate to contact a counselor.

Adaptability

Change is the one constant in life. A disability—whether acquired at birth or later in life—is one heck of an exercise in adapting to change. Being injured means instant and intense adaptation. Being disabled at birth means adapting throughout development, with changing issues in adolescence and as you become increasingly socialized outside of the family. A progressive condition like multiple sclerosis or amyotrophic lateral sclerosis means a continuing process of adapting as the effects of the disability progress, sometimes very slowly. Even people with spinal cord injuries, once thought to be a stable condition after the rehabilitation process, face changes in levels of impairment as they age.

This quadriplegic woman in her 40s is finding that she is being called upon to make new adaptations she didn't expect to face:

> It's depressing. Is this a change? Is this just one step and I get
> used to it and it's going to stay like that for a while? Or is it
> going to be something that's more limiting over time and I'm
> going to have to get used to more and more limitations?

Part of adaptability is the ability to create an environment for yourself in which your disability does not unduly limit you. In many ways, the disability itself is not what "handicaps" you. It is when you can't get up the steps or through the door that you become disabled. You can create more psychological security for yourself by creating an environment that does not unnecessarily limit you. In *Missing Pieces*, Irving Zola asks:

> What happens to all those without sufficient money or
> power to alter their environment, without resources to have
> railings built or clothes custom-made or sufficient influence

> *to have meetings take place in more physically accessible*
> *locations? I suspect that they ultimately give up. Unable to*
> *change or manipulate the world, they simply cut out that*
> *part of their life which requires such encounters, which*
> *contributes to a real, as well as social, invisibility and*
> *isolation.*[4]

Self-advocacy is a critical skill in this process of finding your place in a life on wheels. The very act of pursuing your needs and asserting your rights is itself psychologically supportive. Although Professor Zola's suspicion that some people give up may be true, it need not be. Your resolution of anger, comfort with your identity, gradual release of denial, and the entire process of adaptation—your emotional reality—relies on addressing your physical environment, as well as remaining intellectually stimulated and spiritually curious.

If there is one central lesson that the experience of disability has to teach you, it is how remarkably adaptive we are as human beings. Some people might have fewer obstacles than others, but chances are you can do more than you think you can.

> *Following my disability, I got a college education, accom-*
> *plished a great deal professionally, traveled, made close*
> *friends, loved and lost and loved some more—what I consider*
> *the ingredients of a pretty full life. I wouldn't tell you that my*
> *disability has been neutral in all of this, or that there aren't*
> *things I would love to do that I can't. I'm telling you that at*
> *the time of my injury I could not conceive of doing the things I*
> *ultimately did.*

The capacity to adapt seems to be related to age. Rehab psychologist Ann Marie Fleming sees that children tend to make relatively easy adjustments. Their lives are all about constant change, and their adaptation skills are well practiced. The older a person is, the more difficult it can be to accept a major change such as disability.

As we age, it becomes harder and harder to accommodate major lifestyle changes. We become more fixed in our ways, and we just plain get tired out with the weight of our lives behind us. For some people, the shock of disability can jolt them from a self-destructive path. Fleming states:

> *For someone who maybe used drugs or had trouble holding*
> *down responsibilities, that brush with death is a spiritual*
> *crisis. All of a sudden they want to be alive, they want to be*
> *straight, they want to be conscious, they want to be clear.*

> *They say, "I don't want to die. I don't want to medicate*
> *any more."*

Disability is a chance to be reminded of the universal truth of the frailty of being human. The struggle to adapt to the many demands of disability can increase your empathy for all people, as is the experience of this woman with Charcot-Marie Tooth disease, a form of muscular dystrophy:

> *I believe, too, that having CMT has definitely given me the*
> *sense of being more accepting of others, whether they are*
> *"disabled" in some way or not. We are each so individual,*
> *thank goodness! How boring it would be if not! I try to see*
> *people's insides more than their outsides.*

You will inevitably consider how you previously felt about people with disabilities. You get to revisit your attitudes, now that you have joined the club. Carol Gill sees an advantage in this, saying:

> *You learn a lot about being human from the way you once*
> *looked at people with disabilities and the way you now look*
> *at yourself and others with disabilities. You go through a val-*
> *ues overhaul.*

Interacting With Others

Family

Disability happens to family members, too. They will also have intense emotions and adjustments to make and, in the early stages, be faced with a significant disruption to the daily pattern of their lives:

- Spending time at a hospital or rehab center
- Dealing with doctors and insurers
- Communicating with other family members and concerned loved ones
- Finding solutions for a variety of needs in preparation for home-coming day, not the least of which is making the home accessible and livable

For acquired disabilities in which there is some potential for recovery, family members can become invested in hope, which is also a form of solace that can help them maintain their daily lives with the added emotional and practical demands. Says this young man, spinal cord injured at the age of 18:

I know my disability was very painful for my parents. Their son had been seriously injured. On the day I was admitted to rehab, after weeks in another hospital recovering from back surgery, my doctor told them point-blank that my condition would stay just as it was on that day. Having gone to rehab with hope that I might walk out, they found themselves sitting in the lobby, crying together.

Family members could be afraid to bring up certain topics for fear of upsetting you. Let them know how open you want them to be with you. It might fall to you to draw them out, to start the ball rolling on discussing a sensitive topic related to your disability. Your relationship with them may need to adjust.

Professionals generally advise families not to withhold what they feel. If their injured relative makes them angry or very sad, they might fear that revealing these feelings could overwhelm their loved one. Social worker Joan Anderson of the Santa Clara Valley Medical Center in California writes:

Families seem to believe that if a person has a disability he or she is too fragile to withstand normal human interactions. Such an attitude dehumanizes the disabled person and robs him or her of the normal exchange of feelings that keep our relationships mutual and balanced.[8]

Family members, especially parents, often feel they need to exercise some control, to make sure that you are being taken care of. It might be that they feel the need to accomplish something, since they can't make you well. Regardless of the age of their loved one, the impulse to revert to the caretaker mode of early parenting can be strong.

There was a time in the hospital when my mom was running down the hall saying, "My son hasn't had a shave in three days! Somebody shave this guy!" If I could have moved as fast as she did, I probably could have killed her, but I couldn't. I was too slow, so it was very frustrating for me to feel so powerless about them trying to baby me.

Family members who express doubts about your ability to function or pursue certain goals—for fear of offering what they feel could be false encouragement—might unwittingly weigh you down. Doubt is particularly dangerous when it comes in the form of loving, presumably protective, concern. You can be drawn into self-doubt, giving too much consideration to others' opinions. Or you might feel you have to prove your family wrong, overexerting yourself by ignoring your own realistic limits and capacities.

Just as serious a trap is being overly optimistic, where a family member denies the real implications of your disability and promotes unrealistic expectations. It is easy for you to want to play along, especially in the early stages when the urge is to remain as "normal" as possible. You usually want to please the ones you love, so you might want to match their expectations, pleased that they see you as someone capable of their proposal—whether it is an aggressive schedule of education, travel, starting a business, or returning quickly to a job.

It is natural for you to care about what your family is going through, at the same time as you face your own feelings. You might feel the need to be strong for them or protect them, but, in the process, you risk denying them the chance to know your real experience.

Families usually have a lot to learn about disability. To the degree that you bring unrealistic attitudes about disability into your own experience, you might well have picked them up from your family—not to mention prevailing social messages. You will all have to revisit these assumptions and reconsider how you have allowed society to influence your reactions and views. Many rehab centers offer family support groups for this very purpose.

If family members resist understanding, or if conflict arises, it might be necessary to seek assistance from a counselor to help you work things out. It is not an admission of failure to ask for professional support. When so many changes need to be made at once, it is a hard process for any family, no matter how strong or well adjusted. Your family relationships are one of the most important supportive components in your success at adapting with a disability. It is worth any effort to reach a balanced understanding with your family, to allow them to work through their own needs, and to welcome their support and guidance. Then you can all direct your energies in positive ways and accomplish the best quality of life for all family members. Be a team.

When you and your family find a balance, there is less strain on your relationships and you have a better opportunity to discover your limits and abilities.

> My mother never imagined that I would not be active and independent. She did not try to do things for me that I could do myself, and she was not negative or doubtful about my plans to return to school, drive, or any other goal. It was not a matter of blind ambition, but a balanced view of what was possible. On the whole she did exactly the right thing. She believed in my capacity to have a normal life but did not push me to be heroic.

Support for Families

Family members have very real and important needs that often go unmet during the initial stages of a newly acquired disability. The love and concern is so great for their loved one with a disability—understandably—that all of the family's energy and attention go to supporting her.

Yet there is a limit to what anyone has to give before they begin to become overwhelmed themselves, becoming less and less able to give. Resentments or guilt can arise, on both sides—the family member, feeling that she is letting her loved one down, and the newly disabled family member feeling responsible for being the cause of such overwhelming feelings. The greater the sacrifice the family member makes, the greater the danger of these kinds of wrenches being thrown into the family system.

Says this spouse of a man who became paralyzed from a malignant tumor on his spinal cord:

> *Everyone kept telling me that I had to "be strong for him."*
> *Looking back, I realize they thought they were trying to*
> *encourage me and show me they believed I could handle*
> *whatever he needed from me, but that's not what I really*
> *needed. I was having strong feelings and was struggling with*
> *how completely I was expected to let go of my own needs.*
> *I had no one to express this to, and no way to get any relief in*
> *ways that would have actually helped me replenish exactly so*
> *I could do the best I possibly could. I think I fell short.*

Physical and emotional exhaustion are real risks, involving keeping the home and family logistics going while spending time at the hospital, keeping other family members and friends informed, researching information (like web surfing or reading this book), or beginning complex processes like home modifications for accessibility. The closer you are to the disabled family member, the more your own life is directly affected—and the more you are facing your own losses. You have more to grieve, and to ignore these truths and these needs is to risk your own health, possibly even the strength of key family relationships.

A Tool for Families

The rehabilitation community has come to recognize the need to directly support family members during the early stage of a newly acquired disability. Research departments are studying family needs, and psychologists and social workers are working to develop tools and strategies that will benefit family members, helping them to take care of themselves while giving all they possibly can to meet the needs and potential of their loved one with a disability.

Toward that end, psychologists in the Department of Physical Medicine and Rehabilitation at Virginia Commonwealth University Medical Center in Richmond, Virginia, have developed the Family Change Questionnaire exactly to meet the needs of family members at risk of being overwhelmed, as described above. Says Jeffrey Kreutzer, PhD, of the VCU team:

> *Recognizing the full scope of important family life changes can help you maintain your intellectual and emotional balance. Recognizing change is also a step toward improving family communication, allowing you to work together more effectively and better meet everyone's needs.*

Since it is difficult to pause—or even have the mental or emotional capacity to gain some perspective—the Family Change Questionnaire on the next page helps family members to gain their bearings. It can be used individually, answering the questions in private for your own insight, or it can be a tool used in work with a counselor, who can help you gain even further perspective in a safe and confidential setting.

Communication

Openness and honesty is a challenge for many families. Difficult as it is—because letting people know how you are feeling is often a very vulnerable thing to do, fearing criticism or being misunderstood altogether—there are compelling reasons for everyone sharing the experience of a recent disability to know what each is going through.

This is an easy trap to fall into for well-intentioned reasons. Often everybody is so concerned that they will overwhelm someone with their feelings—especially their loved one—so, from a motive of protection, they hold back. This can leave open the possibility of confusion and assumptions.

It is also often a mistake to imagine that a loved one is so saturated with his experience that he is incapable of handling what others are going through. Yet, one of the greatest fears a person recently disabled faces is that he will no longer be treated as a full family member, that he will be a burden. Keeping him from participating in conversations or hearing information that he would normally have been a part of plays exactly into this fear. Perhaps in the very early stage—or on a certain day—he might not have the capacity to hear what's going on in other people's lives, but he is probably stronger and more aware and more wanting to be part of what's going on outside of his own experience than a family member might assume.

This woman with a T4-5 spinal cord injury describes the unexpressed and unresolved feelings between herself and her mother:

The Family Change Questionnaire

1. How did you feel when you first learned that your injured family member was injured?
2. How did you feel when you realized that your injured family member was going to live?
3. How did you feel when you began to recognize that the disability might have long-term effects?
4. How have other family members reacted to your family member's injury?
5. Have you made yourself available to provide more emotional support to your injured family member and other family members? If yes, how so?
6. Before the injury, what were the most important plans you had for your future and your family's future?
7. How has the disability affected your plans for the future?
8. What responsibilities do you now have to care for your injured family member?
9. In what ways do you help your injured family member get back and forth to appointments?
10. Do you attend therapy and doctors' visits with your injured family member? Please explain.
11. Do you help your injured family member with filling out insurance, registration, medical, and disability forms? Please explain.
12. Do you help your injured family member get authorizations for medical and rehabilitative care? Please explain.
13. Have you taken over responsibilities from your injured family member or uninjured family members? If yes, what new responsibilities do you have related to caring for the house, maintaining the car(s), working, paying bills, and caring for children?
14. Have you changed your work responsibilities or hours since the injury so that you could help your injured family member or the family?
15. How has your family's income been affected by the injury?
16. What new expenses are you facing because of the injury?
17. How have your sports, social, and recreational activities changed because of the injury?

*True to my pattern of discounting what I intuitively knew, I
didn't discuss my feelings or ask what was wrong with me.
My mother was a large woman, often in a take-charge mode.
But she would often come into the hospital room, look at me,
and leave in tears. So I chose to be "strong for my mother,"
with no consciousness that my "strength" was built on a
quicksand of unresolved emotions.*

What could this mother and daughter have gained by talking with
each other about what was happening inside? Perhaps they needed the support of a counselor or to be in support group setting where they could have
observed the benefits of people sharing their experiences. How much could
they have mutually supported each other from the very beginning by being
honest about what they felt? How much could this injured woman have
been able to use her strength for her own grieving and adjustment without
having to be "strong for her mother?" The consequences can be even more
dire, as this man discovered about his father's difficulty dealing with his
son's recent injury:

*My dad was always the one in control, always the one who
was strong and kept it together and never needed emotional
support from any of us. But I came home from rehab to the
news that he was dead, and later learned (just more being
afraid of the truth, of course) that I hadn't been told the real
truth of how he died. My father took his own life just before I
got home, so I'm left having to imagine that he didn't think he
could handle my having a disability. If we had only had the
chance to know what he was going through, to try to reassure
him, to help him, or get him some help, maybe it could have
all been different.*

Letting Go

As you progress through the acute stage of an injury or illness, or grow into
maturity after a childhood with a disability, your family and friends will
need to gradually let go of their roles as caregivers. This can be an especially
hard task for parents, who will once again need to set you off on your own,
afraid for your safety. Fleming states:

*After a while the injured relative will start to say to the
family members who continue to help him, "Get out of my
face. You're driving me crazy!" It's like an adolescent who
starts to test his wings to see how much he can fly on his
own. Parents have to be willing to let their children fall*

*once in a while. I tell the parent, "You've done it before, you
can do it again."*

You need to let go, too. You might be surprised at how accustomed
you had become to people doing things for you during the early stages of
a disability or your childhood with a disability. It is like a repeat of the
young adult experience, when you can't wait to get out of the family home
and have the freedom to do as you please—until you find out that includes
washing the dishes and doing the laundry! Home starts to look pretty good
at that point.

The same process of growth happens with your disability. As you
embrace adjustment, you might continue to face moments that make you
wish your family was still pitching in. Your need to reach for optimal independence is not about your family; it is about defining your needs and the
best way to meet them. If you need assistance dressing or transferring, a
family member could continue to play that role if you are able to maintain
a balanced relationship. But Carol Gill warns that:

> *The deck is stacked against you if you use a family member
> or an intimate partner as a personal assistant. It sets the
> stage for confusing various aspects of the relationship. It's
> hard for family members to just see themselves as providing
> assistance and not being caretakers. Using outside support
> is also easier for the family. It makes it easier for them to
> establish more balanced relationships with the disabled
> family member.*

Letting go might be a matter of identifying how your needs get met,
and that could mean deciding that someone other than a family member
should perform certain tasks.

Dependency

When an experience is difficult, you might feel pressure to give up. You
get tired, or the scale of the task seems overwhelming. Maybe life was
already tough prior to your disability, and now you have the perfect excuse
to surrender.

There are several possible outlets to spare you all the trouble—or
so it seems: reliance on others, over-reliance on government support, or
substance abuse. Each is a trap, a downward spiral that only produces
more grief and pain, less personal freedom, less self-esteem. Each is more
likely to alter your experience from simply having a disability to being
truly unable.

Letting Others Take Care of You

A person with a disability who becomes fixated on the trauma, tragedy, fear, and depression will commonly resort to dependency. Having failed to transcend psychological dynamics such as these—putting yourself into the hands of family or institutions that you expect to take care of you—can seem an appealing and easier path to take.

Perhaps your parents are in that role. But they will get old before you do. Many people who relied on parents are finding it hard to adjust as their parents age and are no longer able to help with chair transfers or other physical tasks.

People who perform necessary tasks that allow you to function are not "taking care of you." They are assisting you. You decide what they do and how and when. It only becomes dependency when you surrender decision making and allow others to have control.

Living on the Government

Some people don't have any choice about taking government assistance. They are unable to work or unable to find work (possibly because of discrimination) or the disincentives are so strong that they can't work, lest they lose their medical coverage, for instance.

However, if you are thinking that you can't work and don't bother to find out what is possible, you might well be underestimating your abilities. Plenty of people with significant disabilities have good jobs or businesses of their own. Corporations are increasingly learning that hiring people with disabilities and making accommodations is profitable for all parties. The front door is now more accessible, and you'll find a wide stall in the rest room. Computer technology makes it possible to work by voice command or with limited hand and arm capacity. Computers also make home-based businesses more viable.

Relying on the government often means a poor quality of life. People with disabilities can tell many nightmare stories of struggles with the bureaucracy, having to fight for benefits, and getting trapped by arcane regulations or incompetent workers. Living on Social Security disability benefits earns you the right to medical coverage under Medicare, but Medicare has strict limits on what it will cover. The power wheelchair that might be ideal for you could be refused. You could need in-home assistance, but a Medicare rule that says that you must be unable to leave the home could mean that volunteering at a local school two days a week might cost you your coverage. It's a mistake to assume your only option for financial support is government assistance or that relying on this aid is the best means for adapting to your disability. For many, this decision carries a high price, including the missed potential to be more financially self-sufficient and contribute your unique abilities to your community.

Substance Abuse

Suppressing painful emotions with substances can be tempting, using them to "self-medicate." Maybe you received a legal judgment and accepted a lump sum that put a lot of money in your pocket. Maybe you don't need to work. Sitting at home drinking or smoking pot could be a hard option to resist.

Substance abuse, be it alcohol, drugs, or food, will compromise your health and hugely amplify the limiting effects of your disability. You will lose strength and need more assistance pushing a chair or making transfers. You will likely gain weight, increasing the risk of pressure sores, and, again, be more likely to need help in transfers. Changes in your health and strength might force you across that boundary of needing personal assistance or even having to move into a "care" facility.

Many other health risks accompany substance abuse, including heart attacks, liver problems, and even cancer, especially if you smoke. You are compromising your immune system when you abuse substances. Drugs and alcohol also compromise your ability to absorb and metabolize nutrients from your food. This lowers your body's defenses and affects your ability to maintain healthy skin and good circulation, recover from an illness, and heal an injury.

Scientists now understand that good feelings relate to chemicals known as endorphins. In effect, your body makes its own drugs—a natural high. When you habitually abuse substances, your body ceases to produce endorphins on its own. After a time, the only way to feel good is to generate endorphins artificially with drugs or alcohol.

Alcohol and drugs affect your judgment and ability to make decisions. At worst, your family might come to believe you are no longer able to make responsible decisions for yourself and may consider taking control of your life. They might even get legal guardian status and have you placed in a nursing facility.

Most of all, drugs and alcohol make things worse. Whatever "benefits" one derives, the benefits of drugs and alcohol are short term at best. Becoming dependent entails a list of liabilities:

1.   Drugs mask the problems in need of real help.
2.   Drugs delay or even prevent your developing more effective and sophisticated strategies of self-management, making repetitive hurts more likely.

3. Drugs can create physical addictions at most, emotional dependence at least.
4. Drugs affirm your sense of being out of control and barely managing, hardly a boost to self-esteem.
5. Drugs can stimulate or aggravate the same neural pathways as depression.[4]

Independence, Not Heroism

Independence does not mean that you have to push yourself too hard and become the stereotypical "supercrip." Independence means using the capacity you have, whether it's your physical ability or your ability to manage resources such as benefits and personal assistance services. Independence is about being willing to take some risks, more than might be comfortable at first.

If your fears of facing life with a disability lead you to escape through various forms of dependency, think again. The results of dependencies are far worse than if you jump in, test your capacity to adapt, and seek support for the process. Yes, this can be very tough to do initially. There are many people out there willing to help, be it the local center for independent living, free community counseling, support groups, or friends and family. Fight hard for optimal health and independence rather than accepting a downward spiral into increased suffering and dependency.

Being Helped

Thanks, at least in part, to the Boy Scouts—do your "good deed for the day"—and the March of Dimes, people have a desire to help those "in need." People are essentially generous in their intentions. Unfortunately, such well-meaning gestures can be more of a hindrance than a help.

There is an art to giving and receiving help. One of the most interesting and never-ending features of life on wheels is to find the balance: to learn to ask for and graciously accept help when it is truly needed, and to teach those close to you how to help appropriately—which often means not helping.

> *I have no problem with people wanting to help me, but on the other hand I need to live my life, so there are certain things that I'm going to have to do by myself.*

How it Feels

The emotions around being helped are amplified for wheelchair users. It is a fact of life that there are now a variety of situations beyond your capacity to handle alone or that are awkward or difficult. An object may be too heavy or awkward to pick up from the floor or put on a shelf. You may need to get down a flight of stairs. No one wants to be dependent on others, but, at times, accepting help is a fact of life for people with disabilities in order to do what you want to do or go where you want to go.

I remember my own notion of disability before my injury. I imagined that these people must be used to being helped. Now that I know better, I continue to get the sense that nondisabled people think the same thing. Why would we resist help? Isn't it part of the disability experience and accepted as such?

Exactly because you must accept some degree of help, the things you can still do yourself become that much more precious. It is sometimes worth a little extra effort or strain to avoid having to surrender control. Says this man with quadriplegia:

> I go out of my way not to ask too many favors of people. Too much of it makes me appear less independent. I'm careful not to accept too many offers of favors. I preserve my asking of favors for those show-stopper moments when I'm completely stuck, no way out.

But going it alone is not worth the extra effort when it wastes precious energy or risks injury. You will need to find your own appropriate balance between doing it yourself and accepting or seeking help in order to ensure your safety or preserve your energy.

The quality of how you relate to people who are helping—or offering—is a poignant exercise in achieving an equal balanced relationship in which all parties feel safe and respected. It's also a built-in opportunity to raise awareness about the disability experience.

> When I get offers of help I don't need, I just say "No, thanks!" in a very positive way. If it's a situation where I think a little education might be a good idea, then I'll explain why. For example, if a neighbor or someone I know offers to help me when it looks like I'm struggling with something, I'll explain that when I'm learning something new I need to struggle with it for a few attempts before I get it down.

But, ultimately, trying to change the world gets old. It takes a lot of energy to get wrapped up in caring whether or not people understand how you function and what independence means to you. As this young woman with paraplegia learned:

*When I was first injured, one of the hardest things was the way
everybody seemed to stare at me and try to "help" me.
Although I was the same person I had always been, I was seen
so differently. While I struggled with this at first, it now makes
me chuckle. I have a whole new perspective. While I try to
advocate for myself and explain my injury to those who try to
"help," I know I'm not going to educate everybody or change
the unfounded stereotypes people harbor about people with disabilities. I have just grown to not care what others think.*

Frankly, we can't always be nice, though this man who had a stroke
struggles with the balance:

*Usually I say, "No, but thanks for the offer." I'm afraid that if
I'm rude, the next time I may need help, or someone else may
need it, people won't be so open, assuming we're angry
because of our disability. Sometimes, I admit, I do respond
with hostility. I may be in a bad mood.*

The line between doing it yourself and asking for help can be a hard
one to straddle. As Irving Zola wrote about his own experience:

*Hardest of all was to ask for something that I knew I could
do. In fact, if I could do it, there was a moral imperative to do
it, no matter how tired I was or what risk it demanded. I did
not want to be put into a position of always asking favors and
thus having to feel obligated. The key was what not doing
something communicated about me. It confessed to all a
weakness. But just because an individual can do something
doesn't mean that he should. By spending so much time and
energy on basic tasks, we eliminate the chance of realizing
other possibilities.*[1]

Personal limits can easily be crossed, as people do not understand that
your wheelchair is essentially part of your body, that you can even sense
when it is touched by the movement you sense through your body. This
paralyzed man defines the boundary and has a creative approach to making
his point:

*Touching my chair is off limits unless you're my wife. For
people I know a bit and like, I'll reach out my gimpy quad
hand and start fiddling with their fly. That usually gets their
attention so I can explain the personal space thing.*

The experience of being helped is inevitably charged on both sides.
Carol Gill observes:

*You have to look at the realistic consequences of being a dis-
abled person who accepts assistance. One study found that
every time you ask for help, there can be consequences. For
the majority of people in our culture right now, if you ask
for help as a disabled person and they give you that help,
there is the risk that they will see you as dependent, incapable, needy.*

Do You Actually Need Help?

Particularly in the early days of a disability, the boundary is not clear about
when to ask for or accept help. For example, it can be easy to fall into the
trap of trying to prove to the world that you are not limited by your disability. "I can do it!" can become a habitual response to any offer of help simply because the identity of having a disability may feel uncomfortable.

It is extremely common to fall into the habit of trying to "prove that
you're not disabled."

*I certainly did this, being the hotshot speedster in my wheel-
chair as a young paraplegic man. I hated letting anyone do
things for me. It was very uncomfortable for me to imagine
that people felt that I couldn't do things like open a door or
push myself up a ramp—especially knowing that I can do
these things myself, and well.*

Many times you will turn down offers of help because you can easily
do the task yourself. The person trying to help actually gets in your way! You
will have gained many skills from your experience of using wheels, but most
people you encounter in public will not know how you adapt. They can
only react according to what they imagine it would be like if they were in
your position. Opening a door from a wheelchair looks very difficult to
them. They don't know how easily you might be able to do it, so they assume
it is hard, and they try to help.

*In the first year after my injury, I was getting into a car,
assisted by the father of a friend who I had known since
before my injury. I opened the door, maneuvered my chair in
place, and lifted myself into the car—all easy for me, and
best done without any help. All I needed from him was to
fold the chair and stow it in the trunk. But during the transfer he kept trying to move me in the chair, lean over me to
open the door, and insert himself in the process. After I
fended him off a few times to do it myself, he finally sput-*

tered in frustration, "Why do you have to be so damned independent!"

No one needs help until they truly need it. Plain and simple.

Who Is in Control?

A helper who helps without asking—regardless of how well intentioned— or who doesn't take no for an answer is invading your independence and actually robbing you of control. Experienced wheelchair users know very well what they need and how it should be done. When someone imposes his will on you, it implies that you cannot decide for yourself. This is frustrating and insulting. For a wheelchair user, the experience can be an almost daily event. You will develop techniques for dealing with such encounters:

> *I notice where people are as I approach a door, and will vary my speed depending on whether or not I want them to hold the door for me. Often I will hang back and wait until they're through and I can just to do it myself. As time goes on, I'm finding it easier to let people open the door and just say thank you as I go through. Once in a while I have to ask them not to stand in the doorway as they hold the door, but then I can joke about running over their toes, and the tension is released.*

At those moments when it is necessary to essentially "fight" for control, it becomes necessary to explain.

> *"No thanks, it's good exercise," is the most reliable way I've found to decline someone's offer to me. It's the loss of control that bothers me the most. I tend to lose my temper if someone tries to push me without my permission, and that's another loss of control.*

> *I find myself using the "It's easier if you don't help, thank you" approach. At my car, that's actually true. People try to lift my wheelchair, which makes it harder to bring into the car. I try to let them know that their desire to "make it easier for me" is actually fulfilled by not helping!*

Being helped does not mean surrendering control, unless you let it. Whenever someone is helping you—whether grabbing an item from a shelf or performing an intimate, clinical task—the assistance should be done on your terms. Their actions are an extension of your own intent—the means of acting on your choices. That does not mean ordering them around. It means letting them know how they can best help you. It means knowing your own needs and being informed, especially about clinical tasks. It means you remain aware of what is happening and teach them how to help you properly, safely, and with dignity for you both. And it means respecting the good intentions of others while you educate them.

Being Pushed Around

Perhaps the most common offer of help to a manual wheelchair user is a push. To an able-bodied person, pushing a wheelchair looks like a lot of work. For them, it may be, but a person who is a manual chair user has gained enough strength and skill so that wheeling a chair is almost as natural as walking. If not, they should be using a power chair. Plus they have the benefit of ultralight, modern chairs, which are much easier to push and coast well. The offer to push is very charged:

> For a long time it was like an insult to me when people wanted to push me. I felt like they were saying, "You can't make it by yourself so I will help you." For me, I think it has to do with trying to be as independent as I can. To have someone push me was losing hard-fought-for independence.

> Once I was crossing some distance with a friend on a fairly level sidewalk. She—more than a little casually—offered to push saying, "Why waste so much effort?" It made me really think about what it was she didn't understand.

> Partly, it's about that difference in perception about how much work it is. She offered because she thought it took much more effort than it does. If she had to do it, it would be hard. It's not hard for me. Offering to push me is not much different—emotionally—from my offering to physically carry her ."Why waste the effort?" indeed.

Being pushed also changes the nature of the interaction between two people. Now, rather than walking abreast where you can see each other and enjoy eye contact during conversation, one person is behind the other in "helper-helped" mode.

If you are being pushed, your public appearance also is affected. Now, rather than being two friends strolling down the sidewalk, you can become self-conscious of being seen as someone getting—and therefore needing—help.

Irving Zola observed this problem of social interaction in his book *Missing Pieces*.[1] As a man who wore a brace and walked with a cane, he walked to the left of people so they wouldn't accidentally kick his cane. This meant he could not always obey the social convention of men walking on the outer street side.

Perhaps most important, the very act of wheeling yourself helps maintain your strength and stamina to be able to continue to do it—the "use it or lose it" principle. It can be a satisfying test of limits and a reassuring reminder that you have the strength to control your own mobility. You might be willing to work a bit harder to push up a gentle slope or even a movie theater aisle. However, there are times it makes sense to let someone push for a while when it is a long distance. This is a choice you will often face. You need to remember that your long-term health is your first priority.

Apart from perceptual, social, and health issues, there are issues of comfort and security. Handling a wheelchair involves more subtlety and skill than an inexperienced helper realizes. A skilled rider is constantly modulating the ride for all of the little bumps and changes along the way and is very aware of their toes—the front-most part of their body in space. A helper pushing the chair is not sensitive to this, so the ride is not as comfortable or secure. A bump in the pavement—and there are lots of them on any paved surface—can be very dangerous if someone is not paying close attention. A wheeler will simply give a little extra push to lift the front casters over a slight rise in surface. A helper who is pushing might wheel right into it, bringing matters to a sudden and surprising halt—possibly even throwing the "beneficiary" of the help out of the chair!

The people who spend the most time with you will develop a sense of when it is appropriate to help, if you take the time to discuss it and give accurate feedback when they offer help. If you accept when you don't need help, or resist help when it would be valued, they can never learn the appropriate boundary.

> My best friend has a great sense of when I prefer help with pushing—often one hand on a handle as he continues to walk next to me. It is clear enough that he doesn't have to ask. And he knows when to stop as well as to start.

Reacting to Offers of Help

You have three choices in how you react to people during the offer to help: passivity, aggression, and assertion. Your response determines the quality of the interaction.

When you are passive, you surrender your own point of view and priorities in favor of another person. Passively accepting what you don't want means that their feelings matter more than yours do. You violate your own rights, often because you are so concerned with that person's acceptance, that you err on the side of caution rather than risk upsetting them. Ironically, passivity is a form of disrespect for other people; it implies that they are unable to handle your disagreement or assertion. By being passive, you will not get what you need, and you will deny other people the opportunity to know you for your own views and feelings.

Aggression does not serve your purpose well either. It may feel like a way of standing up for your rights, but it denies others their rights in the process. Aggression is a way of overwhelming others, not of fostering cooperation and understanding. Aggressive behavior often means humiliating, degrading, or just plain overpowering other people. It will not make them want to be in contact with you, much less care about your views and needs.

The middle ground, being assertive, involves expressing your ideas and feelings honestly as well as being attuned to other people's feelings. Being assertive is a matter of mutual respect. It avoids both the body language of passivity—moving away from the person, nervous gestures, covering the face, a quiet voice—and the body language of aggression—finger pointing, a raised voice, and an intense stare. You speak plainly, making eye contact without challenge, and listen as much as you speak. Acting assertively is how you can develop comfortable relationships with people. You express and protect your personal rights, but at no one else's expense.

Public Attitude

A wheelchair user is necessarily conspicuous in public. People with disabilities are aware of being looked at and set apart as wheelchair users and are often self-conscious about their bodies. For this woman with Charcot-Marie Tooth (CMT) muscular dystrophy:

> *A big part of me wants to say "screw it" to others and what*
> *they see and think so I can wear whatever I want. A bigger*
> *part of me, though, is very affected by the way others see the*
> *outer me and hates negative scrutiny. I thought I'd be past*
> *that at thirty-three years, but I'm not. So, to keep me more*
> *comfortable inside, I wear my sandals, high tops, long skirts,*
> *dresses, and jeans, and only sunbathe in the privacy of my*
> *back yard. I really have no desire, anymore, to wear shorts or*
> *a swimsuit around others, so I will continue to keep my*
> *skinny bird legs hidden out of the sight of others, except*
> *myself, my husband, and our cats and dogs!*

You face all of the attitudes people have about disability whenever you go out in public. People hold doors for you, offer to carry your groceries, grab their children from your path, try to relate to you with stories of other people with disabilities they know, or speak to your companions on your behalf rather than directly to you. In daily life, these kinds of behaviors will inevitably occur, and, as a chair user, you need to develop your own style of dealing with them. As noted in the summary of the 1998 National Organization on Disability/Harris Survey of Americans with Disabilities:

> *Many people with disabilities continue to feel that the rest of the population treats them as if they are different and to have a strong sense of common identity with other people with disabilities. Fewer than half (45%) of adults with disabilities say that people generally treat them as an equal after they learn they have a disability.*[9]

There is work to do to get beyond the emotions these public contacts can bring up. You may not want others to see you as disabled—at least not in the negative image so many people associate with disability. You may want them to know you are really one of them and perhaps to know that you were once able bodied, too. You may be angered by the sometimes patronizing attitudes you encounter and by being suddenly treated as needy, unable, and tragic.

First Encountering Prejudices

There are many new feelings to confront in your early forays in public. What may seem overwhelming at first—potentially to the point of making you not want to go out—becomes familiar. You will learn how to let people have their beliefs and find you don't need to care how they see you. You can demonstrate through your attitude that they don't need to pity you—or make a hero of you. You will learn to check up on accessibility and become familiar with what entrances to use at common locations like movie theaters or shops. These coping tools will help you level your emotions so that your attention can return to the primary tasks of your life—work, play, family, community, love, and spirit.

Teen and early adult years can be very difficult for people with a disability acquired as a child. As children, they may have been very well supported by their families in how to face the attitudes that the wider culture feels about disability. Psychologist Carol Gill notes:

> *I think that a lot of us who were disabled early in life grew up thinking of ourselves as pretty okay and pretty normal. At*

some point in our lives we get disabused of that notion. Our
peers and others in society begin to treat us abnormally. When
we are school age, we don't get picked for the team, people
make fun of us. And it intensifies in the teen years when
dating begins.

Attitudes are Learned

The unfortunate truth is that there are many deeply embedded attitudes in
the culture about people with disabilities. People might be uncomfortable in
an initial encounter with you unless they already have direct experience
with a person with a disability. They'll be wondering if there's some special
way to treat you, or if they'll be expected to help in some way, or if they
might unintentionally say "the wrong thing." They might have an association with someone else, perhaps a parent or grandparent, who used a wheelchair at a time when they were very ill. They might be projecting themselves
into your experience, imagining it as a horrible way to live. These attitudes
can be obstacles in making a satisfying connection with that person. Once
people come to know you well, and witness the kind of life that is possible,
they find out that your personality shines through even the most significant
disability.

Beliefs about disability are planted very early in life. It's evident from
the experience of any chair rider in any shopping mall in America. As you
wheel through the crowd, parents frantically pull their children out of your
path. Of course, parents naturally want to protect their child from a collision
and are likely trying to be considerate so you don't have to maneuver around
the child. But the message the child gets is that something is not OK with a
person using a wheelchair.

Another scenario is more telling. Many children will innocently come
up to you and ask why you are in a wheelchair. They don't yet know that it
is "rude" to ask. The child's interest makes the parent very uncomfortable,
and that gets communicated. Irving Zola wrote:

> The wheelchair is quite visible and of great interest to the
> child, but he or she is taught to ignore it. A near universal
> complaint is, "Why can't people see me as someone who has a
> handicap rather than someone who is handicapped?" Young
> children first perceive it that way but are quickly socialized
> out of it.[1]

Children are not mature enough to understand these boundaries, and
there is a danger of communicating through your actions that people with
disabilities are unapproachable. You can be in the delicate position of want-

ing to demonstrate that disability is a feature of many people's lives and does not preclude a full life, while at the same time being entitled to your privacy and dignity.

> *A child can't distinguish whether I'm in a bad mood, so I am*
> *never bothered by a child's questions. I have a "spinal cord is*
> *like a telephone system" story that I use. An adult needs to*
> *use some judgment, but most of the time I am happy to have*
> *an adult approach me in public and ask why I wheel. I'm*
> *glad to explain it, but I also try to give a picture of my life as*
> *a whole.*

Sometimes parents will give the child their own answers:

> *I cannot count the times I have been in public and have heard*
> *a parent telling their children ridiculous things to explain why*
> *I am in a wheelchair. Things like "Her legs are tired," "She is*
> *taking a break from walking," or "She's resting by sitting*
> *down." I always would rather have the parents have their*
> *kids approach me in these situations with their questions so I*
> *could tell them the truth.*

How you respond to being asked about your disability is a personal matter. In a given instance, you just might not be in the mood! You will have to find your own balance. You can decline politely, by saying that it is a private matter and that you reserve discussions about such things to people you know better. The more someone gets to know you, the more appropriate it becomes to ask such questions. As Carol Gill says, "If you have an intimate relationship, you're allowed to ask more intimate questions." Just as often, people will delay or avoid asking about your disability.

> *In a company where I worked for eight years, there were*
> *people who never knew why I wheeled. They never had*
> *the courage to ask. Many, I expect, assumed I was disabled*
> *since birth, or had been in the Vietnam War, neither of*
> *which is true.*

Attorney Deborah Kaplan is quadriplegic but is able to stand, has full sensation, and is a mother. She also has more than 25 years of disability activism behind her. She says:

> *By and large, it isn't so much a stereotype as the fact that we*
> *just really scare people. People don't want to have to think*
> *about disability. It's very personal. It's very deep rooted, I*
> *think almost cellular. We remind people that we exist in a soft,*
> *vulnerable body and that they're vulnerable. People don't like*

*to be reminded of that. That shows up when somebody looks
at my resume and they go, "Oh!" What are they so surprised
about? I've been on every commission in the world and I
travel all the time. They're telling me something about what
their expectations are.*

The more significant or visible the disability, the larger the attitudinal
obstacle you're likely to encounter. Notes Carol Gill:

*If there is going to be a person with a disability who is
accepted by society first, it's going to be the young white male
who is okay from the chest up. But that's not the majority of
the disabled population.*

*I really feel I have made a contribution. Not only to the dis-
ability community, but to society and to my neighbors and
everybody else. The work that I do. My son that I raised.
I am a valuable person, but I think that the average person
who sees me would think my life is not tenable. I use a ventilator, I need help with all activities of daily living, and I
feel that if I hit a significant medical crisis I am much less
likely to receive aggressive measures to protect my life than
someone else.*

Professor Zola granted the value of his family and support system in
adapting to polio and subsequent auto accident injuries, while at the same
time condemning societal attitudes:

*Had my family been poorer, less assertive, my friends fewer
and less caring, my champions less willing to fight the system, then all my personal strengths would have been for
naught. On the other hand, if we lived in a less healthist,
capitalist, and hierarchical society which spent less time
finding ways to exclude and disenfranchise people and more
time finding ways to include and enhance the potentialities
of everyone, then there wouldn't have been so much for me
to overcome.*[1]

But appearances are not the only thing that counts. Says psychologist Gill:

*A lot of the people we do hit it off with people in the nondis-
abled community tend to be people who are more open.
Sometimes they have what I would consider deeper values
and are people who would critique the same superficial*

*American values that our community does. It gives us a
common bond.*

Perhaps your interactions with able-bodied people are a chance for
them to learn from the experience. Perhaps, as they encounter the truth of
a person living with a disability, they can adjust their beliefs after seeing the
evidence of an active person living fully with their disability.

> *I've heard from many people who say that, after getting to
> know me, their fears about people with disabilities subsided,
> that it was a chance to overcome their misconceptions. I find
> that satisfying.*

You can also hope that children will grow up knowing better because
they are increasingly living in a world where people with disabilities are visible, active, and part of their lives in meaningful ways—including children
with disabilities who are increasingly mainstreamed in the public schools
and our communities.

Disability Pride

You have an important contribution to make to this society. You are in a
position to teach that focusing exclusively on narrow standards of physical
beauty, youth, and conventional athleticism is a problem for all of us. By
continuing to demonstrate that you are not looking to be cared for, but to
be treated as a whole, self-determining person with the right to make your
own decisions and have a full life, society gets the chance to develop values
that respect everyone.

> *My own philosophy is that there is one thing you show the
> outside world: pride. On the other hand, living with limita-
> tions is sort of a drag. That's the reality. But you don't go
> shouting that to everyone in the world.*

Carol Gill expresses her view:

> *I think our Western world in many ways is in a moral crisis.
> Some of the values of the disability world can really help the
> greater world in sorting out this moral dilemma—to look at
> what's important and develop a whole new slate around what
> it means to be human. I think we have an important lesson to
> teach the world because we have to deal with our own acid
> test of what's human. I'm an idealist, too. I'm hoping we will
> win out and be heard.*

References

1. Zola IK. *Missing Pieces: a Chronicle of Living with a Disability*. Philadelphia: Temple University Press; 1982.
2. Morris J. Spinal injury and psychotherapy. In: Yarkony GM, ed. *Spinal Cord Injury: Medical Management and Rehabilitation*. Bethesda: Aspen;1994:223-29.
3. Gregory MF. *Sexual Adjustment: a Guide for Spinal Cord Injured*. Bloomington, IL: Cheever Publishing; 1974.
4. Yapko MD. *Breaking the Patterns of Depression*. New York: Broadway Books; 1997.
5. Shapiro JP. *No Pity: People with Disabilities Forging a New Civil Rights Movement*. New York: Times Books/Random House; 1994.
6. Chödrön P. *When Things Fall Apart: Heart Advice for Difficult Times*. Boston/London: Shambhala; 1997:13.
7. Price R. *A Whole New Life: an Illness and Healing*. New York: Scribner; 2003:55.
8. Anderson J. Psychological issues related to ventilator-dependent quadriplegia. In: Whiteneck G, Lammertse DP, Manley S, Menter R. *The Management of High Quadriplegia*. New York: Demos Publications; 1989:107.
9. Risher P, Amorosi S. *The 1998 N.O.D./Harris Survey of Americans with Disabilities*. New York: Louis Harris & Associates, Inc; 1998.

Chapter 4

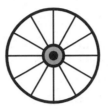

Wheelchair Selection

Selecting the optimal wheelchair is a crucially important process for you. All of the choices you have to make can feel overwhelming if you are choosing your wheels for the first time. You might anticipate that you will recover from your injury or illness, so you wonder why you should even bother to get a wheelchair at all. But the right wheelchair is a liberator, not a prison. When you configure the right chair for you and your abilities, your quality of life increases dramatically. Even people with significant disabilities can have a considerable degree of independence and activity with the right chair—more, in fact, than ever before in history. That's small consolation when you're facing a recent loss of mobility, but perhaps you can appreciate how much more limited you would have been not so long ago, but for the dramatic advances in wheelchair design described in this chapter.

Wheelchair design has advanced tremendously. No longer limited to the aluminum folding chairs you might be accustomed to seeing in hospitals or airports, there is now an immense array of designs and options for both manual and power wheelchairs. Wheelchairs are highly adjustable—or even custom built—available in various sizes, with features that make them easier to drive, safer, and more dignified—even stylish.

Modern chairs are also better-looking; even power chairs have become less bulky and obtrusive and institutional-looking. The visual emphasis on disability has been reduced, bringing more attention to the user of the chair instead of the chair itself.

This chapter discusses the issues involved in selecting a wheelchair, including funding, researching products from various manufacturers, working with professionals who will advise you, the many features and options of manual and power wheelchairs, and criteria to help you navigate the sometimes complex web of choices you will face.

Your Role

The optimal approach to selecting a wheelchair is to work as a team with a therapist (typically an occupational or physical therapist) who specializes in "seating and positioning," and a local dealer who will actually provide the chair along with support services, such as adjusting it properly on delivery. But no matter how skilled and knowledgeable your therapist and salesperson are, you are the leading expert on you. You are the one whose life depends on having the right wheelchair, so it is very, very much in your best interest to take an active role in its selection. Learn as much as you can, and be patient with the process before making the final choice.

Do Some Research

Other chair users you have encountered—possibly from your rehab experience, support groups, participation in athletics, or your local center for independent living—are valuable sources of information about wheelchairs. But keep in mind that experienced chair users tend to be very opinionated and vocal about their choices. You can learn much from what others say, but what works best for them might not work for you. Each person's physical capacities, body type, and lifestyle are completely unique as a set, so your wheelchair must be unique to who you are and how you intend to live.

> My experience with purchasing the best chair for me came
> primarily from my own research, which included talking with
> other wheelchair users. I got a couple of names from the
> retailer, but the best information I got was from the Internet.

Learn as much as possible about chairs and what is currently available on the market. You can request product information for the chair models that are potential solutions for you, which will also be available as a downloadable document from the company website. You should also request or download the order form, which lists the full array of options available for a given chair model.

Check the track record of the chairs you are considering. Although major flaws are uncommon, there could be defects in the manufacture of some chairs, as with any consumer product. The US Food and Drug Administration keeps track of voluntary recalls by wheelchair manufacturers, though not all manufacturers are entirely open about such problems. You can contact the Food and Drug Administration for this information. Newer manufacturers should not be suspect just because they are less experienced, but there is always some risk of unforeseen problems that simply may not have appeared yet. Seek out users of a given product and speak with them about its performance and quality before making your final choice.

Be Prepared for Your Consultation

The therapist and wheelchair dealer will need to know many things about where you live and work. The therapist might visit your home and your workplace to gather information, but you will want to take an active part in making sure your chair will optimize—not limit—your mobility and comfort at home and work. Do your own survey of your home and workplace, and then arrive at your therapist appointment or the wheelchair store equipped with answers to questions such as these:

■ How wide are your doors—main entry, kitchen, bedrooms, bathrooms, etc.?

■ Are there tight angles to negotiate, such as a hallway that turns sharply at the bedroom door?

■ How large is the bathroom? Will it be possible to wheel your chair alongside the bathtub or must you face it directly? Is the door smaller than the others in your house? How much space is available for the chair so that you can close the door once inside?

■ What is the knee clearance of tables and desks?

■ How high are cabinets and shelves that you might need to reach?

■ Is the terrain around your home paved? If not, what kind of surface is it? Is it level?

■ On what types of surfaces will you do most of your wheeling? Carpet, tile, concrete, packed soil?

You must also consider the vehicles you in which you will ride:

■ If you drive, do you have a car or a van? Two or four doors?

■ What is the size of the trunk in the family car, or the cars of friends you go out with?

■ What kind of public transportation might you use?

Failure to consider any one of these points can mean having to live with a constant irritant or insurmountable obstacle and facing the stress of unnecessary restriction of your mobility every day—just because you got the wrong chair. You might even be risking your safety if, for instance, you are forced to make a long transfer to the bath or shower because you chose those fixed footrests, which prevent you from getting close enough.

> *Although my rehab folks were wonderful, my first two chairs did not suit my lifestyle. There were places I might have been able to go, people I might have been able to see, and events I could have participated in if I had had the right chair from the beginning.*

Getting the right chair can also save you from having to make potentially expensive home modifications.

> *It was many years before we could make my home wheelchair accessible. If I had known that there were power wheelchairs out there that could raise a seated person 6 to 8 inches or that had a turning radius of 19.5 inches, my life would have been so much more comfortable. And it wouldn't have cost quite so much for the home modifications that we eventually did.*

You will also want to share critical information about your lifestyle and the kinds of activities you plan to participate in. If you like to be on the go—visiting friends, attending entertainment and sporting events, taking classes—or travel for either pleasure or business, you might need a different chair than if you prefer a more quiet life at home most of the time. Along with the previous lists, make one that includes:

- Hobbies and activities for which your chair will be a consideration
- Relevant information about any "homes away from home." If you like to hang out at your best friend's place, you want to make sure you can get around independently there, too.
- The importance of the appearance of your chair to you. Do you see yourself in something sporty? Eye-catching? Or do you prefer to be as inconspicuous as possible?
- Your usual level of physical activity, including exercise

One rider describes his experience with the selection process:

> *I spent two days with a team in making my decision. The team included a physical therapist and an occupational therapist. The physical therapist spent time assessing my strengths and weaknesses. We then decided on seating requirements before addressing the actual chair selection. We spent a lot of*

time discussing my lifestyle and exactly how and where the chair was to be used.

Once the medical needs were identified and physical measurements were taken, the last thing was to determine the exact model of chair. We were able to narrow it down to five, which I was able to try out for a few hours each. The trial included maneuvering in a simulation of the work area I use and then spending an hour or so outside on a variety of terrain. We also tried them in my van to see how they fit and the method of transfer I would need to use to get in the driver's seat.

Keep an Open Mind

Despite the variety of wheelchairs on the market and the many options available, you may not be able to find every feature and detail you would ideally like in one chair. As with other purchases, such as a car or home, some compromises and tradeoffs are usually necessary. As you work your way through the selection process, try to think about the big picture and how you will use your chair over time. Establish priorities, learn from the experience of others, and value the advice of experts, but place the highest priority on getting what will best meet your needs for mobility, safety, and comfort.

For example, it is common for people to be drawn to the appearance of a chair, but it is dangerous to be overly influenced by the look of a chair, to the possible exclusion of other, more important, functional characteristics. That really cool-looking rigid frame chair might not fit into the trunk of your family car. Doe Cayting of Wheelchairs of Berkeley, California, has seen people become too attached to the appearance of the chair, in lieu of other features more important to their mobility:

You have to think about whether aesthetics is the most important thing for you, because the right chair is always a question of compromise. There isn't an exact right or wrong. But if you want something that looks a certain way, and I know it is not appropriate, it is my responsibility as a supplier to say no.

Fortunately, there are lots of good-looking chairs that fit many needs. Compared to the institutional-style chair that everyone had to use until the 1980s, whatever you choose will be better looking and more to your liking than in "the old days."

The Selection Process

Not only can choosing a wheelchair be difficult emotionally, it can be confusing and exasperating. The professionals who are advising you will talk with you about many issues and options. They will ask you a lot of questions. They may give you catalogs for a variety of chairs that have all kinds of features to choose from. It will likely seem overwhelming. You might find yourself thinking, "Just sell me a wheelchair!" This is a process that takes time, and it is extremely important not to rush it. Too many people have discovered just how huge a mistake that is.

The best advice is to relax and take heart. First of all, your therapist, the supplier, and the facts of your condition and lifestyle will very quickly narrow the choices down to a much more manageable number. If you have taken time to learn about various products, have a good picture of your needs, and have studied the information in this chapter, the entire process will be much less stressful and much more successful. Find the right people to work with, and they will help you identify the chair that will provide you the highest possible quality of life you choose to pursue in the context of your disability.

Who Will Help You Choose Your Chair?

The prescription for your chair will be written by a physician. Ideally she will be a rehabilitation specialist (physiatrist) and refer you to an occupational or physical therapist who will help ensure that you get the right chair. Your lead physician is unlikely to have detailed knowledge about wheelchair specifics but will establish the broad category of what you need and then rely on a specialist to get down to the details in the collaborative process described above. Jody Greenhalgh, OTR, is an occupational therapist with UCSF/Stanford Rehabilitation Services in Stanford, California. She finds that some people end up with the wrong chair because they relied on their primary physician to specify it, and then find themselves in trouble:

> *The primary physician writes a simplistic prescription, and the insurer pays for inadequate equipment. Once that happens, it is very difficult to convince an insurer to pay for a more appropriate wheelchair system.*

A therapist's knowledge of anatomy and biodynamics is inestimably valuable. Your therapist will study your exact disability and do muscle and range testing. He will determine whether you have the physical ability to push a manual chair or whether you should drive a power chair. He will identify how to establish a stable posture that will allow you access to your optimal strength as you push, or study your ability to operate the various types of power chair controls. He will test your eye-hand coordination and cognitive skills. He will measure your weight and height, your knee-to-footrest distance, seat depth, back height, and all of the other specific dimensions needed to configure your highly customized set of wheels.

Your therapist will likely know the best wheelchair dealers to work with, but, if you have to find one on your own, the time you spend locating one with knowledge and experience will be well worth it. You will not be purchasing your chair from a general medical supply store, one that sells all sorts of medical equipment. Such a business will not have the kind of expertise you need or be established dealers of the kind of high-end equipment you need as a full-time user. You will want to find a dealer who specializes in "prescription" wheelchairs.

A knowledgeable salesperson of durable medical equipment can make a tremendous difference in ensuring that you get the right wheels. You'll want someone who has a lot of experience seeing many people with different needs and who has specialized in rehab equipment. A competent salesperson often has absorbed more insight from other users about what worked and what didn't than the therapist has.

Bob Hall is the former head of New Halls Wheels, a custom chair maker no longer in business, and himself a chair rider. He cautions against relying on a dealer who may not be as knowledgeable as one would hope:

> Wheelchair dimensions are often over-prescribed because of lack of knowledge of the dealer. Back heights, in particular, are often too tall and limit movement in the chair. Chairs are often too wide. You can say that you need to make room inside the chair for your winter coat, but if you can't get through the door it isn't doing you much good. The product actually ends up being more disabling, whereas the right chair can raise your self-esteem.

If possible, find a salesperson who has experience with insurance and funding. He can help you strike the sometimes delicate balance between the ideal chair you want—but for which the insurer simply won't pay—and identifying appropriate equipment that will be approved.

You may not always have a choice about the dealer with whom you will work. Your funding source might require that you use a particular supplier with whom they have a contract, and such a supplier might not be well informed about the most appropriate product for you. If you believe you need additional consultation in order to get the best chair, assert yourself with your insurance carrier or agency so that you can work with a local source that is best qualified to consult with you. Once the chair is delivered, it might fall to the therapist to adjust the chair and teach you about its operation and maintenance.

You should be given the chance to try out a close configuration of the chair you will eventually purchase. The supplier should have chairs on hand that can be adjusted fairly closely to your needs and may even allow you to take one out and live with it for a few days. Some manufacturers will actually ship a chair to the supplier specifically for you to evaluate. Larger rehabilitation hospitals have a substantial supply of chairs and accessories to fit you into something quite close to what you will purchase. Some of them are even in the wheelchair sales business—out of necessity for lack of a competent dealer in their vicinity.

Funding Your Chair

Wheelchairs are expensive. A lightweight, modern manual wheelchair can cost as much as $2,000 or more. A fully equipped power chair can reach prices in the range of $30,000, though they generally will cost closer to $10,000.

Because you need the best chair and it costs a lot, you have little choice but to rely on outside payers. Your chair might be paid for by a small or large insurance company, under a Workers' Compensation plan, a health maintenance organization or planned provider organization, a state Vocational Rehabilitation agency, the federal Veterans Administration, or a government plan like Medicare or Medicaid.

Whether private or public, funders are all highly budget conscious and are generally trying to limit their costs. In the current political environment of attempting to control healthcare costs, it is becoming increasingly difficult to get approval for your ideal wheels, though this depends on exactly who is paying. Since the funders have a built-in conflict of interest between your health and independence—which they might sincerely care about—and managing their dollars (and profits) carefully, you will need to be your own best advocate.

Advocate for Yourself

Be serious about advocating for yourself when configuring and purchasing your wheelchair. Read your policies and contracts. Don't be afraid to ask questions or to make phone calls to find out what you need to know. Insurance companies and government agencies are bound under certain laws to give you information.

Don't assume your insurance policy won't cover something you need or even that a refusal of coverage is the final word. It's always worth the effort to check your policy or discuss the situation with your insurance contact person. Generally, justifiable medical need must be established, even for a given feature or option on the chair.

You might even have coverage that you're not aware of, as this long-time wheeler discovered:

> *I spent more years in my heavy E & J hospital-style wheel-chair than I needed to, as it turned out. I was assuming, mis-takenly, that my private insurance through my job would not pay for a new wheelchair. Even though people were telling me that I should get out of my old "tank" in favor of a new lightweight chair, I never did the research. I figured when the day arrived to replace my old wheels, I would have to pay for it myself.*

> *Finally I made the call and discovered that my policy did indeed cover the cost of a wheelchair at least once in the life of the policy. They would pay 80 percent, and I could easily handle the difference.*

There is no reason you can't question a policy that you consider inappropriate or unfair. The worst your funder can do is say no. But if you can make a good case, you just might be able to convince an insurer to reconsider. Dr. Michael Boninger, of the Human Engineering Research Laboratory at the University of Pittsburgh, specifies chairs for people. He advises: "If your policy only allows you a $200 wheelchair, then challenge it. If you fight hard enough, you might get the insurer to make an exception."

Funding agencies and organizations generally do not think proactively. They tend to resist paying for something now, even if it will prevent problems—and save money—later. For example, an insurer might not want to pay for a contoured back to help control the trunk of a rider's body. Contoured backs can reach prices of up to $800, but, for some people, their use can prevent the need for more expensive equipment or corrective surgery later on.

Stanford University occupational therapist Jody Greenhalgh is closely involved in specifying wheelchairs for people. More than once, she has encountered someone with pressure-sore problems who has had expensive surgery. She finds that these problems could have been avoided if a better wheelchair and positioning system had been configured in the first place, as in this worst-case example.

> *We see patients who have severe skin ulcers. They've been on bed rest for months. A specialized wheelchair is medically recommended but denied by the insurer. The patient then requires a $50,000 surgery, after which he returns to the inadequate wheelchair. This causes the surgery to fail and pressure sores recur. The patient has to go back on long-term bedrest and repeat hospitalization.*

The insurance companies seem to be shortsighted, preferring to spend money on surgical intervention rather than paying for the right cushion and specialized wheelchair—which would ultimately save dollars and help the patient return to a productive and independent life. Because the insurer who pays for the wheelchair is likely to not have to pay for future surgeries or extended nursing home stays (since you are likely to move to another company or a government program like Medicare), they are not as motivated to be proactive in this way.

You might need to enlist the help of your physician, occupational or physical therapist, or other medical professional. The initial wheelchair prescription typically includes a "certificate of medical necessity," which is signed by the physician. If your funder denies the chair specified on your prescription, ask for help from your medical team. Your doctor or therapist can write to your funder, explaining in detail why that particular chair is medically necessary for you. Greenhalgh is an experienced advocate:

> *I will write a lengthier justification if a wheelchair prescription is denied. Sometimes I pull up old cases to use as examples and say, "Look, we saved money by doing this." If I persevere, it really does pay off, but the process can extend for months. It means I have to spend a lot of time on the phone and doing paperwork rather than treating patients.*

It is increasingly common for insurance companies and funding agencies to assign your file to a case manager. The case manager should be your advocate, putting your medical interests first above all. He may or may not be a nurse or otherwise medically experienced. Your case manager will talk with doctors and therapists, confirm the policies and limits of your coverage, shop for the best prices (which is part of what makes case managers appealing to the insurer), and even contact social workers to seek out additional sources of funding or equipment if the policy does not cover you.

Sometimes case managers are on staff, or the insurer might have a contract with an outside provider of these services. If there is not a case manager assigned to you, ask for one. You do not have a legal right to a case manager, but it's likely your request will be granted, especially if you are pleasantly persistent. If possible, try to get a case manager with specific background in rehabilitation equipment and your specific disability.

Following are additional suggestions for how to overcome a denial of funding:

■ Submit an official appeal. Your funding contact person should be able to provide you with the appropriate procedure.

■ If coverage is employer provided, enlist the help of your employer's benefits department.

■ Write to the state insurance commissioner.

■ Contact an appropriate advocacy group.

■ Appeal to your congressional representatives.

■ Take your case public. Local television or newspaper reporters might be interested in reporting about a funder who is denying coverage for clearly needed equipment. Funders don't like negative publicity, so they might be persuaded to do the right thing. Even if you still don't get funding, the report could flush out other forms of help, such as a generous donor or someone with a used chair that meets your needs.

Another way you can help yourself is to research a wide variety of manufacturers. For instance, smaller producers are very aware of the need to increase business by making their products a more attractive option to funding sources, so they try to offer good solutions at lower costs. If you can find a less-expensive solution to your needs by doing this kind of research, it might reduce complications in dealing with your funding source and make it easier for you to get approval.

If you are unable to deal with funding problems, perhaps a family member, friend, case manager, or social worker would be willing to invest the effort to overcome resistance you might encounter from payers. Many local centers for independent living offer advice or active assistance with funding issues.

Alternative Funding

If your funding source is refusing to pay for a particular chair or feature, you must decide how long you will fight the good fight. At some point it might make sense to take what they give you and enhance it on your own. The following are some possible sources of funding or finding a chair if you have to "do-it-yourself":

- ■ Your church or other community group might be able to contribute to a purchase or stage a fundraiser on your behalf.
- ■ Many local agencies provide used wheelchairs for people who are not getting proper funding support.
- ■ Your local center for independent living might have surplus chairs or parts or may know of someone looking to donate a chair or sell a used one.
- ■ Some major banks offer special loan programs. For example, San Francisco-based Bank of America offers a longer-term loan with no down payment required if you use the money for medical equipment. Check with major banks in your area.

In every case, you must get proper guidance in identifying what is appropriate for you, including proper cushioning, and have the chair adjusted to your needs.

Manufacturers

Large Versus Small Manufacturers

Wheelchair manufacturers come in many varieties. There are large, corporate companies, small specialized producers, and innovative new companies with a more specialized focus—such as a power wheelchair built for outdoor terrain. You will want to find out what these various companies offer in the process of finding the optimal chair for you. Your therapist and dealer will have a lot of information about the major producers, and, hopefully, between the two of them, they will also have a well-rounded knowledge of smaller producers. No one can know it all, however, so it is in your best interest to do some investigating on your own.

The prescription wheelchair business is a difficult one, so your dealer simply cannot represent all makers. Dealers generally will represent the products that they feel offer the best pricing, the widest array of products and options, and, of course, that provide them with the profit margins that allow them to stay in business and provide you with good service. This means they operate on a fine line of conflict of interest, against the impulse to sell you the chair that produces the revenue their business requires, rather than the best solution from the overall market for your needs. Rather than this being a formula for mistrust, it is simply another reason why you want to be as well informed as possible so you can make the most of your working relationship with the dealer.

Advantages and Disadvantages of Major Manufacturers

Large manufacturers employ more people and operate on bigger budgets. Greater resources mean major wheelchair manufacturers can invest more in research and development than can their smaller competitors. They can afford to build many prototypes and can take a little longer to develop new designs, since these large firms have a steadier stream of revenue from existing products. Following are additional advantages offered by large wheelchair manufacturers:

- They have comprehensive lines of wheelchair products.
- They can offer many options and accessories.
- They can afford to spend time and money on aesthetics.
- They have been in the business long enough to have a lot of experience behind them.
- They will have refined their manufacturing and design over those years and will probably be around for the foreseeable future.
- They are reputable and generally make good chairs, assuming you select the right model, properly configured.
- Your dealer will have greater familiarity with the companies' products and more experience maintaining and repairing chairs from larger manufacturers.

Here are some disadvantages of large wheelchair manufacturers:

- Unless they are highly committed to continual design and development, they might not be offering the most innovative products because it is easy for them to rest on their current share of the market.
- They have less motivation to lower pricing, especially for parts and accessories.
- They provide less personal service.

Find Out What Small Manufacturers Offer

There are dozens of small companies out there making wheelchairs. Since they don't have the marketing budgets of the big firms, it's harder for them to get exposure, so you might not hear about them. However, if you decide a small producer's chair is the right one for you, your dealer should be perfectly willing to call the manufacturer and ask them to sell you one.

- They are generally passionate about their work, concerned with quality, and interested in helping people.

- You are likely to get more personal attention.
- You might find a chair that more specifically meets your needs, even one that can be more aggressively customized for you.
- Since smaller producers don't have huge production schedules, they may be able to deliver your chair faster than can a large company.
- You might be able to find a better price.

Some wheelchairs designed by the smaller companies can look like they were designed by an engineer, whose concerns are more focused on the operation of the chair and the ease of manufacturing it and whose training does not include aesthetics. This is not universally true of small producers, but it is more the rule than the exception. There are, in fact, companies that make image a very high priority, such as Colours. Lasher Sport makes highly artful, beautiful (and extremely expensive), customized chairs.

Ordering Your Chair

The period from your initial consultation to the actual ordering of your chair can take as long as two to three months. This includes taking time to try out one or more models. A more complex chair may take longer. If you encounter resistance from your insurer, that could also add time to the process.

Once you have decided on the model of chair that is best for you, the dealer—using information from you and your therapist—will fill out a specification sheet with the exact details for every aspect of your chair. Ask to see a copy of this list. If you have questions or concerns about anything, ask. Make sure the list is complete and correct, checking for something inadvertently omitted (such as clothing guards) or wrong (such as color). Even if the problem can be fixed, you'll probably have to pay for it. Your therapist will sign off on this list, and it will then go to your physician, who will write a prescription for it.

The prescription and specification list will be sent to your insurance company or funding agency for approval. Once your chair is approved, the dealer will order your chair from the manufacturer. If your chair is not covered by insurance and you are paying for it yourself, a down payment of 50% at the time the order is placed is typical. Your dealer should give you an accurate delivery date so you can plan accordingly.

Have Your New Chair Properly Adjusted

One of the most dramatic changes that occurred in wheelchair design in the early 1980s is that they became far more adjustable. This has allowed people to fine tune their relationship to the seat and the wheels through actual experience, optimizing their comfort and stability and, for manual chair riders, to exert their strength as efficiently as possible.

With this adjustability comes the other side of the coin: a maladjusted chair is going to be even more uncomfortable and difficult to use. So the real trick in ordering your chair is to ensure that, for the features that are adjustable, there is a sufficient range of dimensions that will meet your needs once you fine tune it from experience.

Adjustability is generally more valuable for first-time chair users. Experienced riders come to know what dimensions meet their needs, so they can graduate to a more customized frame with fixed dimensions for such features as seat height or axle position. That also means fewer moving parts, less maintenance risk, and lighter weight. Ironically, the advent of adjustability in the wheelchair industry led to a next generation of product that is increasingly customized and built to fit.

When your chair arrives at the dealer from the factory, you will need to have the store adjust it specifically to your needs. Plan on taking the time to have them fine tune it for you, and don't hesitate to ask them to continue to make changes until it is right. Dr. Boninger, of the University of Pittsburgh, finds that factory settings are not particularly optimal overall. For example, he makes this observation about manual chairs:

> The factory tends to put the wheels far back for stability, but this can force excessive range of motion as you reach back and limit the amount of stroke you can make on the wheel.

Axle position is only one of the many details of chair configuration that have a significant impact on the efficient, comfortable, and safe use of your chair. Remember that a wheelchair is really a complex web of interrelationships. Changing the axle position or caster height affects seat and back angles and the relationship of your arms to the wheels. Placement of a joystick affects overall posture. And so on. With wheelchairs being more adjustable than were early models, this process cannot be overlooked.

Some riders learn—by observing and asking questions of a qualified technician—how to expertly adjust their own chairs, but you should not attempt to adjust your chair until you are confident in your knowledge. Be certain that you understand in principle what you're trying to achieve and have the right tools to protect the chair from scratches or stripping the heads of screws or bolts. It is generally best to make small adjustments and to affect only one thing at a time so you can judge its impact independently from other changes you might make. More than one wheelchair salesperson can tell a story of a customer who called complaining that his chair was wrong or damaged, only to discover that he had made inappropriate adjustments or used the wrong tools.

The Basic Choice: Manual or Power

The first decision to be made when choosing your wheelchair is whether it will be a manual or power chair. Often this decision is obvious or becomes clear after your therapist tests your strength, balance, dexterity, and other abilities. In some cases, though, the choice is not so simple, and, in fact, having one of each type of chair could prove to be the optimal solution.

Two chairs are actually a good idea for everyone—manual and power chair riders alike will want to have a backup manual chair for use in case their main chair is out of commission for a few days. A backup chair doesn't have to be as complete or as customized as one you purchase for daily use. If you aren't able to get your own backup chair, find out if your dealer has loaners available for those times when your chair needs servicing.

Advantages of Manual Wheelchairs

Manual chairs have a number of advantages over power chairs, and most people prefer to use a manual chair if at all possible. Consider the following list of "pros," but also be honest with yourself about your strength and energy—you'll need plenty of both to operate a manual chair, especially if you plan on an active lifestyle:

- Manual chairs are lightweight and getting lighter all the time thanks to modern composite materials, the use of titanium, etc. Lightweight chairs require less strength and energy to push.
- Manual chairs have unlimited range, not being limited by the charge capacity of a battery.
- Manual chairs cost less to purchase than power chairs. Maintenance costs are also lower, thanks to fewer working parts and freedom from having to replace depleted batteries.
- Manual chairs are more discreet than power chairs, being less bulky and, with no motor noise, quieter—assuming the manual chair is well maintained.
- Manual chairs are easier to maneuver for slight rotations or small movements.
- Manual chairs travel more easily than power chairs, whether on an airplane or stowed in the backseat or trunk of a car. Depending on options, a manual chair can be stored more easily when broken down

to its component parts. Swingaway footrests can be removed, as can the wheels by means of the now-common quick-release axles.

■ Manual chairs can extend mobility. For those with the strength and agility to master the art of the "wheelie," many curbs and single steps no longer represent an obstacle in a manual chair, as you can safely "jump" a curb or step either going up or down.

Advantages of Power Wheelchairs

A power chair actually extends your mobility, compared with a manual chair, in many ways. Some riders are also finding that they do better in a power chair as they age. Chronic shoulder pain from overuse or weakness from an illness might make it necessary. Here are some of the reasons you might opt for a power chair:

■ A power chair conserves your energy, allowing you to go whatever distance necessary without exhausting yourself, for work or pleasure activities.

■ A power chair allows you to handle uphill slopes that would be an unnecessary overexertion or perhaps beyond your ability to climb with a manual chair.

■ A power chair frees you from the need for assistance when going a considerable distance or on a steep surface.

■ A power chair leaves one arm free to stabilize an object you might carry in your lap—such as a bag of groceries or books—while operating a joystick control.

■ A power chair can include powered tilt or recline features, which aid in pressure-sore prevention, respiration, and comfort for quadriplegic riders.

Weigh Your Options

Choosing a power chair can be a tough decision. Despite the advantages listed above, there are mobility restrictions that come along with use of a power chair. They are limited by battery life, are too heavy to be carried up a stairway, and don't jump curbs easily, if at all. They make more noise and are less able to make fine maneuvers. Pushing a manual chair keeps the upper body in shape, to a degree, so using a power chair can be an invitation to losing strength.

Some people resist choosing a power chair because it makes them feel "too disabled." But it's important to ask yourself how much of your daily energy you are willing to invest in pushing a manual chair. If you have marginal upper body strength, you can exhaust yourself just getting where you're going. Perhaps you are attending a college that is on a sloping site or live in a hilly town. Consider whether you prefer to trade having more energy in the day against your public image as a power chair rider. Lack of energy from pushing a manual chair around might even make a difference in your ability to hold a job.

Finally, think about how the effort needed to operate a manual chair will affect your health in the long run. Many manual chair riders with 20 or so years of pushing behind them find that their shoulders begin to give out. You are better off using a manual chair if you can, but not at the expense of your long-term health.

Heavy-Duty Outdoor Power Chairs

A special category of power wheelchairs is the outdoor chair. They have stronger motors, bigger batteries, independent suspension for rough terrain, and wider tires all around with deeper tread for traction. Teftec was the first company to develop an outdoor chair, after 14-year-old Jimmy Finch had his neck broken in an auto accident, hit by a drunk driver. It was a high-level injury, allowing Jimmy no use of his hands or arms.

Teftec was born when, after attending a variety of expo shows and wheelchair workshops, Jim and his father took up the challenge of designing an outdoor power wheelchair that could be driven by someone independently who had high quadriplegia. The result was the OmegaTrac® front-wheel drive, heavy-duty wheelchair, first introduced at the MedTrade medical products show in 1995 in Atlanta. Being engineered and manufactured for great strength, Teftec has also found an audience in people who are large. www.teftec.com.

Having a Manual and a Power Chair

Many people with low-level quadriplegia have sufficient arm strength to push a chair, perhaps aided by handrims with knobs that are easier to grasp than rims alone. The development of "power assist" wheels (page 199) makes pushing a manual chair an option for more people, though this chair might not be a final, full-time solution to their mobility needs. Some of these riders use a manual chair at all times, whereas others switch between manual and power chairs, depending on distance and surface and whether they might need to be lifted up stairs, load the chair into a car, and other such criteria. You might use a power chair to go to and from work but use a manual chair at home and at the office. A blend of the two types can be the ideal strategy for your mobility. It is an approach that does not waste your energy or overuse your body.

Yet another solution is a three- or four-wheeled scooter. Scooters are considerably less expensive than power chairs but can give a manual chair user additional mobility for traveling longer distances or climbing steep slopes. They require greater upper body balance, and only certain products can be configured with the specialized pressure-relief seating many riders require. Some users find a scooter preferable as a full-time solution, but, for people unable to walk, this is far less the case.

Power Assist

An option that first appeared in the late 1990s is the power assist chair—in most cases a standard manual chair modified with power assist wheels.

Thanks to advances in computer chips, this design uses small processors and software that read the user's push on the wheels and sends signals to small motors at each wheel hub to "assist" with a little added power to spare the user from having to provide all of the force of the push. The greatest beneficiaries of this are people with low-level quadriplegia, at risk of overstraining from pushing a standard manual chair but hard pressed to resist getting one for the added flexibility it provides. Power assist is for people who don't have sufficient strength or balance to do all of the work of pushing an unassisted manual chair on their own.

The system adds a lot of weight to the chair—battery pack, motors, modified wheels with controls—but the weight is more than made up for by the benefits of the power assist. Compared to a power chair, the weight savings is substantial in comparison. The wheels typically have a switch to choose different gears, since you want more power out on the open road compared to the short distances you'll travel in your home. It is also possible to turn the system off, but then you are pushing a very heavy chair. The wheels can be removed so the chair can be loaded into the trunk of a car—clearly not an option for most power chairs.

The technology is not entirely mature and takes some getting used to. It is not as if you are pushing a manual chair and it's just easier. Power assisted chairs have a different feel. When you first try it, you might find it lurches on you until you get the feel for how to interact with it. And because the chair is battery-powered, your range is limited by how long the charge lasts—shorter when you are handling more uphill slopes. All of this said, many users get the feel of its unique personality and find this is the perfect option for their needs.

Frank Mobility of Oakdale, Pennsylvania offers the E-Motion wheels, and Quickie Designs/Sunrise Medical offers their Xtender power assist option. These systems add approximately $6,000 to the price of the manual chair, in some cases more than the cost of a power chair. Some find it worth the extra expense.

The iBot®

Inventor Dean Kamen has gained a degree of fame for his high-tech design of the iBot wheelchair—which has gotten a lot of exposure in the media for some of the particularly unique abilities it offers, most notably the ability to climb stairs and to elevate and balance on two wheels (Figure 4-1).

Anyone who has gotten good at wheelies knows how secure one can feel once you get the hang of the gentle forward and backward adjustments to the wheels that keep you from falling over. This is what the iBot does when it is in "standing" mode. Gyroscopes and constant monitoring from the onboard computer read your center of gravity and continually adjust, providing for a surprisingly secure feeling knowing you're in a wheelchair that is balancing on two wheels. The benefits: reaching those higher shelves and getting up to eye-contact height during conversations with a standing person. This technology has been transferred over to the Segue™, the two-wheeled standing scooters that are becoming more commonly visible being used by airport security staff, for example.

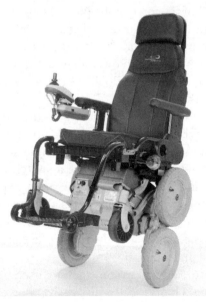

Figure 4-1 The iBot wheelchair.

There are actually six wheels on an iBot, part of a wheel assembly that rotates as a whole to lift the chair in space. It also is how the chair is able to climb stairs; as the assembly rotates under the seat, the upper set of wheels moves to the step below. Stair climbing requires either that the user be able to hold onto a railing as they do it or have a walking helper who assists behind the chair. The iBot is also able to traverse soft surfaces, including sand.

The price tag is very high, and, at publication, the US government had yet to authorize their purchase under the Medicare program. The Veterans Administration, though, has indeed been buying iBots for qualified users. Not anyone can use it—there is an evaluation you must go through to determine if you have the cognitive and physical ability necessary for safe use of this latest, most-advanced wheelchair technology.

Manual Chair Decisions

There are a number of decisions that are unique to choosing a manual chair, beginning with narrowing down the choice between the two primary types—rigid or folding. The wheels are also very different between manual and power wheelchairs, not the least because you put your hands on them with a manual chair. That relationship is crucial for how easily and safely you'll be able to propel your chair—and so how fluid your mobility will be.

Rigid Frame Chairs

It used to be that most manual wheelchairs folded. But a mechanical engineer will tell you that when you push a folding wheelchair, some energy is lost in the flexing of the frame. Less of the force (and effort) of your push translates into forward motion. The loss of energy in a flexible frame led chair designers to come up with the rigid frame chair. According to Doe Cayting of Wheelchairs of Berkeley:

> We like rigid frames because, in a folding chair, 40% of your energy is wasted by the mechanism of the frame. Greater efficiency means you won't tire as easily and you won't have to worry so much about overuse syndrome.

Freed of the mechanism for folding, a rigid chair also has fewer parts and is therefore much lighter and less prone to maintenance problems. With fewer moving components, the frame has more strength. More of the energy of your push translates into motion. The rigid chair design also allows for the angle of the seat frame to be adjustable, impossible with a folding chair because the vertical supports for the chair back are part of the frame structure. The familiar cross-frame structure underneath the seat of the typical wheelchair is not needed with a rigid chair, streamlining its appearance. For those who want to reduce the visual emphasis on their disability and will be pushing greater distances in an average day, the rigid frame design has come to be a de facto standard. Figure 4-2 shows a typical rigid chair.

Figure 4-2 A lightweight, rigid-frame manual wheelchair.

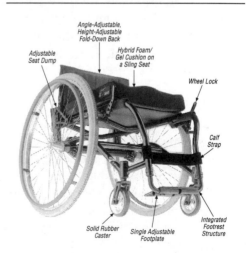

Angle-Adjustable, Height-Adjustable Fold-Down Back

Adjustable Seat Dump

Hybrid Foam/ Gel Cushion on a Sling Seat

Wheel Lock

Calf Strap

Solid Rubber Caster

Single Adjustable Footplate

Integrated Footrest Structure

The front structure that supports the footrest is typically integrated into the frame of the chair, rather than being removable or "swingaway" footrests (although there are some rigid frame products that offer this option). But along with the changes in design fostered by the rigid frame approach, the angle of the footrest has come in closer so that one's feet do not extend out so far from the body. This user has noted the occasional difficulty of fixed footrests but finds a rigid chair necessary because of its more rugged construction:

> I prefer my rigid frame chair. I may be inconvenienced at times when I can't get close to a table, but this is rare, since my chair is quite short and the ends of my toes sit directly below my knees. The durability of a rigid frame is essential, as I am quite hard on my equipment and it must endure Ottawa winters.

However, rigid chairs can be bulky for transporting in a car and do not neatly fold up when they need to be out of the way.

> Even though I tried a rigid frame chair, and, sure, it was easier to wheel and looked better, I found it much harder to put in my two-door car. It wouldn't fit in the trunk either.

You will want to consider what kind of terrain you will be traveling over. Rigid frames are best for hard, reasonably level surfaces. On uneven terrain, a rigid chair will give you a harder ride. And because the frame does not flex, one or more wheels might not be in contact with the ground on uneven terrain, resulting in a possible degree of loss of control, which can be dangerous.

Rigid frame chairs are so responsive that just minor movements of your body can be enough to adjust direction—a technique riders can use to make fine adjustments as they wheel. Some people find rigid chairs a little oversensitive, but many swear by them and will never go back to a folding design.

Folding Frame Chairs

There are a few important reasons why some riders still prefer folding chairs. Folding chairs are likely to fit in most vehicles. On uneven surfaces, all four wheels of a folding chair are better able to remain in contact with the surface because of its flexible frame. The flexible frame also absorbs small bumps and vibrations in your ride. Figure 4-3 shows a typical folding chair.

Some riders prefer a folding chair's ability to fold into a more compact unit important for a variety of reasons that relate specifically to their daily life.

I feel strongly about keeping my chair with me in theaters, and a rigid chair would block the aisles, so I would have to let them take it away during the show. I have enough upper body strength and balance to push a folding chair without tiring myself, so, for these and other reasons, a folding design is still the style of choice for my needs.

Wheelchair makers have put considerable effort into building folding frame chairs that are also ultralight, as well as improving the structure to keep flexing to a minimum and so not waste as much energy of the push. There have also been attempts at alternative designs that attempt to achieve the best of both worlds—rigid-frame performance in a folding frame. Quickie/Sunrise Medical, Kuschall, and Nissin are companies that offer such products. It remains the holy grail of the wheelchair industry.

Chair Weight

The heavier your manual chair, the more energy you will use to push it. This might seem like a good strategy for keeping your weight down, but it's more likely to fatigue you earlier in the day and limit your activities. A heavier chair is also more difficult for anyone assisting you, making it harder to push you a long distance, carry you up a stairway, or store your chair when you're not in it. Although chairs are generally lighter in this modern era than the aluminum frames of the past, there is still considerable range in the weight of various products—especially when you consider (as you must) the addition of various options and the weight of whatever cushion is optimal for you.

Figure 4-3 A lightweight, folding manual wheelchair.

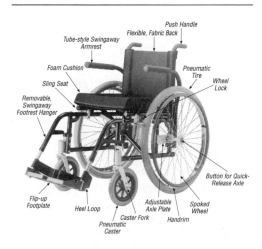

As you make the many choices necessary to define the best chair for you, you will want to consider chair weight versus the advantages of features that will make it heavier. For example, spoked wheels are lighter than molded wheels but require more maintenance. You can choose such items as titanium axles to lighten weight further (though nominally), but they are considerably more expensive. An important safety issue with a light chair is that it has a longer braking distance. You'll want to remember this while getting used to your wheels.

> *When I made the transition from the hospital-style aluminum*
> *chair to a modern lightweight, I discovered that I had less*
> *traction against the pavement and so had to allow for a*
> *greater distance to slow down. It only took one close call*
> *to learn that lesson!*

Titanium frames have become more common, since the company TiSport began marketing chairs in the late 1990s with introduction of the Cross-Sport model. Titanium is much lighter than other metals used for wheelchair frames and also has the qualities of being stronger, absorbing more vibration, and not rusting. TiSport is the American wholesaler of raw titanium, which helps them keep costs relatively lower, although titanium chairs are more expensive—and therefore less likely to be fully covered by insurers. The other major chair makers have since added their own titanium designs to their product lines.

Wheel Size

Your optimal arm reach for pushing will be determined in part by the diameter of the wheels. Manual chairs typically use 24-inch wheels, but wheels are available as small as 20 inches and as large as 26 inches. The combined relationships of the size of the wheels, the height of the seat from the floor, how high you want your feet from the ground, and the depth of your cushion will determine the relationship of your arms to the handrims of the wheels. This is a crucial relationship, defining how effectively you can apply your strength to the wheels and how well your body will endure the repetitive use of your arms and shoulders in this manner.

If your arms are already extended (straight, with your elbows locked) at the beginning of a push—because the wheels are small or you are sitting too high—you will be pushing entirely from the shoulders, rather than being able to engage your triceps muscles, which are the ones between your elbows and shoulders that you use to straighten your arm (and so apply pushing force to the wheels). At the other extreme, if you begin the push with your elbows very bent and your shoulders raised because the wheels are large or you are sitting too low, you will be overstraining your arms and shoulders to get the chair to start moving.

Wheel diameter must be configured in conjunction with seat height and cushion thickness. The sequence of events leading to the decision for wheel diameter goes something like this: first you must ensure proper ground clearance for your footrests based on your leg length. Then you can determine minimum seat height, and from seat height you can determine seat angle. A seat lower at the back will bring your arms closer to the wheels and rims. From there the therapist will determine where your reach falls and determine wheel size from that. Only after you know how high and at what angle your seat will be can you determine your appropriate wheel size. If you want to use larger wheels—which can be easier to push—you might decide to choose a seat height that is greater than the minimum needed to ensure sufficient clearance from the ground for your feet.

Wheel Axle Placement

Two important decisions for chair stability and optimal wheeling efficiency are where the wheel axle will be in relation to the back of the chair and the amount of angle, or camber, on the wheels. With most modern manual chairs, you can adjust the axle position forward or back in relation to the back of the chair. This is the center of gravity, the point of pivot where your body weight is applied against the back of the chair. When the wheel is moved forward on the axle, more of the chair weight is behind the axle, so it will tip more easily, lifting the front casters off the ground. At the least you want to be able to slightly lift the casters with a bit of extra push to lift the chair's casters above bumps in the sidewalk, for instance. But if the casters lift, even slightly, during a normal push on a slight upward incline, then you are wasting energy because some of the force of your push is translating into the upward movement of the casters rather than to the forward movement of the whole chair.

You might learn the technique of doing wheelies to "jump" curbs. The axle position will control how efficiently you can perform these maneuvers without putting yourself at risk of falling backward in your chair. When you get a new chair, you might begin with a more stable rearward position of the main wheel axles and then move the wheels forward as you gain more experience and confidence driving.

Correct wheel position is also determined by your weight and how your weight is proportioned. For example, taller people have longer legs and so have more body weight forward in the chair. More weight forward in the chair allows for a more forward wheel position without risk of falling. If you typically wear heavy shoes or boots, you might take that into account by moving the wheels slightly forward. People with dual leg loss have much less forward body weight, so they must use a rearward wheel position. There are chairs that are specially designed to accommodate this particular type of weight distribution—some even have the axle placed behind the vertical line of the chair back.

If the wheels are too far back, they can be hard to reach for pushing, forcing you to pull your arms farther back. When the wheels are farther back, your chair will be more inclined to veer toward the street on sidewalks, which are always sloped toward the street for water drainage. You will have to push harder on the downhill wheel to compensate for gravity pulling the front end sideways. This is even more true with rigid frame chairs, which are considerably more nimble than folding frames and, so, are more sensitive to issues such as this.

Wheel Camber

Another feature to consider is the amount of "camber" you want on your wheels. Camber is the angle of the wheels toward your body as they rise from the floor (see Figure 4-4). Camber angle is specified when you order your chair, and most products offer you a range of choices. Some chairs have the ability to adjust the camber over a certain range or can be switched between one or two angles, which you would choose when you order. This is an issue to be considered for any manual chair, rigid or folding.

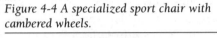

Figure 4-4 A specialized sport chair with cambered wheels.

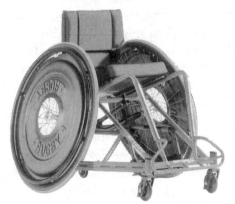

The greater the camber, the wider the wheelbase and, therefore, the greater the lateral stability of the chair as you turn corners or lean over. It also makes the chair more nimble, which is why athletic chairs all use considerable amounts of camber. However, more camber than is necessary for stability will add width at the floor, making it more difficult to pass through narrow spaces.

A different kind of wheel angle—which you want to avoid being improperly adjusted—is "toe-in" or "toe-out." If your wheels were to roll independently of the chair, they would either roll toward (toe-in) or away (toe-out) from each other. Some wheel or caster adjustments can cause your wheels to be angled in one of these ways, making the chair harder to drive and, possibly, applying force on the frame and axles that can cause damage in the long term. Changing the camber of your wheels can impact the toe-in or toe-out, and some chairs have adjustments for this issue. In many chairs, the toe-in/toe-out issue will be automatically accounted for when you switch between available angles. Your technician needs to be sensitive to this issue.

Ultralight Wheels

The standard wheel has steel spokes. Some third-party companies have offered designs that use different approaches to the steel spoke. The goal being lighter and sportier looking.

The X-Core wheel has three "spokes," though they are more like elegant "legs" made of carbon fiber composite. They are easier to clean than having to wipe down each individual spoke of a standard wheel, and it is sometimes beneficial to be able to grab a spoke as you're wheeling or braking. Being a fixed, cast wheel, there is no need for any spoke adjusting.

Spinergy wheels (Figure 4-5) were designed by two recent high school graduates who were bicycle enthusiasts, looking for an alternative to the standard wheel. They discovered an ultra-lightweight material previously available only to the military. This material offered the additional benefit of some degree of shock absorption and the ability to retain its shape under stress. They used this material for the spokes, which do not "kink" when impacted from the side like a steel spoke does. The spokes retain their shape, so they need little tuning.

Figure 4-5 Ultralight Spinergy and X-Core wheels.

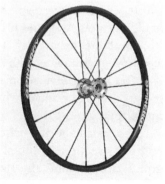

Since the original Spinergy design was created, the number of spokes has been getting smaller and smaller. The company's newest wheel has only 12 spokes. The design of the wheel itself also offers benefits; the company has engineered it to reduce the "moment of inertia"—the amount of force it takes to cause the wheel to rotate—less force, less strain to the hands and arms.

Originally designed for bicycles, Spinergy wheels—though expensive—have become very popular among manual wheelchair users. Some manufacturers offer them as an option on their order sheet.

Geared Wheels

Two recent concepts in wheel design have sought to reduce the amount of force necessary to propel a manual wheelchair and, therefore, put this more lightweight and less costly choice within the range of more people with limited strength and stamina. One of the concepts involves a geared system with which you continue to push on the wheels and handrims in the normal manner. Another adds specialized arms to the chair and the wheels.

MagicWheels® are a geared set of wheels that can be added to most standard wheelchairs. They have two speeds—one that is a normal, 1:1 ratio, feeling the same as standard wheels. In the second gear, the wheels travel twice as far for the same amount of push. In second gear, the wheels also go into "hill-holding" mode so that you cannot roll backward, and, if going forward down a slope, the wheels provide some braking effect. They add approximately 10 pounds to the weight of the chair but are no wider than standard wheels (www.magicwheels.com).

The Wijit system is a set of wheels with geared levers one grasps in order to push forward and pull backward in a motion similar to rowing a boat (Figure 4-6). There is no contact with the wheels or handrims. The Wijit handles can be shifted into forward, neutral, or reverse modes. Pulling the handles inward toward the body brakes the wheels (www.wijit.com).

Figure 4-6 The Wijit lever-operated wheel.

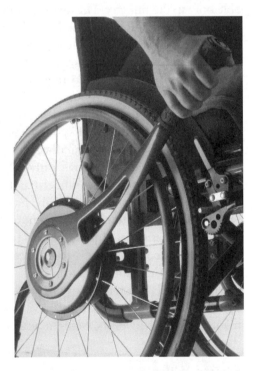

Handrims

The handrim is the circular tube mounted just away from the wheel. You grasp it—and often will simultaneously grasp the tire with your palm—to push the chair. You grasp the handrim by itself to brake the chair while you are rolling.

The basic handrim—circular in cross-section (if you slice through it)—remains the standard that comes by default when you order any chair. They are typically made of aluminum with an anodized, gray coating that is smooth enough not to burn your hands from friction as you brake, but not so slick that you can't slow yourself effectively with minimum grip force. Other options include plastic, foam, or powder coatings. These coatings increase the "gripability" of the handrim but are more easily damaged. Plastic handrims can be very hot when braking and might seriously burn hands that lack sensation.

Standard handrims require the rider to have a reasonably strong grip, but there are other designs that allow for less gripping ability. Low level quadriplegic riders who use a manual chair can elect to use special handrims with added "pegs" or knobs that help compensate for the wheeler's limited grip capacity.

Handrims come in different sizes: in general, the closer the rim is in size to the diameter of the wheel itself, the less force you will have to apply to get the chair moving from a stopped position. Imagine how much force you would have to apply to a handrim about the size of the wheel hub, and you'll get the idea. Some users choose a smaller handrim because, once you are in motion, it is possible to maintain more contact with the smaller handrim, to even get some motion out of the upward movement of your arm—which is otherwise impossible. This is the standard approach for racing wheelchairs. Manual chair riders with only one arm can get a chair designed with a dual handrim on one wheel, allowing either or both wheels to be controlled with one hand.

The design of the handrim has gained considerable attention from chair designers recently. Essentially, the design of the frame has reached relative maturity, so this is a good sign. Designers are getting down to details, and the handrim turns out to be a meaningful component in the efficiency of your use of the manual chair. Its recent evolution indicates that wheelchair design is getting extremely refined.

Natural-Fit™ handrims from Three Rivers (www.3rivers.com) are not circular in cross section but, instead, are a couple of inches wide, providing more surface area to grasp (Figure 4-7). They also provide a surface between the rim and the wheel, which is typically open with a standard handrim. The wheeler can place her thumbs in this curved surface—which is available with a plastic-coated surface—for more "traction" between the hand and the wheel during the push. Braking is made easier because there is more surface with which to make contact as you grip. They also limit the need to grasp the tire, so your hands don't get dirty or as calloused—not to mention the occasional contact with something objectionable you might roll through! Natural-Fit handrims can be installed on most standard wheels.

Figure 4-7 The Natural-Fit handrim.

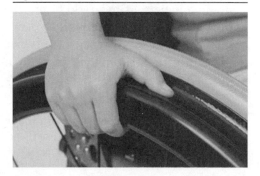

The design of the Natural-Fit handrim came out of the Human Engineering Research

Laboratory at the University of Pittsburgh, led by engineer and chair user Rory Cooper. Three Rivers was able to build its business with support from a federal grant intended to help assistive technologies make the transition from the laboratory to the commercial marketplace.

Another wheelchair user and designer of note is Peter Axelson (yes, that's really his name!) of Beneficial Designs (www.beneficialdesigns.com) in Reno, Nevada. Their design, the FlexRim Low Impact Wheelchair Pushrim uses the standard circular handrim, but it is fused to a flexible, rubber surface between the handrim and the wheel. When the handrim is grasped, it actually flexes slightly, independent of the wheel, reducing the actual impact forces on your hands as you push. It is also possible, as with the Natural-Fit, to lay your thumb in the formerly open space between the rim and the wheel for additional grip and freedom from contact with the tires.

These two designs also protect you from the possibility of jamming your hand or thumb on a wheel brake because your hand is only on the rim and not on the tire where the brake makes contact. For those with long enough arms—and therefore a long enough stroke such that you might make contact with the handbrake—this is an extremely painful experience!

Wheel Locks

Wheel locks, also called hand brakes, are used to prevent a manual chair from accidentally rolling when you want it to remain stationary. The fact is, not much of the world is truly flat and level. Given the much improved engineering of manual chairs, they will move even on the slightest sloping surface—which can be in your house or anywhere out in public.

Some chair riders have eschewed the use of brakes altogether, to the absolute horror of their therapists who subscribe to the belief that a wheelchair must be locked whenever you make a transfer to or from the chair. Just the act of reaching for an object on a table is enough to send sufficient force through your body to your wheels to cause the chair to shift, especially in a hypersensitive rigid frame chair. If you are working at a desk, leaning forward on your arms will cause an unbraked chair to roll backward—and so make you exert your back or have to grab onto something to stabilize yourself to keep the chair from moving out from underneath you.

> *The only people I have seen not use brakes are those that have very low-level injuries and/or have some leg function. They can balance themselves well enough to transfer in and out of an unlocked chair. This doesn't work for me. The one (and only!) time I forgot to lock my brakes prior to a transfer I*

almost ended up on the ground, with the chair shooting off in the other direction!

Use of a hand brake also aids back support. Since you don't have to worry about the chair moving, you can rest your weight against the chair back with confidence.

The standard brakes are a lever placed on the frame just ahead of the tire. When engaged, the brake makes firm, physical contact with the tire and, thus, prevents the wheel from turning. Another design, called a "scissors lock"—meant to solve the thumb-jamming problem mentioned above—mounts just under the seat but engages the tire to lock it in the same way as the standard lock. It is less convenient to reach and requires bending the wrists substantially to engage and release it. It is not possible to apply your body weight to engage it, but some users prefer how this design moves fully out of the way of the wheel when not engaged.

Some brake designs are engaged by pulling backward on the handle rather than pushing forward, for people who have more optimal muscle capacity in that direction. There are also brakes that can be mounted lower on the frame for people who don't mind leaning over more, or who are more likely to be assisted, with the brake being operated by the helper.

Disc Brakes

Brakes that lock against the tire require adjustment, as the support bracket can slightly but gradually slide along where it is attached to the frame from the force of the brake against the tire. And, as your tires lose air (a continual process that needs your attention at all times), the wheel locks become less firm.

To resolve this problem, several companies have developed disc brakes that lock the hub of the wheel rather than push something into the tire. Accessible Designs, Inc. (www.accessibledesigns.com) offers disc brakes with a variety of controls. It is possible to have four different settings of braking force or a single electronic switch that will lock both wheels, for instance.

The downside of disc brakes is that, by locking the hub, the wheel can still move somewhat according to the flexibility of the spokes of the wheels. With some of the ultra-lightweight wheels with fewer spokes, the chair might not feel as stable in the locked position, as you adjust your position in the chair while stopped. This is very much a matter of personal choice.

Power Chair Decisions

The major choices for a power wheelchair are the drive type and the control system. You will need to think about speed—and about stopping. You will need to consider types and sizes of batteries. Finally, you will consider safety and torso stability issues. Figures 4-8 and 4-9 show the various features found on power chairs and contrast some of the design differences.

Front-, Rear-, or Mid-Wheel Drive?

Power wheelchairs have the drive wheels placed either at the front or the back of the chair, or in an increasingly popular "mid-wheel" design, placed immediately under the seat. Each type of wheel drive entails a different style of operating your chair, and it takes a little while to adapt to the feel of it. If the type of drive is right for you, your skill and comfort using it will become increasingly refined, despite any early awkwardness you might experience.

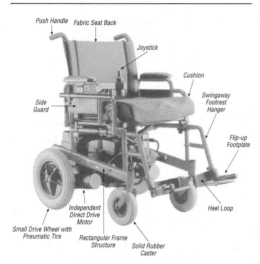

Figure 4-8 A rear-wheel drive, foldable power wheelchair.

Push Handle Fabric Seat Back
Joystick
Cushion
Swingaway Footrest Hanger
Side Guard
Flip-up Footplate
Independent Direct Drive Motor
Heel Loop
Small Drive Wheel with Pneumatic Tire
Rectangular Frame Structure
Solid Rubber Caster

With a front-wheel drive system, you have the sensation of pulling the chair behind you. This sense of pulling means that, in order to operate a front-wheel drive chair, you need greater sensitivity to the chair's movement and control. Front-wheel drive chairs are very agile—capable of making full rotations in a smaller area of space. But, because front-wheel drive takes a little more skill to operate, ability and training issues must be taken into account. People with cognitive difficulties might not be able to safely use front-wheel drive.

One advantage of having the larger drive wheels in front is that you may be able to traverse a change in surface more easily—going over a curb, for example. The larger wheels make contact with the curb first, pulling the smaller casters along behind.

> I live in a rural area where accessibility was initially the major issue. A chair with front-wheel drive would have better suited the terrain that I had to navigate.

If you need a tilt system, you will want to consider whether a front-wheel drive chair will be stable. The tilt system may cause the front wheels to come off the ground, making the chair difficult to operate (Figure 4-9).

Figure 4-9 A front-wheel drive, elevating/ reclining power wheelchair.

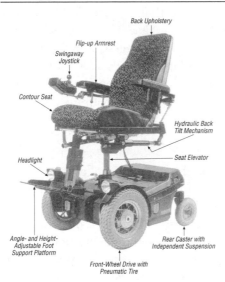

Back Upholstery

Flip-up Armrest

Swingaway Joystick

Contour Seat

Hydraulic Back Tilt Mechanism

Headlight

Seat Elevator

Angle- and Height-Adjustable Foot Support Platform

Rear Caster with Independent Suspension

Front-Wheel Drive with Pneumatic Tire

When you operate a chair with rear-wheel drive, you feel as though you are being pushed forward. There is a greater sense of control over the chair, but rear-wheel drive doesn't afford as much agility.

Tipping is also a concern with rear-wheel drive. You may need to use anti-tippers with a rear-wheel drive chair, since it's possible for the casters in front to be lifted off the surface by the power and weight of the drive wheels in back when you accelerate the chair. (Anti-tippers are optional small wheels that attach to the chair frame at the rear and float a few inches above the ground. If the chair begins to tip backward, the anti-tippers touch down and stabilize the chair.)

If the rear-wheel drive mechanism extends out of the rear of the chair and is low to the ground, you might have the opposite problem—not being able to tip back enough. This could limit your ability to climb over an obstacle or negotiate a ramp or curb cut.

The mid-wheel drive design uses six wheels altogether: two casters in the rear, the two drive wheels, and two more caster-size wheels in the front that are not in continual contact with the ground but are there to help prevent forward tipping. These front casters are usually spring loaded and adjustable. The main advantage of mid-wheel drive is its tight turning radius; it can almost turn in place, making it helpful for people who must navigate small spaces at home or be able to turn around inside a van.

Mid-wheel drive helps to improve traction because more body weight is over the drive wheels, but forward tipping is a concern. Newer models have each pair of front and rear casters in contact with the ground, adjusting to the terrain with shock absorbers. They have worked to optimize stability, but, necessarily, mid-wheel drive chairs are prone to some degree of forward tipping if the chair or your torso leans forward enough. Sudden stops or going down ramps are more likely to bring the front wheels in contact with the ground. Mid-wheel drives should only be used by people with good upper body balance.

Mid-wheel drive chairs do best on firm surfaces. To use them on rough terrain, the front wheels need to be raised and then more rocking occurs.

Whichever placement of wheel drive you select, there will be a range of wheel sizes from which to choose. The advantage of larger wheels is that they will enable you to drive more easily over changes in grade, possibly even small curbs. The disadvantage is that larger wheels add width to your chair. Use of independent suspension—which allows each wheel to shift upward separately with a change in surface—can make up for the loss of maneuverability in a chair with smaller wheels.

Control Systems

Power chair controls are available in a number of designs, allowing for varying degrees of customization and programming. The most common power chair control is a joystick device, mounted on the armrest. The joystick should be positioned so that it can be comfortably reached by your dominant hand while you are sitting in a well-supported, stable upright posture with your shoulders relaxed. Improper positioning of the joystick would force you to compromise your posture in order to put your body in the right orientation to the control. If the joystick is not accurately positioned, using the joystick can strain your hand, arm, shoulder, and back. If you need to sit close to a desk, you will need a joystick control that is able to swing away to the side. Not all joysticks are designed to do this.

For those unable to use a joystick, several other kinds of controls are available:

- Breath controls (sometimes called sip-and-puff) respond to an in or out breath, as if you were sucking on or blowing into a straw.
- Chin controls use a small rubber cup placed just below the chin. A chin control works essentially the same way as a joystick.
- Head controls employ head movements to the back and side, with nothing obstructing the face.

The settings of your control are crucial, and you will need to work with a competent technician who understands your activities and needs. If you set too slow a deceleration rate, for example, but don't have sufficient dexterity or skill level, you might find yourself running into your furniture a lot because the chair keeps rolling once you have let go of the joystick.

How Fast?

Safety should be the most important consideration when determining maximum speed. What will happen if you are going fast and a dog or a child suddenly steps out in front of you? A sudden stop might throw you out of your chair if you do not have sufficient upper body balance or are riding without the use of restraints. You might also lose your grasp of the controller in such a situation. Both maximum speed and stopping distance (deceleration) can be programmed in modern controllers, and you would be well advised to err on the side of your own safety—as well as that of any being or anything that might accidentally get in your way. Some of the more sophisticated controllers even allow an automatic acceleration adjustment when you are making a turn.

For use indoors, a maximum speed of five miles per hour is a recommended standard. When you are inside, moving in smaller spaces, a slow speed can feel fast. Traveling the short distance from your desk at work to the restroom, or from your living room to your kitchen, seems to go quickly even though you may actually be moving slowly.

A speed that is comfortable inside feels extremely slow once you are out on the open road. Outside, you usually travel farther, and you are more conscious of how long it takes to reach your destination. Traveling from your home to the corner grocery store four blocks away would seem like an eternity using the same speed you were using inside your home.

Yet, outside, you might be with another person who walks. Walking speed always seems slow to a wheelchair rider, yet you don't want to make your companions run to keep up with you. Average walking speed is three miles per hour, whereas a moderate running pace is eight miles per hour, numbers you can take into account when choosing your chair. Some chairs are capable of traveling as fast as eight miles per hour.

User definition of speed is now typical of power chairs and scooters. A common feature of modern power controls is a switch that lets you alternate between two programs so you can have a maximum indoor speed and a higher maximum outdoor speed. Another approach is a knob that allows you to adjust maximum speed. The amount of force you apply to a joystick also controls your speed, just as with the accelerator pedal on a car.

Cushions

Although your wheelchair and cushion are separate purchases, which chair you choose—and the specifications when ordering it—is significantly affected by the type of cushion you will use. Chair and cushion are a team, each influencing the other. The proper combination of chair and cushion will enable you to sit in a neutral and stable posture and drive the chair safely.

Cushions come in various depths and sizes, which need to be accounted for in the size of your wheelchair frame. The length of footrests, the height of the chair back, the position of armrests, and other features are influenced by how high or low you will be sitting on a cushion. You need to decide which cushion is best for you before you can make a final decision about which chair is best. You must know the depth of the cushion before you can specify the exact dimensions of your chair.

Pressure Distribution

A critical function of the wheelchair cushion for those with paralysis is the prevention of pressure sores. Since, when we sit, only one third of the body's surface is supporting all of its weight, blood flow is restricted. In the presence of muscle atrophy—which is experienced in particular by many people with spinal cord conditions—circulation is limited further by the loss of muscle that once served as a sort of natural cushion. An additional risk of sitting is shear force, as we tend to slide forward on the cushion, causing stress across the surface of the skin. Resulting pressure sores (decubitus ulcers) can be very serious, leading to hospitalization, surgery, and—though rare—even death. The right cushion is a primary tool for maintaining the health of your skin.

"Pressure-mapping" technology has become widespread in rehabilitation centers, now that it is extremely affordable and runs with a laptop computer. It is a simple mat that is laid over your cushion—or one being considered for you—that produces an image on the computer screen detailing where the pressure points are located and how substantial they are. Using this extremely powerful tool, the therapist doing the fitting can ensure the correct cushion and chair configuration, evenly spreading pressure across your vulnerable points.

The other crucial role of the cushion is postural stability. Even if you are able to walk or are an amputee with sufficient built-in ischial cushioning, the right cushion helps to position and stabilize your spine. If you already have some asymmetry in your body, you need to be supported in a way that will not increase any spinal deformity. For manual chair users, greater stability in your chair also means you can push the wheels with more confidence and strength.

It can't be repeated often enough—posture is key. Bob Hall puts it well:

*The wrong seating system leads to poor posture, which leads
to physical problems, which lead to becoming more sedentary,
which leads to a negative emotional and personal experience.
It's a dangerous chain of events.*

Foam Cushions

Foam technology has come a long way. No longer just the soft, airy stuff of the past, foam now comes in a range of densities and with varying degrees of "memory," holding its shape as you sit, and contributing to your stability. The new foams can adapt to any shape and still provide even support, spreading pressure across the sitting surface. Different types of foam are often used in combination, layered for their various properties of softness, even support, and memory.

Foam is relatively inexpensive, and it is easy to cut. A therapist can experiment with shapes free of financial risk. If you have an area of skin that is broken down or on the verge, pressure can easily be reduced by cutting out a portion of the cushion. (You should not do this on your own, though, because only a doctor or therapist can identify the changes in your cushion that will help relieve pressure while still maintaining appropriate support.)

On the downside, foam wears out faster than other materials and loses its shape, but, because of its lower price, this might not concern you. It simply means you must be more earnest about checking on the condition of the cushion, and pay attention to your body if you feel some pressure or notice your posture has changed. If you choose a foam cushion, be sure to replace it when its time is up. Old foam that is compressed can allow pressure points to form that can lead to a sore. If you choose a gel or air flotation cushion for daily use, it is a good idea to have a backup foam cushion, since gel and air flotation cushions can leak.

Gel Cushions

Gel cushion designs attempt, in effect, to replace the consistency and support of atrophied muscle tissue. Highly engineered gel fluids are placed in pouches and usually attached to a foam base so that the cushion conforms to the pressures placed on it. As a result, gel cushions provide excellent pressure distribution and are very comfortable. Many gel products also offer supplemental inserts to stabilize your legs. Your knees might tend to fall together (adduction) or apart (abduction), so such an accessory can help keep your legs straight, which also aids your overall posture.

Gel cushions are much heavier than other types, which can cancel out some of the benefits of your lightweight wheelchair. If you will be taking the cushion in and out of the chair often—transferring into a theater seat, getting in and out of the car, etc.—then weight becomes a consideration for ease of this much handling.

If you jump up and down curbs using wheelie techniques, or commonly experience similar impact in your chair, a gel cushion might not be ideal. When you sit in a gel cushion, there is no further "cushiness" to absorb impact, a concept known as impact loading. Other cushion types are better able to absorb impact.

Another drawback to gel cushions is the possibility of them "bottoming out" as the gel is pushed aside by your weight. You can help prevent this distribution problem by kneading your gel cushion once a day, keeping the fluids loose and spread evenly. Look for a design that divides the gel portion into several sections so that all of the gel cannot push entirely to the sides.

There is also the chance of the gel leaking. Although cushions arrive with patching kits, patches are ineffective when the breach is at a seam, which is often the case. A leak might be very minor, or it could be an extremely messy affair.

Air or Dry Floatation Cushions

Air floatation cushions support the body entirely on air. A typical example is the ROHO® cushion, designed with a group of small, interconnected rubber balloons arranged in rows. Pressure is balanced by air shifting out to surrounding balloons, spreading pressure evenly against your skin. The whole system is closed, so air floatation cushions can't bottom out the way gel cushions can.

If you have a pressure sore, you can tie off individual balloons to reduce contact under that area, allowing you to spend more time sitting as the sore heals. Air cushions are relatively lightweight and are waterproof, allowing for double duty in the bathtub or on a boat.

Air cushions can be less stable for those who move around a lot in their chair, but recent designs offer either low- or high-profile options that minimize this problem. Some allow halves or quadrants of the cushion to be inflated separately, which also helps ensure optimal posture if there is some asymmetry in your body. The balloons used in air cushions can be punctured, of course, and leaks do occur, although a fairly heavy-duty rubber is used, similar to the rubber used for tire tubes. Patching them is easier than with the gel design. The hard part is submerging the cushion under water to find the leak (look for escaping air bubbles).

The biggest drawback to air cushions is that they require more maintenance. It is necessary to check the pressure frequently, especially if you have pressure sores.

Urethane Honeycomb Cushions

Thermoplastic urethane honeycomb cushions, such as those from Supracor®, are the most recent development in the world of cushions. Because there are many individual cells—like a beehive—these cushions are able to distribute weight evenly, but there is no risk of leaking gel or of an air bladder being punctured. The many open spaces in the beehive structure of the cushion allow air to travel more effectively. This design helps to protect against skin breakdown because your skin is kept cooler and moisture is prevented from collecting.

Urethane honeycomb cushions are very light and absorb shock, and a low-profile cushion can provide significant support. These cushions can even be thrown into your washing machine and dryer, making them attractive for people with incontinence problems, during which the cushion will be soiled from time to time despite best efforts at bowel and bladder management. Urethane cushions are available in standard or in contoured shapes and can also be purchased for use with a bed mattress.

Alternating Pressure

In this design, an air pump creates alternating pressure in various chambers of the cushion, of particular interest to those with more significant disabilities who are unable to perform their own weight shifts to relieve pressure. Sitting for extensive periods of time without pressure relief causes the muscle and fatty tissues to separate, putting the delicate skin layer in closer contact with the bone. This creates even more pressure on the skin. Lack of air circulation increases the temperature between you and the cushion. Moisture collects and is trapped against the skin. All of this further increases the risk of a sore.

One alternating pressure solution is the ErgoDynamic™ Therapeutic Seating System from ErgoAir in New Hampshire. This system pumps air into and out of alternating portions of the cushion. The product is contoured for pelvic stability. Special vent holes serve to allow the flow of air and moisture. In a five-minute cycle, compartments are inflated and deflated to shift support alternately between the ischial (sit) bones and the hips. Both areas get regular periods of complete pressure relief. The manufacturer likens it to a massage while you sit, with the resulting promotion of blood flow. In some cases, the makers suggest that a pressure sore can even heal while you sit. This cushion system can be plugged into some power chair batteries or charged in a cigarette lighter in your car.

Alternating pressure products are of course heavier—given their use of batteries and air pumps—and, like air floatation cushions, are prone to puncture. However, the technology for these innovative systems is likely to evolve further in the future as new materials and batteries are developed.

Seats and Backs

Although we usually think of a seat as a single unit—such as a couch or recliner—seats, backs, cushions, and armrests are distinct when you are choosing your wheelchair. Seats, backs, and cushions have a number of interrelationships, so, to some degree, you will need to think about them all at the same time. For instance, how high you will sit on the chair and where your feet are in space will be determined by the seat-to-floor height of the seat pan plus the thickness of the cushion. ·

Seat or Chair Width

Your chair should be as narrow as possible for your body size without creating contact points that can cause pressure sores. A seat that is too wide limits mobility. Even an additional fraction of an inch in the width of the chair can make the difference between being able to get down an aisle in a store or past a couch at the home of a friend. You don't want to squeeze yourself into the seat—if you wear a heavy coat in the winter, or typically work in a business suit with a jacket, the width of the seat should take this into account—but you also don't need the wasted space or mobility limitations of a chair that is too wide. A wider chair is also heavier, given the extra metal in the frame.

A seat that is too wide will promote poor posture. If you have extra space, you are more likely to slump to one side or the other. You might think that because you would have more room to shift your position, extra seat width would be helpful in the prevention of pressure sores, but this is not a good strategy for skin management. You don't want to protect your skin by risking damage to your spine with twisted sitting postures. Rather, your skin management program should consist of proper cushioning and diet, as well as push-ups while you are in the chair. Put a high priority on good postural habits.

A wider chair also means that the wheels will be wider apart, making it necessary for a manual-chair wheeler to reach farther, extending the arms out to the side. Wheeling with the arms extended is a less efficient way to wheel, will be more fatiguing, and puts your shoulders at a great risk of overstraining. If the chair has armrests, they might further interfere with the process of wheeling if the chair is too wide for you, or the armrests may rub against your arms as you wheel.

A wider chair does provide better lateral stability, which will help prevent a manual chair from tipping over sideways, but, frankly, unless you are reckless or wheel on rough terrain, tipping sideways is highly unlikely. Stability can be similarly achieved by proper adjustment of camber (discussed above), determined by the axles and plates that are typical on most chairs today.

If weight management is difficult for you, you will want to take the possibility of weight gain into consideration when determining the seat width. You don't want to find yourself ultimately squeezed into a chair purchased when you were lighter. Your risk of pressure sores—particularly at your hip bones—will increase considerably. If you become heavier and truly need a new chair, you might have to fight with your funding source for approval or be forced to dip into your own savings or credit limit to buy new wheels. But do you want to purchase a wider chair on the assumption that you will gain weight? Is that risking a self-fulfilling prophesy, inviting weight gain? The best solution is to reach a stable weight, whatever is normal for you, and then specify a chair that will remain appropriate to your needs while you practice the best weight-control habits you can.

Seat Depth

It is critical to get the depth of the seat pan right when you specify the dimensions of your chair. The seat pan should be deep enough so that the seat is in contact with as much of the bottom of your thighs as possible without making contact behind your knees.

When the seat pan is too shallow, your upper legs extend beyond the front edge and more pressure is placed on your ischial "sitting" bones. This additional pressure increases the risk of skin breakdown. You are also giving up greater stability. The chair can't "carry" you if it can't make full contact with your body. Without full seat support, your body might be prevented from being in its neutral position, risking spinal curvature or muscle and tendon strain. A too-shallow seat pan also means that your feet will not rest properly in the footrests, which will be located further back underneath your legs instead of under or just ahead of your knees where they belong.

On the other hand, when the seat pan is too deep, you will be unable to sit properly against the chair back. You will be kept from sliding back fully in the seat, stopped behind the knees. When the seat is too deep, the only way to make contact with the back of the chair is to rotate the pelvis backward and round the spine. In other words, you will have to slump. Slumping is potentially dangerous for the spine, as it can cause degeneration, and is also a source of chronic back pain. This posture also makes it difficult for you to wheel efficiently in a manual chair and, so, contributes to the risk of chronic shoulder strain as well.

A seat pan that is too deep can interfere with the position of your legs if you use calf supports with your footrests. Calf supports keep the legs in a more-forward position. The seat pan might need to be shallower to compensate.

A deeper seat means a heavier chair due to the added metal in the frame. When more of the chair is ahead of the axle, you will feel as though you are pushing even more weight. If you require extra depth in the seat pan, you will need to adjust the forward position of the main wheel axles so the chair is not too front heavy, particularly if you rely on doing wheelies in your wheeling style.

> I am very tall and recently purchased a chair that is two
> inches deeper than my past wheels so I could have more con-
> tact with my legs along the seat. It has worked very well, and
> it was not a problem to adjust the chair for wheelies and for
> ease of wheeling, although it did feel slightly heavier at first.
> Now I can't tell the difference, partly because I have nothing
> to compare to anymore, and I probably gained a little
> strength to compensate for the additional weight just by
> using the chair.

A crucial element that must be taken into consideration before you can determine the appropriate depth of the seat pan is the type of seat back you will use. A fabric-upholstered back requires you to sit a little farther back in the chair and tends to loosen with time unless it is equipped with adjustable tension straps. A rigid back will not change much over time, but some are quite thick and cause you to sit more forward on the seat.

Seat Height

The minimum height you can sit off the ground will be determined by physical factors. The main considerations are the length of your legs and the clearance needed for footrests. Whether you'll choose to sit higher than the minimum—and how much higher—will depend on environment, such as the height of standard tables or other surfaces that your knees must go under, and on personal preferences.

The seat-to-floor height of a chair (typically specified separately for the front and back of the seat) will be part of the frame dimensions ordered from the factory. It can also be adjusted in a manual chair in which the axles are installed relative to the frame. By lowering the axles, you essentially raise the frame and, so, the higher the seat. On a modular power chair, the seat structure is installed on top of an independent drive unit and so does not depend on the wheel position. The seat will often be adjustable within a range of a certain number of inches. The manufacturer will offer either a specific set of height choices or a variety of height ranges if adjustability is a feature of the chair.

The minimum seat height for your wheelchair is determined by how much space your footrests need to clear the floor. How high you sit, how long your legs are, and the angle of the seat will determine where the bottom of your feet will be in space. To decide minimum footrest ground clearance, you'll want to account for bumps in sidewalks, table-leg bases, or any other kinds of changes in the surface you might encounter. Two inches of clearance for footrests is recommended as an absolute minimum, but, depending on where you will be riding, you might need more.

Footrest clearance is also an issue when making a transition from a sloped surface—like a ramp—to a level one. If you are moving forward down a somewhat steep surface (the world does not necessarily conform to the recommended 1:12 standard), then your footrests could potentially make contact with the level surface while the rear wheels are still coming down the slope. This contact at the footplate will stop you cold. This would cause the chair to tip forward, dumping you out, lying on your face or your side! In other words, don't tempt the issue of footrest ground clearance. It is extremely important.

Whether you want your seat to be higher than the minimum needed for footrest clearance depends on a number of factors. The higher you sit, the better you can reach your cabinets in the kitchen, shelves in stores, or a bookshelf at work. Your visibility will also be a little better. Be sure, though, that your knees will be able to fit under tables and desks. On the other hand, it might be important for you to be closer to the floor, perhaps for your work.

You might be a user who doesn't use footrests—common for people who have had a stroke and have the use of at least one leg. Your seat height, then, will be determined by being able to get your feet in solid contact with the floor so you can use them to help propel the chair while you are able to sit fully back in the chair. This is also therapeutic, allowing you to continue to make use of all the physical capacity available to you.

For people who have less agility and strength, being at the same level as the surfaces you transfer to—such as your car seat, your favorite chair, or your bed—would be a higher priority. When the chair seat is at a different height, you or someone assisting you, must exert some extra strength to deal with that change in height. Your body will need to be lifted somewhat onto a higher surface or kept from essentially being dropped onto a lower surface.

If you sit too low, you might strain your neck in conversation with people who are standing next to you. Some people feel that, when they sit low, they are less charismatic or appear inferior to those around them. They feel "looked down upon." However, seat-height preference is an individual matter. Some folks are just happier at a higher or lower level. Make sure you take time to consider all the practical, psychological, and personal aspects brought to bear by the height of your chair. Remember that the height of your seat has an effect on the optimal relationship of your arms to the wheels of a manual chair, and that you must account for the thickness of your cushion during this part of the process.

Seat Angle

Your chair seat does not necessarily need to be parallel to the ground. Seats can slope down toward the back. The angle of the seat compared to the ground is sometimes called "seat dump" or "squeeze." (For an example of extreme seat dump see Figure 4-2.)

Having some degree of seat dump means that more of your weight presses against the chair back, making you feel more stable in your seat. People with higher-level spinal disabilities—and therefore less control of muscles in their torso, which would provide greater stability—gain security and safety by using some seat dump. Manual chair riders use whatever amount of seat dump they need to exert the most push with less effort through their arms and shoulders while remaining stable and symmetrical in their seat.

Many chairs allow you to adjust seat dump. Raising the rear axles to a higher position has the effect of lowering the rear of the chair and, so, increases the seat dump. It might also be possible to raise the caster height, achieving the same effect. Many rigid frame chairs are customized with fixed front and rear seat heights, so changing the casters would be the only way to adjust dump once the chair is delivered.

There are trade-offs for the advantages of seat dump, however, including health risks such as an increased possibility of spinal curvature and back strain. The more your knees come up relative to your thighs, the more your pelvis rotates backward. Your spine, attached to your pelvis at the bottom, then gets rotated to the rear, flattening out your lumbar curve, which helps the spine do its remarkable work of flexibly supporting your torso and head and shoulders. Too much dump can also make transfers more difficult, your body wanting to slide back down the angle of the seat with gravity. Consult carefully with your therapist and dealer about the best seat angle for your needs.

Back Support

Until recently, cloth or vinyl sling backs that necessarily had to fold with the chair were the only choice. Flat backs provided no lumbar support, lateral trunk stability, or accommodation of people with more advanced ortho-pedic or neurologic needs.

Aware of the need for better postural support, chair and cushion designers directed their efforts to making other options available. Designers gained more freedom with the advent of rigid frame manual chairs and mod-ular power chairs. Rigid frame chair backs pivot down against the seat, rather than closing sideways, so the back upholstery does not need to col-lapse. Power chairs used to be folding chairs with motors and controls tacked onto them. Now the back can be designed as an independent ele-ment with more shape, support, and upholstered comfort.

The folding chair, however, as we've seen, has not completely disap-peared and has its place for some users. A now-common design enhances the traditional cloth back by adding a series of horizontal straps down the inside of the chair back (Figure 4-10). The straps are tension adjustable so that each strap can be individually tightened or loosened according to the need for sup-port at a particular point in your back. A tension-adjustable back can still provide support only as far forward as the vertical sup-ports of the back, but it is a vast improvement over a back that is simply a piece of material.

Figure 4-10 A chair back with tension-adjustable straps.

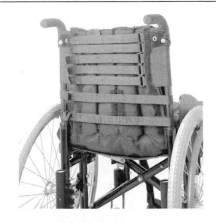

Another approach to back support is a rigid back with deep upholstery. These products typ-ically allow you to adjust lum-bar support. To install this kind of chair back, the standard cloth back is removed entirely, sup-port clips are added to the verti-cal canes of the chair, and the new back is hung on these clips. For a folding chair, this back must be lifted off before the chair can be folded.

If you will be pushing a manual chair, you'll want to compare the ben-efits of improved back support against the additional weight of a more sup-portive back. Keep in mind that, with extra back support, you will be able to maintain more firm contact with the back of the chair as you push, enabling you to exert more force on the wheels. You will also want to take into account whether the back can remain on the chair when you collapse the back down. If you drive a car (as compared to a ramped van), you prob-ably break the frame down to its smallest components, so a back that can remain in place would be desirable. Other back designs involve special clips that the back slips onto and off of.

If your strength and balance are more limited, your need for other back support features increases. For instance, if you have limited side-to-side stability, you can choose a back cushion that wraps around you, curving to your sides to help support you laterally. If your balance is precarious or you tend to slip easily from neutral posture, you might require additional lateral-support accessories, a hip or chest seat belt, or both.

For people whose bodies are not symmetrical, the chair back might need to be customized by a rehabilitation engineer who works closely with your therapist and wheelchair supplier. This more-advanced approach can involve making molds of your body to make a highly specialized support system specifically for your needs. Some positioning centers have newer technology that can actually take a computer model of your body shape by having you sit in a special device loaded with sensors that can map your body's shape. The data are then used to manufacture a support system for you.

Back Height

You need sufficient support for your upper back, not just the lumbar curve. If you are unable to use your legs, your balance is limited and your center of gravity is higher up your trunk. Simple physics is at play here—if your center of gravity is higher up, you are going to fall over more easily. If you are paralyzed as high as your abdomen and trunk, without control of those muscles to stabilize your upper body, you will need a higher back to provide you support and stability. Too low a back might leave you unnecessarily fatigued from having to balance yourself rather than allowing the chair back to carry you.

If you use a power chair because of a lack of strength or stamina but have normal control of your torso muscles—such as would be the case for users with multiple sclerosis—then you would need less height. You would be able to preserve the free range of motion of your upper torso and shoulders. Some people who have higher spinal cord conditions and are using a power chair will need their back fully supported, maybe even a headrest. Since your ability to move your upper torso is limited, being more fully carried is going to be the higher priority. Use of a tilt-and-recline system certainly requires a full-height back with a headrest.

At the same time, lower chair backs have become popular on manual wheelchairs, partly as an image issue because they lessen the presence of the wheelchair. Your chair back should be high enough to provide the support mentioned above, but not so high that it limits your ability to rotate your upper body at the shoulders. There will be times you need to reach for something beyond and just behind you, but the most important thing is that your arms and shoulders have unobstructed range of motion for the process of wheeling a manual chair.

Many current wheelchair designs allow the vertical support rails of the back of the chair to be set at various heights so that back height can be customized. The upholstery has the ability to adapt to the support heights, with any extra material folding back underneath or running along the seat pan beneath the cushion. It is then held in place with Velcro.

When you order your chair, you will usually specify a back height that is then adjustable within a range of a few inches. A third-party rigid back can be installed on the chair rails at the specific height desired. They also come in different vertical sizes.

Footrests

One of the risks of using a wheelchair if you are not able to move your legs or experience significant spasticity is to have your foot fall off a footrest, or be improperly supported to begin with, and then be injured by getting caught on an object or literally run over by the chair itself. That's especially dangerous for power chair users. To achieve good support for your feet while maximizing mobility, you'll want to take care to choose the right footrests—including hanger angle, type of footplate, and type of supports—for you.

Fixed or Swingaway?

There are essentially two types of footrests—fixed and swingaway. Fixed footrests are increasingly common, spurred by the growth and popularity of rigid frame wheelchairs. They are integrated into the frame of the chair and are held in place by telescoping tubes that slide into the frame to be adjusted for your leg length.

A fixed footrest typically has a single metal plate that holds both feet, rather than a separate plate for each foot. The single footplate either attaches between two tubes that extend from the frame or is clamped onto a tube that is part of the frame itself. The single footplate is therefore a design that can add to the structural rigidity of the chair. And, since it involves fewer moving parts, there is less maintenance risk. For an example of a fixed footrest, see Figure 4-1.

Swingaway footrests are the historical norm and remain an option for most folding wheelchairs that would be specified for a regular user.

Individual footplates are attached to the bottom of hangers—metal tubes that attach onto the frame structure. A spring release allows the hanger or footrest mechanism to be held in place but easily released to swing the whole unit aside or remove it completely. The ability to remove your footrests can help when sitting at a table with a large base, getting into a very small elevator, approaching a bathtub, or putting your chair into an automobile trunk. For an example of swingaway footrests, see Figure 4-2.

The footplates of swingaway footrests usually flip up to help you transfer to or from the chair. Flip-up plates are mandatory for folding chairs or the chair would be prevented from closing. (If someone else folds your chair, be sure they know the footplates have to be lifted first, to avoid damage to your chair.) Some folding chairs offer the option of a full-width plate that can also flip up as a single unit to allow the chair to fold. The single plate offers added structural stability—helping a folding chair to perform more like a rigid one—as well as more freedom for the positions of your feet.

As you wheel, your feet are kept from sliding off the footplates by heel loops—strips of sturdy material attached and looped across the rear of the footrests. Instead of heel loops, some chairs—usually rigid frame chairs with single footplates—use a support strap that passes across the frame behind the calves, keeping your feet in place by preventing your legs from sliding backward. Some people find their feet are less stable with a calf-support strap, particularly if they have a tight hanger angle. Feet can more easily slide off the footplate. Adjusting the footplate at more of an angle—or specifying an angle when you order the chair—can help.

Angle and Position of Footrests

The angle of your footrest hangers—the support that goes from the frame of the chair down to the actual footplate—determines where your feet will be in relation to your knees. A tight angle will put your feet more toward the knees than forward from the knees. Some footrests even angle backward, so that feet are farther back than the knees. A wider angle, of course, will bring your feet forward so that they are more forward, ahead of your knees. Which angle is best for you depends on a variety of factors, including leg length, physical limitations, and personal preference. The wheelchair order sheet is also likely to offer you the option of "tapered" footrest hangers. These angle inward toward each other and can help when you're trying to turn in or pass through a narrow space. They also bring your feet closer together because the footplate width is narrower.

Recent designs have brought the angle of the footrests closer to the body, putting the legs into more of a perpendicular position. Table legs become less of an obstacle, removing the need for flip-up footplates for some people. A tighter footrest angle means a shorter "wheelbase" from rear to toe and, so, allows you to turn around in smaller spaces. You need sufficient range of motion to bend at the knees and ankles to use these closer footrest angles.

Some people like to be able to see their toes so they can tell where their feet are. If you are conscious of your posture and concerned about your feet being even and flat on the plates, you might want to choose a more forward angle. If you have long legs, you might choose a more-forward angle to bring your feet up away from the ground. This is an alternative to an even greater seat height, which can bring your knees too high to clear desks or tables.

For people with flexion contracture, in which the knee will not open to a 90-degree angle, the feet need to be supported underneath the leg. Some chair producers have an optional footrest that can be adjusted back underneath the chair. This is generally available only for manual chairs, since batteries and motors usually take up this space on power chairs.

The angle of the footplate itself can be either fixed or adjustable, raising or lowering your toes relative to your heels. The more forward the angle of the hanger, the more upward an angle the plate needs to be at to accommodate the natural posture of your feet. Most manufacturers offer an adjustable footplate as an option. This is especially useful for people whose feet are different, who go through changes with contractures in the legs, or who have progressive conditions that affect foot angle.

Tires

Tires influence the comfort of your ride and the amount of maintenance your chair will need. Some riders also consider the choice of tires an important aesthetic consideration. Generally, wheelchair tires are made of a gray rubber designed not to leave scuff marks on floors, as compared with the black rubber used for car or bicycle tires. Your choices range from pneumatic, air-filled-tires, to solid rubber tires, to solid inserts that replace the pneumatic tubes inside a tire. As you decide which type of tire will serve you best, keep in mind that larger tires will add width to your chair.

Pneumatic tires have inflatable tubes in them like bicycle tires, so they offer a more cushioned ride. Like bicycle tires, they can be punctured by a tack or piece of glass picked up on the street. The risk of punctures is greater for power chair tires because the extra weight of the chair against the pavement can help a sharp object pierce the rubber. Obviously, getting a flat tire means you might find yourself stranded away from home or going back for a repair, riding on the deflated tire. Riding on a flat tire can cause damage to the rim of the wheel. Flats can be minimized by using heavy-duty, thorn-resistant tubes or Kevlar tires. (Kevlar is a material used for bulletproof vests.)

Pneumatic tires must be kept well filled. Soft tires cause the chair to coast less, and that means more pushing for a given distance of rolling. This fatigues you sooner and puts more strain on your shoulders.

Pneumatic tires need replacement more often, since the depth of the rubber before reaching the fiber lining is thinner than that of a solid tire. The rubber wears down from normal use, particularly the more shallow treads of most manual chair tires. Knobby tires with a deeper tread are also available. They will last longer and provide better traction on unpaved surfaces but are harder on the hands of manual chair riders.

Thin-profile pneumatic tires—used on manual chairs when you expect to primarily travel on paved surfaces or in buildings with solid flooring—have less surface area in contact with the pavement, so there is less friction when turning. This makes the chair more agile, critical for sport use and preferred by some riders for daily use. The treads are substantially thinner, so if you plan to wheel on unpaved surfaces—or shoot baskets in the driveway, causing a lot of friction between tire and cement or asphalt—the thinner profile tires might not be for you. They also typically inflate to 100 pounds per square inch, so you need access to a strong pump or a gas station that goes up to that pressure.

Solid rubber tires make for a rougher ride. You will feel each bump of the pavement, but your tires will never go flat. You might value the security of knowing you will not get a flat, like this power chair user:

> I found, when I had air tires on my chair, I would get flats
> an average of two or three times a month. It happened at
> very inopportune times, like when I was alone or on vaca-
> tion. Switching to solid tires has been a godsend. Now I
> don't have to avoid that broken glass. I can go right
> through it.

Many power chairs have solid tires with a deeper tread that lasts longer while providing better traction. Solid rubber tires tend to be slightly heavier than other options, since they contain more rubber.

A recent variation that is a compromise between pneumatic and solid rubber tires is a rubber insert. The insert is placed inside a tire as an alternative to an inflatable tube. The tire doesn't need to be pumped up with air, so obviously it can't go flat. Manual chair riders will find that the resulting apparent tire pressure is softer and that the chair won't roll as easily. The wheels will also lose momentum faster, which means having to push more often—or burn up your battery charge sooner. However, some power chair users swear by rubber inserts, which continue to be improved in the efficiency of their ride.

Casters

Casters are the smaller wheels at the front (usually) of your wheelchair that allow the chair to turn. Casters rotate on their forks as you change direction in your chair. They can be large or small, soft or hard. The kind of casters you choose has a lot of impact on your comfort and mobility. You will want to weigh the advantages of small casters against those of large casters.

Small casters allow tighter footrest angles, thus the reason for their popularity on rigid frame chairs. Small casters are less likely to get in a position that prevents them from rotating when you turn. Greater agility has made small casters very popular, but, since they are hard—typically made of solid plastic or rubber—they make for a bumpier ride. Some small-caster wheels are the same type as those used on rollerblades or skateboards. You will feel every crack in the sidewalk, you will need to lift the casters by doing a mini-wheelie to clear thresholds at doorways, and you must pay close attention on sidewalks for joints that are pushed up by tree roots or any other kind of change in the surface as you travel. They might get caught in a sewer or ventilation grate on the street. The smallest types of casters can even be stopped by very small obstacles, like a stone on a sidewalk. These kinds of sudden stops, as you know, can mean being thrown out of your chair.

Pneumatic casters are larger, at least six inches in diameter. They will provide a very soft ride. Any air-filled tire is at risk of being punctured, but it is also true that a flat caster will not strand you the way a flat main tire will. The chair itself will also last longer with larger, soft casters, as the vibration from harder tires causes more wear and tear on the frame.

Large casters can handle obstacles and rough terrain more easily. Picture a hard caster approaching a three-inch curb, and you can sense that it would require more force to roll over the curb than would a softer, larger tire. This is why front-wheel-drive power chairs typically have larger front, main wheels.

Before choosing a large caster, you'll want to consider your ideal footrest angle. When larger, pneumatic casters are used, your heels must be moved forward with a greater footrest angle to clear the rotation of the casters, extending your overall length, "wheel to toe," if you will.

Larger casters can also obstruct your movement suddenly if you are close to a wall or some other raised surface. As the caster begins to rotate, it becomes blocked by the wall, stopping your movement. You won't be trapped; you'll simply have to maneuver so that you get the caster free of the obstacle. Some people find this stressful, but many users learn to avoid these situations.

A compromise between the two extremes of caster options is the four-inch solid rubber caster. It cannot be punctured and is not stopped by small obstacles, but it does still transmit more vibration through the chair.

Suspension Forks

A manual wheelchair is more agile with smaller caster wheels. They also allow the footrests to come in closer—your heels have to be more forward to allow for larger wheels and the space they need to rotate around the vertical axle. Having your feet closer in means your overall length is reduced, so you can turn around in a tighter space.

But small caster wheels mean you can feel every little bump as you wheel, meaning cracks in the sidewalk, joints between paving tiles, or the cracks between floorboards. You can imagine that there are many surfaces you would wheel on that are anything but perfectly smooth. And if you're a wheelchair athlete, you get banged around enough, so anything to absorb some impact is welcomed.

It was after seeing wheelchair rugby that Mark Chelgren decided to design a shock-absorbing caster fork for manual chairs, and Frog Legs were born (Figure 4-11). Integrating shock absorption into the caster fork makes it possible to use smaller, harder caster wheels and still have a soft ride. For some users, that has meant freedom from inflatable caster tires, which are always going soft and, sometimes, flat. Frog Legs are available for manual chairs and in a heavy-duty version for power chairs. They have been so popular that the major manufacturers have begun to offer them as options when ordering a new chair. Some have designed caster shock-absorption forks of their own, mostly for power chairs.

Figure 4-11 Frog Legs shock-absorbing caster forks.

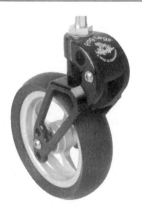

One cautionary note: there are choices for how soft or firm the caster shocks are. If you go with something softer for a smoother ride, it will also mean that the caster fork will flex if you lean forward, for instance if you are picking up something from the floor. The chair could conceivably tip in this case, so take care to specify the caster forks properly.

Suspension Systems

Cars have shock absorbers to soften the ride, so, why not wheelchairs? This thought is occurring to an increasing number of chair designers. Outdoor terrain and vibrations from wheeling on sidewalks with all of their bumps and potholes have an impact on the tissues of the body. It is not good for us to be shaken up every day, so a soft ride is protective for people who encounter lots of vibration when they wheel. If you have back discomfort that is exacerbated by the bounce of your wheelchair, adding a suspension system can reduce the impact enough to spare you some back pain.

Several manual chair designs are based on shock-absorber designs, notably the Colours Boing and the Quickie XT. The manufacturers have worked with makers of shock absorbers for bicycles, engineering specialized shocks that address the specific kinds of forces and vibrations that are inflicted on a wheelchair and its rider.

As we've already discussed, one concern about rigid frame chairs is that they are less able to keep all four wheels in contact with surfaces that are not level, such as an outdoor trail or a city sidewalk with bumps and dips. This instability can mean a temporary loss of control, which potentially could be disastrous. Independent-suspension designs enable rigid frame chairs to have better contact with the ground.

Shock absorption is common to many power chair designs, especially those with independent suspensions. Heavy-duty outdoor power chairs particularly rely on shocks.

Tilt and Recline

Spending the better part of the day—especially if you plan on a serious education, working full-time, or traveling—means that there is continuous pressure on certain parts of your body. Some people also have limited ability to remain in an upright position, at risk of fainting without intermittently reclining.

Your doctor or therapist will no doubt recommend such tilting and reclining features if:

- Your upper body balance and stability are seriously limited
- Your disability involves structural deformities, spinal curvature, or muscle contracture

■   You are at risk of fainting or developing dysreflexia
■   You do not have the strength to shift your position on your own

Make sure you have expert assistance when choosing a tilt or recline system, lateral supports, and head support. It's important to make sure that you have the optimal system for your needs and that the specific models you choose are compatible with the rest of your chair.

"Tilt-in-space" and "recline" systems are distinctly different. With a recline system, only the back of the wheelchair changes its angle, whereas a tilt-in-space system brings the seat and foot rests along for the ride. There are some specific reasons why you would consider one or the other.

Reclining adds "shear forces" to your back and to your bottom. Shear pulls along the surface of your skin, which is stressful to your tissues in the same way that direct, prolonged sitting pressure puts your skin at risk of breaking down. Tilt systems involve no shear forces.

When reclining, your posture is more likely to shift in the chair. Those unable to adjust their posture once back or forward are better candidates for tilt systems. Likewise, reclining opens up the angle of the hips, which requires that you have the range of motion to be able to accommodate the open angle. Hip flexors or the hamstring muscles in the back of the legs can be tightened enough to preclude the use of a reclining system.

A recline system can also elicit spasms. A need to maintain consistent physical relationships to items, such as chair controls or ventilators, could also be compromised with a recline chair.

Tilt-in-space is not ideal for persons who work or spend time at a table, since the full tilting of the seat and legs would be blocked by the table or may even knock it over. This system would also not work if you keep a tray on the chair that must remain flat.

People with circulation issues or edema benefit from tilt, or a recline system combined with elevating leg rests, bringing you closer to a position of laying flat.

Some users find that tilt-in-space is inappropriate for social situations, where extending their legs and feet forward as they lean back is obtrusive or likely to make the user feel self-conscious.

A power chair product unique to the market is the Redman© Chief. It is a rear-wheel drive chair that is capable of reclining back to a fully lying down position, reclining only the back, and is also capable of putting the rider into full standing position. Armrests and positioning supports are designed to stay in the same relationship with the body as these changes are made (www.redmanpowerchair.com).

Armrests

Power chairs always have armrests, but many riders of ultra-lightweight manual chairs find that armrests interfere with their ability to push the chair comfortably and effectively. It's true that armrests can interfere with wheeling when you want to get your body into the push by leaning forward, and people with shorter arms in particular might find that armrests interfere with a comfortable relationship with the wheels. Armrests can also get in the way of reaching to the side or to the floor or may prevent you from being able to get close enough to a table at work or in a restaurant. In addition, armrests add weight to the chair—a significant amount in some cases. But, before you decide against armrests for your manual chair, consider the following benefits of having them:

- Armrests can help prevent spinal problems. When you put the weight of your arms on armrests, you relieve some of the load on your spine.
- Armrests may be important for transfers into and out of the chair.
- Armrests are helpful for shifting your weight in the chair, a crucial habit for the prevention of pressure sores.
- If you have limited upper body balance, your safety may depend on having the added stability that armrests provide.

Generally, armrests are removable, so nothing says that you have to use them all the time. Many chair users purchase armrests and then use them only when it is appropriate. As always, the choice depends on your individual needs and activities.

> *My habit is to get dressed while sitting in my chair, and I rely on armrests to lift myself high enough to pull up my pants. More recently I've been spending more time at the computer and find that armrests offer some relief to my neck and shoulders. Otherwise, I leave them off.*

There are several types of armrests. The typical armrest is wide enough to support the arm, padded, and covered with vinyl upholstery. This type of armrest can be ordered in the desk style—which has a shorter upholstered section allowing you to pull closer to desks and tables—or full-length, which might be important to support a lap tray if you use one.

Some armrests lock down and can be used as a grip to carry a folded chair or by people who might carry you on a stairway. If the armrests on your chair are not fixed, be certain to let people helping you know this before they attempt to lift your chair. Locking the arms of your chair will ensure that the armrests will still be with the chair when you reclaim it after an airline trip.

High-level quadriplegic riders can choose sculpted armrests, possibly with straps, to keep their arms in place. Some riders may have enough dexterity to operate a joystick control on a power chair even though their arms are generally weak. Sculpted armrests can aid them in keeping their arms in place while driving the chair. Sculpted armrests might also include supports for the hands and fingers to keep them from curling into contracture.

Many modern manual chairs have tube-design, swingaway armrests that can easily rotate away from the chair. The horizontal portion is covered with a soft, water-resistant material. These armrests tend not to be comfortable for resting your arms because they are round and not very wide. Tube-design armrests are more appropriate for doing push-ups and correcting yourself if you feel off balance.

There are also flip-up armrests, a good solution for those who need or want armrests only part of the time, but who don't want the bother of taking the armrests off and putting them back on.

Whatever type of armrests you choose, it is important to adjust them to the correct height. Armrests that are too high will lead you to elevate your shoulders, which can cause tight muscles and pain in the neck and shoulders. If armrests are too low, you will be encouraged to slump to the side to make contact, increasing the risk of developing spinal curvature.

Clothing Guards

Clothing guards—also called side guards—protect clothes from being soiled by or getting caught in the wheels. They are optional, but, if you will be riding your chair outside very much, clothing guards are a practical choice. If you live in a rainy environment or a place where it snows, these are mandatory equipment. Some armrests have built-in clothing guards. Those people who do not use armrests, or who prefer the tubular type that include no side panel, can use separate side guards. Clothing guards can be made of fabric, plastic, or metal.

The advantages of using cloth side guards are that they are lightweight and can be easily loosened when you need to move them out of the way, during transfers, for instance. The disadvantages are that the flexibility of cloth side guards makes them tend to bend outward from general use. When this happens, your clothing will not be completely contained.

Since plastic side guards do not get crushed down as the cloth ones do, they are more effective in holding in your clothing. The main disadvantage of plastic side guards is that they require extra care during transfers. You can injure your skin by hitting the hard edge, potentially causing a sore. You might also break the side guard. Finally, plastic guards can be an obstruction if you sometimes sit cross-legged in your wheelchair.

Maintaining Your Wheelchair

Whether you can physically work on your chair or not, it is extremely valuable for you to have at least some basic knowledge about the way it is put together and how it functions. The better you understand how your chair should be working—including how it should feel and even sound—the better you are able to notice early signs that something might be going wrong. This can mean the difference between a simple, inexpensive repair and a serious breakdown that could severely limit your mobility, have you waiting potentially months for a part, and cost a great deal of money. If you can't handle tools on your own, then you can ask someone else to do it under your guidance.

Your chair should feel solid. If a nut and bolt are getting loose, you'll feel a little bit of movement in the frame, for instance, which can put great stress on the overall structure of your chair and lead to significant damage. A squeak or any unusual sound or vibration can also indicate something on the verge of breakdown. The better you make note of how your chair feels when it is maintained and well-adjusted, the better you'll be able to catch situations that can be dealt with easily.

Power chair users should know where connections go—for the batteries and for the control unit. This can also be handy at an airport if your chair arrives back at the airplane door with something in the wrong place. Since power chairs have more parts than a manual chair, more things can potentially go wrong, so knowing your chair is of even greater value.

For manual chair users with the dexterity (and tinkering aptitude), basic skills like being able to change tires, tighten up a sling seat or adjustable back, and clean and adjust brakes are very useful. Everybody should have an air tank or small battery-operated pump on hand to keep tire pressures full.

Your chair is a vehicle and, because it is customized to you and your needs, is simply not replaceable during a period of disrepair or being "in the shop." It's just like a car—you should take good care of it with regular basic maintenance and not delay getting it attention whenever something doesn't seem right.

Wheeling Style and Technique

It is the nature of the body to become highly coordinated simply from the act of doing—the more you perform a particular task, the better your nervous and muscle systems integrate the very fine movements and myriad decisions that add up to mastery. Wheeling becomes as natural and second nature as walking. All of us can remember learning a skill that was awkward at first, whether it was tying shoes, playing a musical instrument, or cutting vegetables. This "practice-makes-perfect" principle applies to driving your wheels.

Optimal Wheeling

In order to become adept at maneuvering your wheelchair, you need the right chair, properly adjusted for your needs and well-maintained. Time and practice will lead naturally to expertise in how you and your chair move through space. Style and grace will distinguish you as a true master of your wheels.

Need for Speed

Faster isn't always better, for the obvious reason that you could be thrown from your wheels. Too much speed makes it harder to control the chair, as you must brace your body against the various forces and sheer momentum of traveling so fast. Turning corners at high speed is a maneuver of extra risk, with centrifugal forces trying to keep your body going straight as you turn the chair.

Some manual chair riders wheel quickly to demonstrate their dexterity and agility to the outside world:

> Looking back, I can see how much I was invested in being the hotshot wheelchair rider in the early years of my disability, which happened when I was a teen. Wheeling slowly somehow made me feel more disabled, a purely psychological response to how I imagined the public saw me. Surely, I seemed to think, if they see how agile and strong I am with my wheels, they won't think I'm a "cripple" and everything I imagined to be associated with that image.

Although it's only human to consider how others perceive us, it doesn't really matter what others think or what their cultural assumptions might be in regard to disability. If your first concern is how you appear to others, then you are less focused on where you're going and are using your body inefficiently, making you more likely to bump into something or jam a thumb on the brake.

For manual chair wheelers, frenetic wheeling wastes energy, is more fatiguing, and even puts the body at risk, such as for developing shoulder tendonitis. If you allow brief breaks between pushes, bringing your arms back in an unrushed manner, you will do fewer pushes for the same distance and expend less effort. A well-adjusted chair with well-inflated tires will coast more easily, helping ensure that you won't have to exert yourself unnecessarily.

By taking your time, you also reduce the cumulative strain on your shoulders, elbows, and wrists, which could ultimately cost you the ability to use a manual chair. Some people who are aging with disabilities are losing the ability to push a manual chair. Slow down just a bit, and you will have more grace and more energy for your day and will preserve independence throughout your lifetime. You can certainly still have fun in your wheels.

> I have a favorite block in San Francisco with a really wide
> sidewalk. It doesn't slope too steeply toward the street but has
> a great downhill slope at a moderate pitch. It's perfect because
> I can build up some good speed, but not so fast I lose control.
> Better than most amusement park rides!

Negotiating Curbs and Obstacles

Certain wheelchair features aid in negotiating curbs and other obstacles. Larger, air-filled wheels and casters go over curbs more easily than hard, smaller wheels. Shock absorbers or an independent suspension system also help in getting over changes in surface level. Some power chairs with front-wheel drive are better able to handle a modest curb.

Wheelies?

For manual chair riders, riding over obstacles can often be accomplished with wheeling skill, using the wheelie technique—tipping back on the two main wheels. Occupational and physical therapists teach the technique to chair riders who they feel have sufficient strength and balance. The chair will need to be properly adjusted so that the axle is not too far forward—which makes the chair prone to tipping over backward too easily during normal wheeling—or too far backward.

Knowing how to do a wheelie makes it possible to wheel up or down (jump) curbs (Figure 4-12). A highly skilled wheeler can hop curbs several inches high. Some riders can even wheel down a series of steps, assuming each step is wide enough to stop on and allow the riders to check their balance. In some situations, the ability to do wheelies might make the

Figure 4-12 Using the wheelie technique at a curb. Photos A and B show going up a curb; C and D show going down a curb.

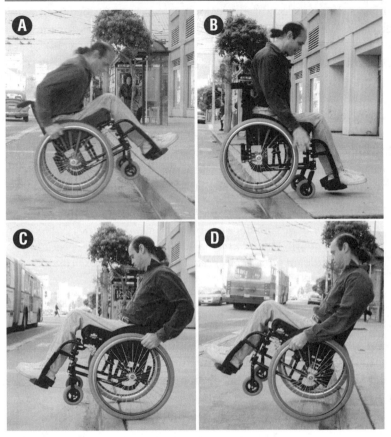

difference between doing it yourself and asking for help, may make it unnecessary for you to have to go out of your way to get to a ramp, and may allow you to independently escape in an emergency.

Wheelies can help even when there is a ramp or curb cut. When you approach a ramp going upward, a good push at the base just before the incline gives you momentum to get started up the ramp, saving you much energy. If you raise the casters slightly at the same time, you will maintain better momentum. You will not have to overcome the resistance of the casters against the upward-sloping pavement.

If you must wait for a light before crossing the street at a curb cut, don't go down the curb cut until your way is clear. That way you can use the momentum of going down the curb to help you get back up the crown of the street. Use whatever downhill energy you can, rather than wasting it by stopping at the bottom and having to push uphill with your own power. Doing a slight wheelie as you go down the curb cut will also help you use your momentum to get up the rise in the street. Techniques like this take some practice and, of course, depend on your strength and balance. If you are still working with a physical therapist, you can discuss developing these skills.

Another advantage of the wheelie is that it gives you an opportunity to change your position. Reclining by doing a wheelie changes the pressures on the spine and allows muscles of the upper body to relax, since the back of the chair is now carrying more of your weight. As one chair user notes:

> I'm fond of tipping back against a wall and putting my
> brakes on because I find the change in posture to be a
> great relief.

Each rider has to find his own limits and account for the dangers of any wheeling technique. Going down stairs alone entails obvious risks. Don't attempt such methods until you've gained confidence through practice with someone to check you against a fall. First, explore your abilities and limits.

Zen Wheeling

Zen Buddhism is a practice in which you bring your full attention into the present moment, instead of reviewing the past or planning the future. Wheeling can be like a Zen meditation exercise. The principle of mindfulness—observing the forces at play right now—can be applied to driving your wheelchair. For instance, riders often encounter very tight spaces. The more patient—or present and observing—you are, the less likely you are to bump into one side or the other, jam a finger, or damage your chair in the process.

Similarly, when you are wheeling along a sidewalk—which is typically sloped toward the street for water drainage—the downhill wheel needs to be pushed a bit harder or the joystick pulled a bit to the side to keep you on a straight line. The more aware you are of the sometimes subtle forces at play on you or your chair, the more accurately you can respond with just the right amount of effort at the right time to keep yourself traveling on a steady path. The better you observe the cracks, potholes, slopes at doorways, metal plates, and various other features of the terrain, the better you can make the fine adjustments in wheeling that they require of you.

When there is a slight rise in a section of concrete, you will want to give a little extra push to raise the front casters very slightly over it, or you will want to slow your power chair just a bit as you approach, then accelerate over it.

You can also use your body weight, gently pushing against the back of the chair to slightly lift weight from the casters.

When you are pushing a manual chair up a slope, take your time and feel the forces you are working against. You can waste a lot of effort if you try to go fast, maintain a consistent speed, or always travel in a straight line. If you use your arms fluidly with the shoulders, apply your upper body weight as your balance allows, and note subtle changes in sideways slope, you can find wheeling uphill a calming experience. Sometimes you will even need to allow yourself to slow substantially or stop completely for a moment as you reposition your arms for the next push. The climb will be good exercise, and it will seem that you got up that slope pretty quickly because you stopped worrying how long it was going to take.

When you pay attention and your chair seems like an extension of your body, you will be amazed at the sensitivity to your surroundings you can develop. For example, you will find you are able to judge curb heights or spaces between cars in a parking lot by fractions of an inch.

Riders of both manual and power chairs develop elegance in the way they move. The relationship of your awareness to your terrain and your sense in your body of what you feel through your chair is exactly the kind of integral experience taught by Buddhist masters. Wheeling with mindfulness will preserve your energy, reduce stress, and even protect you from the chance of an accident. You might even find that the quality of attention to other aspects of your life will improve.

View a series of brief, video examples of wheeling techniques at www.lifeonwheels.net/wheeling.

Chapter 5

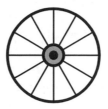

Intimacy, Sex, and Babies

Whatever your situation—newly injured or living with a disability all your life, young or mature, single or in a committed relationship—sexuality is a part of your nature and a component of your intimate relationships that need not be sacrificed, regardless of the degree of your impairments. You can find a way to express your sexuality in a way that is satisfying and meaningful for you and your partner.

Adjusting to a new disability has its difficulties. Some loss of sexual function occurs with many injuries and disabling conditions. However, this is a matter of adaptation. You are fully deserving of love and sensual experience. Understanding the physiological impact of your disability is crucial to knowing your limits and, therefore, your possibilities. Unrealistic expectations are far more destructive to your sensual life than are the actual physical limits.

Advances have been made that allow paralyzed men to participate in intercourse and fathering a child. Women's experience of sex—a topic largely neglected in the rehabilitation community until recently—is getting more attention, in addition to the question of having babies.

Sexual Beings

Is sex possible for a disabled person? Absolutely.

Is childbearing possible for a disabled person? That depends.

These are big questions. It is human nature to desire intimacy and to reproduce. These needs are in no way diminished by a disability.

243

Sexuality is different from "normal" for a person with a disability, often in dramatic ways. You will need to ask questions, experiment, and perhaps readjust some of your notions of what sexuality means. There are physical limits and adjustments you might face that can affect your sexual options.

At the Baylor College of Medicine, the Center for Research on Women with Disabilities conducted an extensive study, drawing from the responses of 475 women with disabilities and 406 able-bodied women. Margaret Nosek, PhD, principal investigator in the Baylor study, says about that study:

> We found that women with and without disability had the
> same level of sexual desire, but the women with disabilities
> experienced a lot of frustrations and barriers in having sexual
> activity at the level that they wanted. They had trouble find-
> ing partners, and so the rate of marriage and of living with a
> partner was much lower for women with disabilities.[1]

Ultimately, the study is reassuring.

> What we also found is that many women with disabilities
> have overcome the effect of those [negative] stereotypes and
> have had wonderful success in developing relationships, fami-
> lies, and satisfying lives.[1]

Especially interesting is the finding that level of disability is unrelated to the level of sexual functioning or satisfaction. Other factors were found to be the cause of limited dating, relationship, marriage, and childbearing options.

Even for the most confident women with disabilities, it was harder for them to find partners. Nosek observes about the Baylor study:

> There were many, many women in our study who were very
> self-confident, had high self-esteem, had a positive body
> image, and yet they still experience big problems finding part-
> ners. The reasons they cited were that potential partners were
> afraid of their disability, couldn't handle physical limitations,
> or assumed the woman was not interested in sex.

This woman has been with her partner for the last 20 years:

> Many things have changed. When I was young, I defined
> myself as a sexual athlete of sorts. I liked playing around
> with everybody. I enjoyed experimenting with wild posi-
> tions, etc.

> *Well, that ain't me no more. Now, most intercourse positions*
> *are simply too painful or too fatiguing for me (including*
> *some of my former favorites). The medications I take to*
> *keep the depression at bay also make it difficult to achieve*
> *orgasm. I've begun to get my gut around the notion that*
> *sex is 99% mental, and that the point of sex is to share*
> *love with someone.*

In a study on sexual response in women with spinal cord injury (SCI) conducted by Marca Sipski, MD, and Craig Alexander, PhD, at the Kessler Institute for Rehabilitation in New Jersey, they found that:

> *When questioned about activities and preferences, there was*
> *no significant change pre-SCI and post-SCI in the types of*
> *activities, nor was there any relation to the extent of injury.*
> *Where sexual satisfaction significantly decreased after SCI,*
> *sexual desire did not diminish.*[2]

The study goes on to conclude that those who had a greater number of partners pre-injury had more partners post-injury. Sexual experience and confidence have been found to correlate with successful sexual adaptation for those who acquire a disability. Someone with a disability since childhood will face unique adjustments, in contrast to the way their peers will experience puberty.

There are indeed challenges, but most chair users still have many options for sensual contact available to them. You can discover that you are not only still a very sexual being, but that sex in the context of disability can offer some surprising and gratifying new experiences.

Intimacy and Sexual Pleasure

Sexual function actually plays only a partial role in the overall experience of authentic intimacy. Caring touch by itself can be truly satisfying—loving and being loved, giving and receiving it—and still rich with erotic possibilities is a powerful human exchange in and of itself. Love can be expressed in an infinite variety of ways, as simple as a touch or a kiss or cuddling together. These experiences do not necessarily require genital contact, are clearly available to anyone, and in the context of disability often rise to higher levels of preference and satisfaction.

At its ultimate, sexual intimacy is an experience of unity, of joining, of feeling as if there is no longer any boundary between you and your partner. For couples who don't have this deep a romantic connection, sex is nonetheless an act of trust, a choice to make yourself vulnerable, and an opportunity to share the incredibly powerful experience of human sexuality. The remarkable sensations, the sense of bliss, the shift in consciousness, and the quality of relief and clarity are all life experiences possible in sexual intimacy. These qualities are no less available to people with disabilities. They might simply take other forms. The emotional, in fact, is a necessary foundation, as for this woman:

> *While I enjoy the physical experience of sex, for me it is more*
> *an emotional experience than a physical one; if I am not emo-*
> *tionally/psychologically/spiritually engaged, then I am not*
> *physically aroused.*

Sexuality is about fun and trust and sharing pleasure with another person. Sexuality empowers you with self-worth and reduces the stresses of your daily life. It can even be healing.

Mitch Tepper is the founder of the Sexual Health Network and holds a doctorate in human sexuality education. Tepper—himself quadriplegic, married and a parent—has noticed that, although there is much written about issues of erection, ejaculation, pregnancy, and disability in marriage, there is little said about sexual pleasure for people with disabilities.

> *There is growing evidence that sexual knowledge and*
> *sexualself-esteem are related to the ability to experience*
> *sexual pleasure. It seems that knowledge is power, power*
> *fuels self-esteem, and self-esteem opens the door to sexual*
> *pleasure.*[3]

Getting It On

Although love in an intimate committed relationship contributes in its own particular way to sexual pleasure, it is by no means a mandatory ingredient. Erotic experience comes in many, many forms, including casual sex— an activity in which some people with disabilities find that society somehow doesn't believe they are entitled to participate. A different set of possibilities arise with someone you don't intend to partner with in life, but with whom you share a desire to explore sensual experience in a safe, consensual interaction.

Naturally, your personal values or perhaps religious views will inform your choices regarding with whom you choose to have sexual experiences, but, remember the most important rule: ensure your safety, both physically and emotionally. Your greatest potential for sexual pleasure—and all the benefits of self-esteem, physical release, and sense of personal wholeness— happen when you are with someone who equally wants to share the benefits of the experience. If you've found a sexy friend who is game for respect-ful, consensual sex, you're entitled.

Culture and Sexual Mechanics

Modern culture places so much emphasis on the mechanics of sex that the range of sexual possibilities becomes very narrow. Advertising, media, and the easy availability of explicit materials on DVD and the Internet focus on the clinical act of intercourse. This focus places undue strain on sexual adjustment to a disability, as this woman with traumatic brain injury says:

> *Results-oriented sex—he gets one big O [orgasm], I get one*
> *(or three), then we've "had sex"—is not very compatible with*
> *what my body likes right now. Too bad I've grown up in a cul-*
> *ture that trumpets this sort of sex above all others.*

Men are expected to maintain an erection and complete the sexual act in ejaculation. For women, the ability to move their hips and to control the vaginal muscles seem indispensable.

Orgasm is particularly glorified as the indispensable goal of sexual con-tact. Glorya Hale, in *Sourcebook for the Disabled*, says:

> *Although the aim of most sexual expression may be reaching*
> *orgasm, it's clearly not necessary to have an orgasm for both*
> *partners to achieve intense sexual satisfaction.*[4]

Initially, any sexual limitations at variance with "norms" as described by the culture can appear to mean a life sentence of loneliness and sensual depri-vation. This is simply not true, unless you allow yourself and your options to be defined externally rather than by your own desires and imagination.

Cultural pressures are hard on everyone. Able-bodied persons also struggle to find true sexual identity amidst this cultural noise and the emphasis on externals—large breasts, sculpted muscles, the right car, etc. For a person with a disability, the challenge to find sexual identity can seem horribly amplified. False cultural myths promoted for commercial motives can rob you of self-esteem and incorrectly lead you to believe that you have no sexual identity.

Recent Disability

Immediately after an injury or the onset of a disabling disease, your previ-ous sense of self remains intact, although it might not feel that way at first. It takes some time for sudden and dramatic change to be integrated, and it may not be an easy process. Redefining your sexual identity is part of the larger process of finding your identity as a person with a disability. It is natural and understandable that concerns about sexuality would arise early after the onset of a disability.

Sandra Loyer, clinical social worker at the University of Michigan Medical Center, works in the Department of Physical Medicine and Rehabilitation. Loyer is part of the team that is immediately involved with patients with SCIs. She says:

> There are guys who come out of surgery and their first question is "Will I ever get it up?"

People also labor under their existing beliefs, as reported by women studied by the Baylor College of Medicine.

> For women disabled in adulthood, it is often a realization of their worst nightmare. The have grown up absorbing the social stereotype that women with disabilities are asexual and are a burden to their families, and they feel that this type of life has now been thrust upon them.[5]

It is equally true that a strong male role is presumed, where men are the protectors and seducers of women. A disability forces a core reassessment of what it is to be a man or a woman in society and tests your ability to disengage from socially implied roles and find your own way.

Often, medical personnel, counselors, family, and friends find the topic of sex and disability uncomfortable. They avoid the issue and unintentionally reinforce the notion that sex is not an option. Yet there are people who are familiar with sex and disability—an increasingly well-studied topic—who can comfortably answer your questions and guide you in your efforts to achieve an integrated sexual identity.

In their book *Enabling Romance*, Ken Kroll and Erica Levy Klein tell of a man with quadriplegia who had been told by his doctor that he could not be sexual. Then he met a woman with whom he had an immediate physical attraction.

> Much to Gary's delight, he found that, despite his being paralyzed, his relationship with Beverly awakened feelings of sexual excitement he never thought he'd experience again.[6]

They achieved a long-lasting marriage and satisfying sex life. A 23-year-old woman born with cerebral palsy recalls:

> I think the toughest thing about sex with a disability you are born with is the assumption that you are so innocent and

*childish you don't think about that stuff. I didn't date in high
school. I ended up being good friends with people, but none of
the guys would have thought to date me. I met my first when
I was 19. He's also disabled, and we had a very passionate
relationship.*

There is often not time in rehab to address sexuality when other medical and rehabilitation tasks must take priority. Staff might also be lacking sufficient training in sexuality. Sexuality educator Mitch Tepper gives seminars on sexuality and disability to professionals and observes:

*I am surprised at how little training rehab staff have received
about the unique needs of people with disabilities with regard
to their sexual identity.*

The problem is more pronounced for people who acquire their disability at a young age:

*I learned nothing about sexuality or reproduction in rehab
because I was in a children's rehab hospital and I guess the
powers that be didn't think young people should know about
sexuality.*

In the Baylor study, only 59% of women felt that they had received adequate information about how their disability affects their sexual functioning.[5]

Don't allow anyone to convince you that sex is no longer an option, regardless of your disability. Success is possible in ways you may not have yet explored.

In *Enabling Romance*, Randi—a nurse who discovered a deep relationship with Tom, a quadriplegic, while he was a patient in rehab—describes his change after they became intimate sexually:

*It is in this one area that I've seen Tom change from a shy boy
into a confident man. These changes have carried over into
other parts of our relationship and into his ability to cope
with his disability and the world in general.*[6]

The process of exploring your capacities for sexual function, your sexual style, and your sexual identity is one that takes time, as your body reaches medical stability and as you begin to learn from your own experience. Time is on your side. According to Mitch Tepper:

*Time since injury is associated with a general increase in self-
esteem; however, an increase in sexual self-esteem often lags
until people face the issue of their sexuality. That is the point
where there is growth potential.*

Putting Sex Aside

You are not obligated to be sexually active, as people who practice abstinence by choice will tell you. You might be engaged in work or a have community of friends and family that is intimate and satisfying, that provides
you with affection and fun and affirmation. Intimacy takes many forms, and
not everyone needs to be sexually active in order to feel whole.

It can also be understandable to choose to set sexuality aside when
your disability demands so much of you in addressing day-to-day matters.
Reasons to abstain might include the difficulty of finding a partner, pain,
medical challenges, or the simple loss of the urge—more likely repressed
than actually gone. You might be taking medications that suppress sexual
impulses. You may need to integrate these other issues of adaptation into
your life first, moving on to sex when the time is right for you.

Some people may use their disability to avoid sexual issues that have
no real relationship with the disability itself. Disability can be a convenient
excuse to simply give up the game, driven by fears of which you may not
even be fully aware. However, not addressing fears or other feelings means
that you might miss out on the potential for greater personal fulfillment
through discovery of your sexual identity—all the more in the context of
your disability.

Past abuse, failure, or adjustment to your disability might simply feel
overwhelming. A period of recovery and healing might be necessary and
entirely appropriate before you can address your sexual identity. Just
remember that, for many people with disabilities, these issues have been
surmountable.

Emotional Struggles

All of us face the work of sorting through our sexual psyche. The challenge
of discovering your identity as a sensual disabled person can bring new levels of exploration to this universal life process in which absolutely everybody
is engaged. Ultimately, our deepest needs are for intimacy, affection, trust,
and love. Some people find that they are able to live a lifestyle abstaining
from sexual activity yet rich in these affirming qualities in relationship. In
the *Journal of Rehabilitation*, A. Frankel notes:

> *Most people have unconscious conflicts about sex which they
> keep buried. A devastating injury or disease serves to unearth
> these conflicts.*[7]

Loss of sexual function—multiplied by the burden of inaccurate messages from some healthcare providers, family, and the broader society—

can erode your self-confidence. If you were already struggling with issues of sexuality prior to your disability, they will certainly not just disappear. They will have an impact on your overall adjustment and so need to be addressed as directly as are the physical or social aspects of your disability experience.

Even if you accept that you will have some sexual limits, and you want to relax and have as much pleasure as possible for yourself and your partner, there can be a feeling of having been left on the sidelines. You might find yourself experiencing feelings of resentment toward your partner for having what seems to be a more substantial sexual response than you experience. Despite the advice of many rehab professionals or well-meaning loved ones, "thinking positively" is not necessarily easy, independent of doubts or painful emotions, nor is it automatic. You may want to take pleasure in your partner's enjoyment and in providing your partner with sexual satisfaction, but you may still struggle with other feelings. If negative feelings can't be worked out through trusting communication, the support of a counselor may be called for if you want the relationship to succeed.

Able-bodied partners may find themselves feeling guilty over the fact that they are capable of sensations that are not possible for you. Just as you may struggle with emotions unique to your sexual experience, the feelings an able-bodied partner might experience are natural and deserve to be recognized and discussed. Often these feelings can be brought into perspective, if not altogether resolved. A partner experiencing guilt, for example, can learn that his pleasure actually reinforces your confidence in yourself as a sexual partner. The real issue is equal pleasure, not equal intensity.

Overemphasizing Intercourse

For those who were sexually active prior to their disability, the memory of sexual sensations remains, amplifying their sense of loss. They know what they are missing, so the idea of redefining their sexuality might feel like nothing more than compromise and loss. These feelings need not last as you discover what previous—and new—pleasures are available.

People disabled prior to the loss of virginity might carry an unresolved curiosity about intercourse—feelings that might never be satisfied in their lifetime. They might envy the general able-bodied population and imagine an able-bodied sex life to be more ideal than it actually is.

Losing the capacity for intercourse in adolescence includes some unique issues, coming at a time when the anticipation of a first sexual experience is extremely high. This grand sense of expectation can linger for a long time. A meaningful rite of passage has been missed. Experience ultimately teaches us that our maturity is based on values and accomplishments—and pleasures—other than genital intercourse.

Staying stuck in what you want to happen increases the distance between you and your partner. It reinforces your association of tragedy with your disability and costs you the pleasures that remain.

For a person with a disability, sex may become more precious precisely because of the existence of limitations. Once you have lost certain options, those that remain become more valued. If you experienced early fears that sexual activity might not be an option—or worried that sex would be complicated—the discovery of deep intimacy in a relationship becomes all the more treasured. Changing the emphasis from intercourse to sensuality and caring intimacy—wherever it may lead—is key.

A 1993 study of men with SCI performed by Drs. Craig Alexander, Marca Sipski, and Thomas Findley of the Kessler Institute for Rehabilitation in New Jersey found that

> Post-injury there was a dramatic reduction in the percentage
> of subjects engaging in penis-vagina intercourse. The majority
> of subjects preferred penis-vagina intercourse pre-injury. Post-
> injury, however, subjects seemed to prefer a wider variety of
> sexual activities with not as strong a preference for one activ-
> ity. Moreover, preference for penis-vagina intercourse
> decreased substantially while preference increased for oral
> sex, kissing, and touching.[8]

Once you gain sexual experience in the context of your disability, you will find that your relationships are not defined by your disability as much as you might have imagined.

> I'm blessed with having had a relationship with a very won-
> derful and loving woman. Although we are no longer together,
> it is not because we failed as a couple, but that the circum-
> stances of our lives did not allow us to make a commitment at
> that time. This experience left me with a very great gift: I can
> no longer doubt that someone could ever be attracted to me
> because of my disability.

Redefining Orgasm

Orgasm is different for everyone, defined in each individual's terms. If you have acquired a disability later in life, you should know that you can redefine what orgasm is for you, even if it is different from what it might have been in the past. As this married C5 quadriplegic man found:

> An orgasm is really in your mind. Sure, before my accident there were sensations that felt good, but it feels just as good in my mind.[9]

Orgasm is not exclusively either physical or mental. Or emotional. The feelings and chemistry if you are being sexual with a partner—as compared to stimulating yourself—are all part of the formula as well. All of it is part of the whole, all of it interacts, and all of it is brought to bear in the course of redefining orgasm—toward the goal of allowing yourself the most optimal experience and pleasure your body allows. As this woman with an SCI learned:

> I had to relearn HOW to have an orgasm. The physical sensation of orgasm changed for me—different post-SCI than pre-SCI—and I had to learn to recognize the physical sensations of arousal (in my "New Body"). I needed to allow orgasm to occur emotionally, to feel the building of arousal, to emotionally and psychologically participate in the arousal, and to LET GO and ride the tide, as it were. At one point it was much less a physical process than an emotional one; having a lover who had a vasectomy—which totally relieved me of ANY fear of pregnancy—had a very interesting effect; I could really relax and revel in the physical sensations. It took me a while to realize how much fear of unplanned pregnancy had inhibited my enjoyment of sexual intimacy.

The Macho Problem

There are a lot of ways that a man identifies himself as manly. Physicality is a big part of this, whether it's about being a construction worker or an athlete—in bed or otherwise. Loss of physical capacity is a major adjustment when your very identity is substantially based on it. That is where men's sense of power resided, that's how you impressed and attracted your intimate partner. It's a real loss.

In fact, men are wired by evolution and culture to play the role of protector and provider. As much as historically recent social changes point men toward being more "sensitive" and women are sharing more of the financial load, the expectation to protect and provide is deeply set in men. A disability is a direct threat to that part of what the male psyche thinks it is supposed to be.

Is it just as manly—and attractive—to be a person who has a strong sense of yourself, who believes in values that are infused throughout your life and actions, that you mean your word and are reliable, are decisive, and are able to do your share in getting your needs met and those of the ones you love? Try to look beyond the physical, and you might well find that there is plenty to base your masculine identity on, and that you're anything but "crippled."

Which brings us to the penis. Granted, it may not be up to its usual performance, and perhaps you are no longer capable of ejaculation—something you and your partner might have valued a great deal. More real loss, absolutely.

When it comes to erection, though, you probably don't have much to worry about. The pharmaceutical solutions that are out there—be they pill or injection—work really well once you learn how to use them. In some cases, men with higher level SCIs are prone to dysreflexia that preclude the use of these drugs, but that is something to be explored and possibly solved working with your urologist.

Which brings us back to the question of what it is to be a man. In heterosexual relationships, at least, many women report that their men are in too much of a rush for insertion, and, once that happens, ejaculation is not far off. All done, lovemaking over. Too quick for a lot of women. Ask around, and women will tell you it's true.

Since you don't have to rush—either because you know your erection is not going to suddenly go limp or because you've learned to love the kind of foreplay that your partner wants more of, you might just find your new sexual style is actually—in some truly meaningful ways—more appealing to your partner. You might find yourself being considered more of a man, not less.

It's no small adjustment. Letting go of such a strong basis of your sense of self as your current masculine identity is heavy stuff. But it's doable, and there is an even stronger self on the other side, with plenty of pleasure to go around.

Partners

You might already be in a committed relationship, have a sexual partner and wonder if it's going to last, or be thinking about embarking on a search for a new partner. Each relationship has its particular dynamics, but all involve how you feel about your body.

Your Body Image

The body goes through certain changes—depending on the given disability—about which you might feel insecure or self-conscious. Muscle atrophy that results in very thin, sometimes skeletal limbs is common with SCI. Amputees have their stumps. There might be scars from surgeries, leftover effects of skin rashes, burns, or other skin conditions. Higher-level spinal disabilities can result in a distended stomach and loss in tone in the abdominal muscles. People with quadriplegia have curled fingers and thin hands that they cannot use for handshaking or for certain sexual activities. Spinal fusions or the insertion of rods in the spine can impose a very upright posture that others may misinterpret as an uptight body language. You might adopt a stiff posture for fear that movement will induce muscle spasms. Your disability might entail different shapes or proportions in your body or limbs. These physical realities all affect the signals put out to potential partners. They also influence your sense of self. For this woman with paraplegia, this was a central part of her sexuality and disability process:

> I had to work through the emotional process of growing into
> the belief that my body is a way to be in the world three-
> dimensionally, but is NOT the ultimate expression of my
> being. I came to the belief that my metaphysical self is more
> ME than my physical self. My body is a way of manifesting
> who I really am, not the TRUTH of who I am.

Over time, you will adapt to your "new normal" because you will no longer have the point of reference to what your body looked like prior to your disability. You become accustomed to your new shape, and it is just your familiar body. This might sound like it's another quality of loss, but, in fact, it's a feature of the amazing adaptive capacity of your being human. This, of course, has something to do with how well you take care of yourself: remember, body-image issues are not unique to disability but affect everyone. Your body-image issues are different and particular to your disability, but take care not to fall into the notion that someone who is able-bodied is confident in their body simply because they don't have a disability and you do.

Your wheelchair becomes part of your body image and is part of what people react to when they first meet you, so body image is a factor in your choice of wheelchair—although it shouldn't outweigh function. Choose a chair that fits your personality, but make sure that optimal mobility and safety get the highest priority.

Body image is a powerful force in how the world views you as a sexual person, as this paraplegic woman in her 30s found out in the early years after an SCI:

> It wasn't easy at all to develop my sexual identity as a dis-
> abled teenager. I was 14, so I never got to wear hose or walk
> in high heels. Our culture defines so much of a female's sexu-
> ality by the appearance of her legs.

She went on to marry, have children, and discover a clear and satisfying sexual identity for herself.

> *I don't have time to feel sorry for myself as a woman in a wheelchair because I'm embracing life now.*

The Baylor study reports:

> *Women with disabilities who had a more positive sexual self image and who perceived themselves to be approachable by potential romantic partners also had higher levels of sexual activity.*[5]

It's not hard to imagine that these things would be true for men as well. As one woman explained, "The sexiest thing to me is self-confidence." Feelings of shame and embarrassment can be overwhelming, yet, again and again, people with disabilities have found that these feelings become irrelevant in the presence of a trusted, intimate partner.

Existing Couples

There is a cultural assumption that an able-bodied person who stays with someone after the occurrence of a disability is either masochistic or heroic. This is among the most inaccurate of cultural assumptions about disability. Ultimately, people stay together because of love and loyalty, not obligation or sacrifice. Some couples will stay together, some won't. Staying together is more about people and their values and what they mean to each other, not any social notions about being an "invalid" or a "caretaker."

> *My doctor told me that I would have to forget about my girlfriend and move on to others. It turned out that he was right, but not especially because of my acquired disability. It was getting time to move on anyway. She might very well have made the transition with me if she were the right partner for me in the first place.*

When love is real, it shows, as this wheelchair user discovered:

> *I had a conversation on an airplane with an accomplished businessman who told me about a young couple who were recently married. The man had become a quadriplegic during the engagement, and they still got married. My flying partner said that many people doubted her motives or their chances of success. They saw a woman giving up her future. I asked what he saw. He answered, "Two people in love."*

A sudden disability can be a strain to an existing relationship. Some couples might have allowed sexuality to be so much the foundation of their relationship that, in the presence of a sudden disability, they don't have enough of a foundation in the other aspects of their relationship to carry them through. The issue of changes in their sexual relations can be the final straw that breaks apart a couple whose relationship was not strong to begin with.

In the Baylor study of women with disabilities,[5] several issues with existing partners were reported.

- A woman with a disability may blame herself for everything that goes wrong in a relationship.
- Her husband may take advantage of her self-blame and collude in blaming all their marital problems on the disability.
- Nearly half of women with partners responding to the study sometimes felt like a burden to their partners.
- Nearly half also felt that their relationship suffered because they were less able to contribute to housework or participate in previously enjoyed activities.

Baylor's Dr. Margaret Nosek states:

> *You find relationships that go beyond the physical. Many women reported they found new kinds of activities they can do with their partners. If the relationship is good, they'll find other doors that can be opened.*

Some reported cases of later-onset disability, in which the men they were with just couldn't deal with it, and it broke up their marriage. In other cases, it didn't, it made them significantly closer. Success in marriage didn't depend on when the disability happened, whether they were born with it, or if it happened later in life.

Some couples don't succeed. A man who broke his neck 10 years into his marriage recounts the subsequent breakup of his marriage. His wife had been very supportive during his rehabilitation and return home, but then they ran into severe difficulties:

> *The only thing that I was so disappointed about in her was she was so fearful of making love to me again. And I wanted to please her needs, not worried about my pleasure. Maybe 5% curious to find out if I could do more than I was told. For 14 months, every time I would bring up the subject she would say, "I'm not ready yet," and end of discussion!*

Then two months later, her reply would be, "I don't know if I'll ever be ready." Before I was injured, our sex life was great; we did just about everything to please each other.

In October, we had our 11-year wedding anniversary. The first Friday of November, she came home later than usual and said, "I don't know how to tell you this, but I want a divorce. If you hadn't broken your neck I wouldn't be leaving."

The statistics about couples staying together are encouraging. The rate of divorce after disability is only slightly higher than in the nondisabled population. Successful couples have achieved a bond that goes beyond simple matters of sexual function. Though important, loss of sexual options have less impact than you might think on an existing relationship that is strong. Such a couple is capable of accommodating the disability and enjoying each other. A woman in her 40s describes her relationship:

I married my partner because we communicate so well. Talking about sex is not easy to do, but it's critically important. At first, all discussions had to take place well away from the bedroom because there's lots of potential for hurt feelings and misunderstanding in the heat of the moment.

Now I treasure the intimacy that we share. I appreciate the cuddles and the sensations that aren't painful. Hand-holding and kissing have always been wonderful. I've learned to stop thinking of these as "foreplay" and enjoy them for their own delights.

The right partner—married or not—can make an important difference in one's overall adjustment to a new disability, as this paraplegic man with an SCI says:

Fortunately, for the year prior to the accident, I was in a relationship with a strong woman. She helped me through the hard times and showed me that my sexuality—now different—could be enjoyable. She was there for me and this was very important in my recovering with a reasonable amount of sanity.

According to the University of Michigan's Sandra Loyer, men have a greater challenge adjusting to a disabling injury to their wives. She says:

They're afraid they'll hurt her, that they have nothing to offer, whereas women are more naturally nurturing. Sure, there are more sensitive men these days, but it's still harder for them.

Adjustments are possible. The following 40-year-old woman has C5 quadriplegia and has been married for 22 years. She became injured by a gunshot 18 years into her marriage.

> *We had a great sex life before my injury and we still do. My disability has never turned off my husband. We had the Big Sex Discussion while I was in rehab and had our first post-injury sex there, too. I assured him that he wasn't going to "break" me or anything. One of his concerns was about doing something wicked to the catheter. So for us, aside from the physical changes, our sex life has remained the same. I have a theory why this is: We were very much in love and very close before this happened, and we still are.*

Finding Partners

If you don't currently have an intimate partner how do you get started?

Finding love is tough enough for anyone these days. Single Americans complain more and more about the difficulty of finding companionship, much less a mate. Personals ads and Internet dating sites abound, flooded with people on the hunt for a partner. Bringing a disability into these environments is hardly an advantage.

This 23-year-old man with an SCI struggles with finding a partner:

> *My hormones are raging, but I have no outlet. I go out a lot with friends, but even friends who were potential lovers before are now certainly just friends. I can't seem to shake that "Wow, you are a great person" line. I know that in the long run I will end up with someone who is great, but I could really just go for a one-night stand or two! I'm a pretty good-looking guy, so the prospects are there, but what do I do!?*

Likewise for this woman born with a disability:

> *I would like to be involved again, but I know that I can't meet people sitting around the local bar, like many of my fellow college students. Frankly, I'm clueless.*

Women have a greater challenge finding partners. The culture has historically promoted the idea of the male as aggressor. Women were supposed to wait for men to approach. This has changed somewhat, with women more able to make the approach, but some disabled women still find that men are less likely to approach a woman with a disability.

This woman born with spina bifida found that growing up with a disability had its challenges:

> *I felt really inadequate next to my female friends. I thought they were inherently more attractive simply because they didn't use a wheelchair. I think I got around it by being more assertive. The stereotype of the woman waiting for the man to make the move didn't work for me. If I was attracted to a man, I would make the first move.*[9]

According to the Baylor study,[9] women with disabilities reported their perceptions of the obstacles to dating:

- Someone who is interested in me might not ask me out because of what others might say.
- Many people do not ask me out because they assume I am unable to have sexual intercourse.
- People seem surprised that I might be interested in sexual intimacy.
- People I would like to date see me as a friend, not as a romantic partner.

Margaret Nosek elaborates on the cultural differences that women face:

> *The nurturing role is the role of the woman. So if the woman is the one who needs the help, they're up a creek. There are very few male partners or male family members who are willing to make the sacrifices necessary to provide the kind of assistance needed by a woman with a significant disability. The man with a disability has many more resources than the woman. The man gets it because it is the traditional role of women.*

When it comes to attracting partners, women in the study found themselves in a paradox: you can scare off potential partners by aggressive pursuit, but, if you don't pursue partners, they're gone.

The good news in the search for partners is that there are more singles on the market now. People are marrying later. Women have more options for a profession and independence than society once allowed. Life expectancy is much longer as medical advances preserve our health; making a commitment when you are still young can mean being together for quite a long time, so what's the rush? With later marriages and the increased divorce rate, there are a lot of unattached folks out there looking for love.

You certainly won't meet anyone by sitting at home. You can meet people through volunteer activities, political groups, clubs of all sorts, classes at the local college or community center, or professional organizations and trade shows. Centers for Independent Living sponsor activities, including social and educational events. Although the percentage of success is not high, people do find partners through personal ads and on the Internet. It's worthwhile to say hello to someone interesting at the grocery store or movie theater. You never know. There are dating resources specifically for persons with disabilities (see the Appendix).

It is not unusual for couples to meet in hospitals or clinics. Therapists, nurses, volunteers, and other staff get a unique chance to know the person beyond the disability. Friendships form, and sometimes romance results. These can be equal and sincere meetings of people for whom the opportunity to see each other regularly allowed authentic intimacy to develop. Mitch Tepper notes:

> *These people are professionals with less fear of disability, so*
> *some are capable of forming authentic relationships.*[3]

At the same time, these relationships have no guarantee of success. Says Tepper:

> *Some people also need to control or take care of someone.*
> *That might be why they're in the health profession in the*
> *first place.*[3]

Its just reality: there are extra challenges when you have a disability. In *Enabling Romance*, a 36-year-old man used a personal ad to seek a partner. He was open about his disability and received no response, and then:

> *As an experiment I placed an ad in a magazine without*
> *mentioning I was disabled. I received three responses. I was so*
> *thrilled! But then, when I replied to their letters and explained*
> *that I was in a wheelchair, I never heard from any of them*
> *again.*[6]

This is really the only approach—be honest. It can work to first discuss other areas of interest, but don't wait too long to identify your disability. Allowing the connection to go deep before you reveal your disability is risky and can be taken as a violation of trust. Then, if the other person is unable to accept you, it is best to move on with no regrets, possibly having made a friend in the process. Yes, it can be painful and disappointing, but try to remember that you're looking for a partner with the ability to see and respect you on a deeper level than your disability.

Women can have a more difficult time finding a male partner. There is more social pressure on women to fit the supermodel image; men tend to be more attached to the public image of having a beautiful woman on their

arm. Margaret Nosek doesn't think that media images make people with disabilities aspire to fit those images so much as they lead others not to consider a person with a disability as a potential partner:

> *I think that the media have a more damaging effect on the*
> *general public than women with disabilities. I think it's very*
> *similar for men and women.*[1]

Trading Signals

Humans give out certain cues to attract a mate: a deeply ingrained, evolutionary system of physical signals. In *The Anatomy of Love*, Dr. Helen Fisher
writes that:

> *Men tend to pitch and roll their shoulders, stretch, stand*
> *tall, and shift from foot to foot in a swaying motion. Some*
> *women have a characteristic walk when courting; they*
> *arch their backs, thrust out their bosoms, sway their hips,*
> *and strut.*[10]

These signals are hard to give while sitting down, so a person on
wheels can be at some disadvantage. They must exaggerate their body language and use other signs to transmit the message of interest to someone
they might see at a party, a museum, a restaurant, and so on. According to
Fisher, the ensuing stages include getting close enough to begin a simple
conversation, achieving those first subtle touches of a forearm or shoulder,
and getting into a body synchrony, in which two people begin to mirror each
other's movements and posture. You will need to find other ways to overcome your physical limits. For instance, eye contact is very powerful and
gets the message across just fine.

The impact of your sitting in a wheelchair is undeniably powerful, and
you might find yourself drawn to circumvent its effect as did this quadriplegic woman in her early 20s:

> *I will transfer out of the chair just to break the contact to*
> *make it easier for other people to approach me.*[11]

In some cases, the message that a wheelchair sends—that the person
in it has a physical limitation—can be welcome. A man who uses a chair
because of his difficulty walking found that his awkward gait had been an
obstacle to meeting potential partners:

> *I never get the girl if she sees me walking. But if we meet*
> *where we're sitting and she gets to know me first, then*

*she realizes I'm a nice guy and it doesn't matter to her if I
walk weird.*

If you doubt someone showing signals of attraction could be interested in someone who uses a wheelchair, you might miss important cues. Be open to signals, while taking care not to mistake friendly signs for more than they are. Go gently, and allow things to take their course. Respond subtly, and if a relationship is meant to proceed, it will.

Who Are You "Limited" To?

Some people believe that they must find someone to "match" them physically. University of Michigan social worker Sandra Loyer incredulously remembers a young spinal-injured male who asked her:

*Because I'm like this does it mean the only girlfriend I can
have has to be like this too?*

Other people assume that a disabled partner will need an able-bodied partner to provide care. Relationships based on dependence may not be satisfying. Sex researcher Mitch Tepper warns:

*Be wary of relationships based solely on dependence because
they have a tendency not to succeed or be enjoyable in the
long run. Seek interdependence. You must have things to offer
the relationship, too.*[3]

You aren't limited to disabled partners nor are you limited to able-bodied partners. The goal is to be with the right partner. There are many examples of successful relationships between a person with a disability and an able-bodied partner, just as some people find advantages in being with another person with a disability. There is a pattern emerging from the various writings and studies on relationships and disability. When people let their personalities shine, take care of their health, assume interest rather than rejection, and are able to communicate openly and honestly, they are attractive human beings, disability or not.

Able-Bodied Partners

There are many more able-bodied persons out there than there are disabled persons. The odds alone seem to suggest that people with a disability need to take their search for love into the wider world. Yet, many able-bodied persons who meet a disabled person will doubt that you have sexual inclinations at all. Don't let that stop you. You might get the chance to set them straight!

Some potential able-bodied partners might have unresolved issues about disability that they could impose on you, such as insisting that you use braces rather than a wheelchair or remain under the covers in bed because they are uncomfortable with seeing your body. Unless they're willing to reassess these beliefs, they will not be an empowering partner for you.

Disabled men might consider it good news that many women are nurturing and open minded. However, according to Loyer, there are also women with less-than-ideal motivations:

> *There are women out there who find guys in wheelchairs*
> *very appealing. They might not be healthy reasons, for*
> *example, they may feel they "have them where they want*
> *them," or they are looking for men who won't mistreat them*
> *the way other men might have. It can also fulfill the need*
> *to be needed.*

There is nothing wrong with finding a nurturing person—male or female, straight or gay—but you need to know that you are recognized for who you are, not that you are only seen as "safe."

There are reasonable concerns someone could have about involvement with a person with a disability. Given the same situation, you might ask the same questions. "Will he be dependent on me, now or later in life?" "Are their emotional traumas too complex for me to deal with?" "Will it limit my freedom to do things I enjoy that she can't, like hiking in remote areas? How important is that to me?" "Will there be resistance from my family and friends?"

Mitch Tepper has an approach he calls "inoculation against rejection."

> *The answers aren't always based on you, but on their own*
> *previous experience with relationships and with people with*
> *disabilities. It might be more frightening because they're just*
> *unaware.*[3]

To build a solid relationship with an able-bodied person, these reasonable questions need to be addressed. Tackling these questions is not just for the other person's benefit; you want to know what you're getting into and whether your commitment to the relationship is based on reality.

An able-bodied woman in her 30s, asked if she imagined a disabled partner would be necessarily dependent on her, says:

> *No, not if the person was independently minded (and my*
> *impression is that most handicapped people fight very hard*
> *against the image of dependency). My concern would be that*

*they would be limited in certain activities I would want to
share with a partner (like hiking, for example). I would also
think that it would require a certain basic patience that I'm
not sure I have. I like to move fast, and I might have a problem slowing down my pace to match that of a disabled partner. But we're talking about a hypothetical partner here, so it's
hard to say.*

She has reasonable questions, knows her needs and desires, but realizes that she can't know until faced with the actual situation. It is exactly this
opening that creates the opportunity for two people who are interested and
attracted to explore how their relationship might work out. She might be
surprised to find that there are plenty of hiking possibilities they can share,
and that she might be the one who has to keep up with her disabled partner! Perhaps she might even find that hiking becomes less important in
exchange for a loyal and loving partner who enhances her life in many other
yet undiscovered ways.

Finding a comfort level around how much help an able-bodied partner will provide in day-to-day life is an important question you will face.
Given the greater degree of accessibility in the world today, and the availability of adaptive devices and technologies, couples can have less to work out
than they might think.

Often, a person with a mobility disability will imagine more reluctance
on the part of an able-bodied partner than the partner actually feels. This
able-bodied single woman in her 40s says:

*I can imagine disabilities that would be an impediment, and
others that would not. I suspect the difference would come
into play at the point of attraction, not at the point of "choice
to be sexual," though. For instance, I had no problem imagining myself in Jane Fonda's place with Jon Voight (in the film
Coming Home). Once attracted to him (hell, he's Jon
Voight!), I imagine no insurmountable problems.*

Nondisabled partners usually find out that their concerns are
unfounded. This woman in her early 40s is in a relationship with a paraplegic man and says:

*From the beginning I was attracted to him, both physically
and emotionally. Somehow I just knew that his disability
would not be an issue. For one thing, he didn't call attention
to it. As we became involved, I learned certain details like
how I can help with the wheelchair at the car and not get in
the way! But he helps me as much as I help him. It's not an*

issue. His "limitations" are not a burden, since we are so close, have such a good friendship, and are such wonderful lovers.

It is nonetheless important to ask yourself whether you might be trying to reinforce your self-image as a complete person through an involvement with a nondisabled person. It is not unusual to want to reduce your association with the identity of disability in this way. This doesn't mean that your motives are therefore suspect or tainted. A certain satisfaction can come in strengthening our connection to the broader world through a healthy relationship with an able-bodied partner. It is simply important to be aware of the degree to which you might be motivated by this issue and whether it may be distracting you from focusing on the characteristics that constitute a healthy relationship—love, trust, commitment, and shared values.

Devotees

There are people in the world, you should understand, who are stimulated by a person with a disability. You might be repelled by the thought of this as something that is unhealthy.

Everyone has something that they find more compelling about someone to whom they are attracted. Someone attracted to women might be drawn to breasts or curviness or long hair; those drawn to men might like someone muscular or with a deep voice. Anyone might like a shapely bottom or be drawn to eyes. How much different is it for someone to be drawn to a disability feature?

Consider that the issue is actually about honesty. Some of these people—and it's well-advised to take care around this—will not be open about their motives or could be more inclined to want to keep you playing a certain role, possibly a submissive one. Any relationship—short or long term—needs to be based on honesty and mutual respect for each other's preferences. If these are present, then honestly ask yourself what is actually healthy or not? As this paralyzed woman says:

We have a great friendship, really enjoy our sexual life, and he's turned on by my disability. I can't see anything wrong with this picture!

Two-Disability Couples

A couple in which both partners have a disability is a mixed blessing. It might be easier to find a partner who also has a disability, whether through disability-specializing dating services, involvement in the local disability scene or Center for Independent Living, or getting to know someone on the Internet. You might imagine that another person with a disability will be more of a kindred spirit or that you won't have to take time to explain ways that your disability impacts your life.

Such an alliance can make for a uniquely powerful intimate connection, both of you having faced the particular questions or tears surrounding sexuality in the context of your respective disabilities. They can be more sensitive to the necessary changes of a redefined sexual style, free of performance pressure and focused on the simple enjoyment and real erotic potential of touching, kissing, and the many sensual options that remain.

There are many couples with disabilities in successful relationships. But, in public, a disabled couple might not be seen in intimate terms, as this married couple found.

> *People usually assume that you're together for something other than a relationship. We've had people ask us if we were brother and sister.*[9]

But, just as an able-bodied partner might be cautious, this can be just as true for another person with a disability. After all, they have their own stuff to deal with. Why would they want to take on more? Sharing the fact of having a disability can mean camaraderie and increased intimacy, or it can be an increased burden.

It goes both ways for Cindy McCoy, writing in *New Mobility* magazine. Now in her 40s, she has had multiple sclerosis since the age of 21. McCoy is now in her third marriage, this time to a man with cerebral palsy. She writes:

> *If the compassion and camaraderie between us are deeper and more satisfying due to the shared challenge of coping with disability, then perhaps that balances the times when double disability equals double distress.*[12]

Relationships are always relationships, no matter who is involved. They can succeed or fail. It always begins with one question. Do you love each other? And then a few others. Do you communicate well? Do you have complimentary skills that you can combine to create a home and manage your day-to-day affairs? Can you build a shared social community and be confident in the individual friendships each of you should have? Are you willing to work on yourself at the same time that you are committed to working on your partnership? No matter how many disabilities there are in a relationship, those are the questions that matter.

Prostitutes and Surrogate Partners

Since it is can be difficult to find a partner, being with a "sex worker" might help address the need for sensual experience. Some have explored the use of prostitutes, such as this 26-year-old paraplegic man quoted in *Enabling Romance*:

> *Despite my paralysis, I wanted and needed sex, and prostitutes seemed like the easy way out. I was a virgin, yet I had this driving need to find out what sex was all about. I started going to this very kind and sincere call girl who taught me a lot about sex and about my own physical capabilities as a man.*[6]

The book relates that he ultimately found a steady lover.

Mitch Tepper notes that there are risks in interacting with a prostitute. At the worst, it is possible to acquire a sexually transmitted disease such as HIV from a person who has that much sexual contact with many different people. There have also been cases of a sex worker luring people into situations in which the people can be robbed. A prostitute—despite the experience noted above—is also unlikely to be sensitive to the emotional aspects of your disability experience. They might be insensitive about issues such as ability to attain or maintain an erection, scars, scoliosis, or spasms.

Some have pursued more formalized experiences using professional surrogate partners in association with sex therapists. Mitch Tepper explains:

> *It's a three-way relationship. The sex therapist assigns you a sex surrogate who helps you develop your sexual and relationship skills. They also teach you about dating, anatomy, giving and receiving pleasure. The relationship is about building your comfort level with a partner. Usually there is sex with the surrogate, but it could be toward the end of the series of meetings. A typical example would be an older person who has never had sex and feels too much pressure to succeed on their own. Their nervousness prevents them from being able to establish a sexual relationship, so the surrogate helps them over it.*[3]

These possibilities are mentioned here only as options that some disabled people have explored.

Going It Alone

Masturbation can play an important role in your discovery of a new sexual identity as a person with a disability. It might be easier than starting with a partner, no matter how recent or long-term your disability might be. The emotional demands of being with a partner at this time can be overwhelming. This is not to say that the right partner couldn't share the process of exploring your sexuality with you in an atmosphere of deep and giving acceptance. Especially if you have a recent disability and are without a partner, self-stimulation is an option that can help you find your sexual identity, preparing you to ultimately find a partner, if that is your desire.

Some redefinition is called for here, as well. Ejaculation or orgasm is not the only criterion for being sensual with yourself. Masturbation does not need to be fixed in those terms. Touching yourself, fantasizing, using vibrators, magazines, videos, or the Internet to enjoy stimulating erotic material—any of these can be a means of expressing yourself sexually. Self-loving can give you a break from sexual loneliness—an experience hardly limited to those with a disability.

There are many ways to provide pleasure to yourself. For men, a penis-sleeve—often in the form of and designed to act and feel like a vagina—is widely available. As psychologist and sexuality counselor Dr. Linda Mona recommends on her web site, MyPleasure.com:

> Try rubbing your body up against a pillow, a couch arm, or a
> portion of your wheelchair. Perform this type of stimulation
> on all parts of your body, including your penis or vagina.

Even if you don't have normal hand strength or dexterity, there is a way. Objects that can be used to stimulate the body—be they vibrators, pieces of satin, or anything you imagine would feel good against sensitive parts of your body—can be strapped to your hand.

Pornography

A special word on video and Internet sexual content. Very little of it portrays good sex in the context of authentic personal connection. The quality of interaction between the participants is extremely basic—if not base. Unwittingly, you can get drawn into the belief that anyone is secretly just waiting to get it on with you or that you're supposed to be attractive enough that they should. Your disability self could well end up feeling less validated, rather than getting the enjoyment and release you're seeking through this content.

This is not to preach that adult materials are bad for you, simply that there is a boundary to which you should give some attention, observing how you feel after you watch something erotic, and take your feelings into account around the material you choose. There is, in fact, some adult content that depicts more authentic relationships—and so more authentic sexual connection in which people are really wanting to please each other and really having satisfying sex instead of just performing for the camera. Good Vibrations (www.goodvibes.com) has a rating system for adult videos that allows you to make choices along these lines.

The Sexual Experience

When you can't feel parts of your body, or have a reduced sexual response, your priorities are a result of what is possible, and you will learn what your personal "top 10" list of intimate preferences includes. Your favorites are your favorites, and what might have been your favorite prior to an acquired disability moves to a lower priority in relation to those activities that provide you with optimal pleasure—often found in more subtle sensations. This paraplegic woman in her 30s observes:

> I'm very present when I'm having sex. I'm not thinking
> about peanut butter sandwiches. I don't know if I would
> have been that way without a disability. I know that what
> I've experienced has really helped me to be present. I can
> imagine that my disability has actually enhanced my
> overall experience.

Sexual experience can also be better for your partner. Studies have found that many women prefer a slower, more romantic style of sexual sharing and that genital intercourse is not their first priority. A disabled man may be a more satisfying lover in many ways because he may not be as physically or emotionally driven to accomplish intercourse.

Roberta Travis, writing in *New Mobility* magazine, says that the best lover in her experience was a paraplegic man.

> He was completely in touch with his body (and mine) in spite
> of limited sensation, a moderately functional erection and
> inability to ejaculate. It just didn't matter since neither of us
> cared to focus on these so-called "negatives." He immersed
> himself in the moment of intimacy, all fears and pretenses
> swept aside. He was not, like so many men, primarily penis
> oriented and in a hurry to climax.[13]

Getting Started with Someone New

Having met a new partner, it will be necessary to have "The Talk," during which you'll explain your unique sexual style. At first, this can be a daunting task. Describing catheters, a weak bladder or bowels, levels of sensation, and other details is not very sexy. But, by demonstrating your willingness to be open and honest, you will set the tone of mutual intimacy needed in a healthy sexual relationship. If you show you are unafraid, you will help your partner—who will certainly have questions in mind—relax into the process with you.

This is the chance to demonstrate that you are attracted to and excited by this person. Once you know the feeling is mutual, then you are in for a wonderful experience, and your partner is likely to be open and accepting about understanding your needs.

> One time I had become romantic with a woman, and we had enjoyed some very satisfying kissing on several occasions. The opportunity arrived for her to stay the night, and—wanting to have a "normal" sexual encounter—I did not explain that I had limited penile sensation and did not ejaculate. Inevitably, we reached a point where her expectations were not met. She felt she was perhaps not attractive enough, and suddenly there was an emotional obstacle that we never overcame. I learned clearly that the pre-sex talk is crucial for a satisfying and mutual experience.

You may need your partner to assist with clinical tasks such as changing a catheter or helping in the bathroom. This can have a negative effect on creating a romantic mood, but it can also be a shared process that enhances intimacy, even as an opening to sexual intimacy. Once these duties are addressed, a couple can enter into the space of closeness and passion just as any other couple must—with patience, gentleness, and doing those simple things that begin the process of arousal.

The style with new partners is to relax into mutual discovery, to discuss and learn about each other's needs, to find every possible touch and contact that is pleasurable, and to separate from the various cultural pressures that create skewed expectations. Getting started with honest discussion and exploration puts the focus where it belongs: on people loving each other and expressing that love through sensual touch, trust, and sincere giving. Pretty damn sexy.

First Revelation

Revealing your body intimately—despite the fact that you may be very accustomed to being naked with a physician or a personal assistant—is a very vulnerable encounter. It can be a poignant test of trust with a person you choose as a sexual partner.

First exposure deserves to be handled with care. But success with well-chosen intimate partners who will show you acceptance will expose the invalidity of your fears. Your partner is able to make the same adjustment as you are to your "new normal," though you may need to allow him or her time. Everyone—even those who fit the cultural models of what's beautiful and sexy—tends to be self-conscious about their bodies on some level. As always, remember to keep the real effects of your disability in proper perspective with the whole of your shared life experience.

Bodily appearance, although meaningful, does not play as large a role as you might suspect. Besides, while in the act of intimacy, lying next to or on top of each other, we are not seeing much of the body anyway. We are reveling in touch and intimacy.

Your body-image concerns can simply be overridden by what you find stimulating and sexy:

> It does feel awkward for me the first time I reveal my body to
> a new partner due to the Foley catheter and skinny legs, not
> to mention the scoliosis. Once her clothes are off, nothing else
> comes to mind (ha) really.

Be in Good Health

Your general level of health has a direct impact on your sexuality. If your body is pressured with physical and emotional demands, you are less able to enjoy your sexuality. Depression and stress have specific physiologic effects through hormones and enzymes that are released in response. They can impact your immune system, reduce your capacity to relax and be open to sensations, greatly lessen orgasmic response, and draw your attention away from your partner.

Eat a good diet, balanced with a range of foods that are whole and free of chemicals. Control the amounts of sugar, alcohol, tobacco, and caffeine in your diet, all of which deplete the quality of your blood and circulation, promote fatigue, and lessen sexual response.

Control your weight. If you are substantially overweight, you will have to work harder if you use a manual wheelchair and will increase the risk of pressure sores. If you are fatigued and wearing dressings on a sore, this will limit your feelings of being attractive as well as limit possible positions.

Use of drugs—prescription or otherwise—can impact sexuality. Ask your doctor about the possible effect on your libido of any prescription medications you take. If you see different doctors, make sure that each of them knows what the other has prescribed. Some drugs—particularly spasticity control, pain management, or tranquilizing medications—can directly interfere with sexual arousal, ejaculation for men, or menstruation for women.

Always learn the detailed effects on the body of any medicine or substance you elect to use. For example, some disabled partners have an interest in the drug MDMA, also known as Ecstasy, to heighten their sensual responses. Although it may have this effect, it also impedes sexual function. MDMA contains an amphetamine, and the aftermath can include prolonged fatigue and headache. It is also very dehyrdrating, and people endanger themselves by not drinking substantial amounts of water during the experience. Use extreme caution if you are considering the use of any drug that has not been prescribed for you.

The Physiology of Sexual Function

Genital function varies greatly according to the particular disability, its degree and type. The stage of a degenerative disorder such as multiple sclerosis, the level and completeness of a spinal cord lesion, nerves attacked by the polio virus, the area and extent of an infectious disease of the brain or spinal cord—all are examples of what will differently determine functions, including lubrication, penile or clitoral erection, ejaculation, and orgasm. The effects on these of a given disability could be significant—or nominal. The better you understand how your body works, the more realistic your expectations will be of your sexual capacities. Know your body, be aligned with your objective possibilities, and you will be freed of unnecessary frustrations and more open to the many enjoyable options that remain available to you.

Some physiologic features of your disability will not change. An SCI, depending on the level and completeness, will affect penile or clitoral sensation and response. Weakness and spasticity from advanced muscular dystrophy, cerebral palsy, or ataxia may disrupt the ability to tilt the pelvis. Examples like these are a fact of your body and its disability.

Sometimes, your physiology can change, even for presumably stable conditions. Take the example of this 40-year old spinal cord paraplegic:

> I gained a capacity for ejaculation some 20 years after my spinal cord injury. I can't say what changed. Perhaps my own belief, since I remember very clearly my doctor telling me at the age of 18, just after my injury, that I was not capable of ejaculation. It was a shattering piece of news, and I wonder how much my very acceptance of his statement limited my actual ability.

Belief is a very powerful thing; this is being increasingly proven scientifically. "Psychosomatic" doesn't just mean "in your head." Clear and measurable connections exist between what we think and our body chemistry.

Those who experience muscle spasms will need to identify sexual positions that are less likely to bring them on. For women, spasticity of the perineal muscles can interfere with vaginal penetration. Lying on your back with the knees bent or on your side are positions that some have found less likely to promote the occurrence of these spasms.

Orgasm is a response that men and women generally associate with peak sexual experience. But orgasm occurs in stages, a sexual response cycle marked by increases in blood flow and muscle tension. Changes in the body you might experience include erection of the penis in men, enlargement of the clitoris or vaginal lubrication in women, sex flush (blood flow to the skin), an increase in heart rate and blood pressure, a focusing of the mind to the body, and a deep quality of relaxation.

Orgasm is very much a matter of where you put your attention. Sexuality researcher Mitch Tepper says:

> Orgasmic sex is about being in the moment and forgetting
> about quad bellies, atrophy, catheters, and making embarrass-
> ing sounds. What's right is what works now.[3]

What kind of sexual response you are capable of depends on the nature of your disability and nerve damage. It is also a question of time. Most spinal-injured men will be capable of erection within six months of injury, some sooner. Both women and men recover varying degrees of sensitivity and response after injury. In the case of a progressive condition such as multiple sclerosis, loss of response—and interest—is not unusual and might come and go over time.

In a 1995 study at Kessler Rehab in Orange, New Jersey, 25 women with SCI were asked to attempt to achieve orgasm in a laboratory setting. Partners were allowed to provide stimulation if needed. They found that level of injury was less of a factor and that education was significant.

> Neurological pattern of injury did not preclude the ability to
> have orgasm; thus both women with complete and incomplete
> injuries should be considered candidates for sex therapy
> aimed at improving their ability to achieve orgasm. Women
> who experienced orgasms were significantly more knowledge-
> able about sexuality and had a higher sex drive than did
> women who did not experience orgasm. Sexual education
> would seem to be an important factor in overall sexual
> responsiveness and satisfaction.[14]

There are two ways in which genital arousal takes place in the body. A psychogenic response is brought on by sensual thoughts—-the presence of your partner or fantasies, for instance. Psychogenic response relies on a connection from the brain to the lower thoracic/upper lumbar area, between the 10th thoracic and 2nd lumbar vertebrae. For example, for those with complete spinal lesions at or above these levels, sensual thoughts are unlikely to produce erection in men or clitoral enlargement and lubrication in women. With impact below this area or incomplete lesions, the psychogenic response is likely to remain.

Reflexogenic stimulations work from the other direction. They travel a direct route from the genitals to the T10-L2 portion of cord and back. They can occur in the presence of varying types of genital stimulation, intended sexually or not. Some men experience reflexogenic erection during catheterization or from the weight of bedding. Persons with complete lower lumbar and sacral injury to the spinal cord will not have a reflexogenic response.

Discovering your capacity for orgasm is a matter of experimentation, time, and patience. Your body might even go through changes over longer periods of time after a disabling trauma. In this case, it is true that practice makes perfect. If orgasm is difficult or seems doubtful, don't give up trying. You'll discover how best to stimulate yourself and what kinds of sensations are possible. The right moment might arrive when you least expect it.

Sexual Options

If genital sex with orgasm is impossible, difficult, painful, or just not satisfying for you, what's left? There are many adaptations and options to consider. You are a sexual being, not a sexual body part.

What's Possible for a Disabled Lover?

What sexual activities remain possible? Start with kissing—an extremely enjoyable and underrated pastime. Don't limit yourself to each other's lips. The face, the ears, the neck, the shoulders, the back—so many places that even the most significant disabilities leave capable of sensations—are extremely erotic. For example, many men find great pleasure in having their nipples licked.

Touch alone is very powerful. A gentle touch of a hand on your face or the slow exploration of each other's body is very erotic. Caressing expresses loving feelings and promotes the relaxed, take-your-time approach to lovemaking that helps a couple reach deeper levels of passion and intimacy.

Sensual massage—in which you incorporate erogenous zones such as nipples and genitals—is an excellent way to sidestep the pressure of performance. People with limited grip strength can use vibrators or gloves. You can take turns with this and allow each other the absolute luxury of receiving totally, knowing that you will be able to return the favor. Sensual massage is also a great way to continue to find those previously undiscovered areas of sensitivity.

There are usually many undiscovered places, such as the palms of the hands, inside the elbow, or behind the knee. There are thousands of nerve endings in places like this that light up when kissed or touched but that many people take for granted. Research has shown that, when parts of the body lose sensory function, the brain turns up the volume elsewhere. Parts of the body that still have feeling become more sensitive.

> My chiropractor and my massage therapist both say that my
> upper body is much more sensitive than other people they
> work with. They share the theory that it is a compensation for
> my paraplegia, that the rest of my body became more sensitive
> because of the lost sensation in the lower part.

Women usually have the option of sharing genital intercourse, even if they might not perceive sensation from it. There may be a need for additional lubricants. Water-soluble products such as K-Y Jelly should be used rather than petroleum-based lubricants, which can promote infection. Men having intercourse with a disabled woman might experience less friction as a result of weakened vaginal muscles. Yet the reverse may also be true: a woman with spasticity could have very active vaginal muscles during intercourse.

Women's fear of not pleasing a partner because of lack of tightness in the vagina can interfere with pleasure, just as men can be concerned about maintaining an erection. However, less friction might extend the amount of time a couple can participate in intercourse before male ejaculation occurs; if intercourse becomes tiring, the couple can use other options to achieve satisfaction. Regardless of the muscle tone of vaginal muscles, intercourse is a very intimate experience but doesn't have to be the final act of a lovemaking session.

Options change, of course, over time as we age, or according to the progressive nature of certain disabilities. Just as with your disability in general, a continuing mind of adaptation and exploration—and acceptance— is what will allow the most options to remain open to you. (Acceptance, it is understood, is not immediate but demands going through some associated feelings of loss. The process of grieving, as discussed in Chapter 3, The Experience of Disability, is part of the challenge of keeping sexual options open and appealing.)

Oral Stimulation

As preferences shift, oral techniques can rise in priority in the context of disability. Oral sex may not have been part of your sexual repertoire; you may imagine it is inappropriate or unpleasant; you may even feel it is taboo. Younger persons might not be comfortable with the idea if they have never participated in this kind of contact. Yet, once over their initial hesitancy, many consider oral sex as enjoyable a form of lovemaking as they would ever experience.

Some women report that intercourse is less stimulating than genital stimulation with the mouth, tongue, or lips. This may be exactly the forte of a partner with a disability.

There has been some concern expressed that oral contact can transmit sexually transmitted diseases such as AIDS. Mitch Tepper explains:

> *This is considered a low-risk activity for acquiring the HIV virus, but if fluids reach an open sore in or near the mouth, it is still possible for a virus to enter the bloodstream.*

Changing Your Style

New sexual possibilities open up when you are willing to reconsider previous beliefs, redefine your sexual priorities, and keep your focus on what is pleasurable. You might discover new levels of gratification as the giver of pleasure and perhaps discover a surprising degree of stimulation in that role. You can use sex toys, view adult videos, or read erotic material together.

If you are with a fully orgasmic partner, you can "ride the wave," drawn into the intensity of their climax. The deep, shared connection with your lover is itself an orgasmic experience, a shifted consciousness. If your attention is fully with them, and not thinking about what you aren't feeling, very rich levels of emotion and sensation open up to you.

Although some more of your attention might shift to your partner, that doesn't mean giving up the idea of being the recipient of direct pleasure for yourself. Mitch Tepper writes:

> *The possibility and benefits of receiving sexual pleasure still need to be pursued. Reciprocal sexual pleasure is seldom impossible.*[3]

The visual experience is often amplified for the disabled lover. Choose positions in which the partner with the disability can see what is going on, with enough light for the purpose. Perhaps leave your glasses on or your contact lenses in place. A man with limited genital sensation who cannot see what is happening might not be certain of the state of his erection. This can be discouraging and distract from the ability to relax into the moment. Being able to participate in intercourse at all is gratifying, and being able to also witness intercourse is particularly stimulating.

Anything that is pleasurable is fine. You are in the privacy of your own relationship. Whatever you choose, in any order, at any time, is entirely up to you, just so it is consensual and safe. The more you can drop your expectations and assumptions, the more possibilities will reveal themselves to you, and the more satisfying your sexuality can be.

Take Extra Care

Sex can be physically demanding. Your disability may preclude your ability to move in certain ways. For example, without the ability to use your legs, hips, and bottom to assist in pelvic movements, the typical movements of intercourse become tiring very quickly. An able-bodied partner needs to understand that certain motions have a time limit. The partner can take on more of the physical work, and you can relax and enjoy, moving as your capacity allows.

Use pillows or various sized cushions to help get your bodies into comfortable positions—and within reach. Pillows can also help stabilize you so that you can remain in a given position longer. The strain of needing to shift your weight or fatigue from bracing with your arms can distract from your pleasure.

Educate your partner about your ability to balance yourself and in what directions and positions you are able to bear weight. If your upper-body balance is limited, your partner will need to know when not to lean weight against you, such as when sitting up, straddled together. This position can work with the proper support, possibly even in your wheelchair.

You need to change positions regularly to prevent pressure sores. This takes attention, since you may not have sensations to tell you when to move. Hugging with your partner in the wonderful aftermath and glow of lovemaking, you might not want to break the spell to shift positions. But, at some point, you must; this is an important point for your partner to be aware of. You can just say, "It's time," and find another lovely way to lie together.

Toys and the Setting

Explore the world of sensual products, which are now quite easy to acquire without the stigma of being in poor taste. If you are uncomfortable going into a shop, there are catalog suppliers who are very discreet in their packaging.

Sensual products include:

■   Vibrators. Available in many shapes and sizes and can be sexually satisfying or used to give massage to either partner.

■ Penis stiffeners. Worn as a supplement to ease the pressure of having to maintain a full erection.

■ Dildos. An artificial penis that a female partner might enjoy as a supplement to whatever capability a disabled male partner may have for erection. Lesbian relationships benefit, too.

■ Books and videos. For private stimulation, to share with a partner, or for instructive purposes.

You can make simple modifications to these products—such as a Velcro strap for a vibrator or dildo—to accommodate limited grip strength that might otherwise be needed to use them.

Pay attention to the setting for romance. Set soft lights or burn candles. Choose music that will enhance the mood. Wear sexy clothes that are fun to take off of each other or to caress each other through. Use perfumes or incense (we are biologically built to respond to sensual aromas), or surround yourselves with flowers. Remove items that could detract from romance, like prescription bottles at the bedside. Pay attention to the setting and have fun with romance.

Bowel and Bladder Issues

In a scene from the film *The Waterdance*, a recently injured quadriplegic man is with his female lover for the first time since his accident. During their lovemaking, his catheter slips, wetting the bed. His reaction is embarrassment and frustration while she attempts to reassure him that it is not a problem. But the moment has been lost. They were caught by surprise in these new emotional dynamics of their sexuality.

Certainly loss of bladder control can interrupt the romance of the moment, but the couple in the film was facing the shock of their first encounter with the issue. When a couple develops a true intimate bond, their bodily fluids need not be repelling. We all deal with body fluids— urine, semen, menstrual blood. Experienced, committed couples are not troubled by such slips. They could even laugh it off—or, if there is stress in their relationship, perhaps it could bring up some conflict. Again, the disability is not the issue; it's about the nature of relationship and the kinds of stressors that any couple must manage.

A brief spasm of urination or movement of the bowels might occur during particular motions. Some of the same reflexes triggered during sex also control bladder and bowel activity. Choose techniques or positions that are less likely to exert pressure on these areas. Go easy on liquid intake and empty yourself fully before lovemaking, and time such activities earlier in your lovemaking before the bladder begins to fill again.

Then keep a towel handy just in case. A regular bowel management program will help prevent surprises.

An indwelling catheter—which remains in place continuously—can be bent over and worn inside of a condom during intercourse, taking care to not exert any tension on it. Use of an internal catheter increases the risk of urinary tract infection, which can be passed on to a sexual partner. Emptying the bladder after intercourse will help prevent infections.

Women with indwelling catheters may be able to leave them in during intercourse, depending on the size of their vagina and the positions used. Some have found that a catheter is able to remain in place more easily when the man enters the woman from behind.

Men who wear a condom-like external catheter need to remove it before genital contact, cleaning the area to remove traces of adhesive and urine. Some men develop a sensitivity to latex and experience drying of the skin of the penis or open sores, particularly on the head, which is very delicate. A high commitment to cleanliness, the use of creams, or switching to a silicone type of catheter helps manage this problem. It is unwise to have intercourse while the skin of the penis is irritated or broken down. A normal prophylactic condom might be used at such times.

A partner or spouse who aids you in bowel and bladder care may come to have a difficult time seeing you in sexual terms. If personal-assistance duties are placing stress on your sexual relationship, take some time to explore ways to shift the responsibility from your partner by doing more yourself, if possible, or perhaps by employing a greater degree of outside attendant assistance. Perhaps there are portions of your support that you had not thought you could perform or that were unknown to your original therapist. There might be products available to aid in grip and dexterity that you were not aware of or had only thought of for other purposes, like feeding. Be creative and open minded, and possibilities will increase.

Male Erection

Although there are many options for satisfying sexual expression, it is the desire of most men to be able to reliably participate in intercourse. It is psychologically gratifying for a man to perform intercourse. As much as their partner might not begrudge a limitation on erection, most partners enjoy this form of sexual contact. More to the point, it is a lovely experience to share.

How erection occurs and is maintained is complex and depends on the physiology of the specific disability as well as psychological factors. Men with a disability experience either psychogenic or reflexogenic erections or some degree of both. More spinal cord impairments occur above the area of the spine at which psychogenic erectile function is processed in the hypogastric nerve plexus between T10 and L2. This means that fewer men experience erection psychogenically, since their erotic thoughts cannot stimulate that area of the spine, but their reflexogenic processes remain intact. In either case, surface sensation is not necessary to accomplish erection.

But loss of penile sensation might limit the ability to maintain an erection if a man's expectation is that the sensation of intercourse is what stimulates erection. Loss of sensation (not always the case in a disabled man) might lead to doubts about the ability to maintain the erection, especially in positions in which the man cannot see his penis during intercourse. To the degree that a psychogenic process is involved, such mental distractions will affect the ability to maintain an erection.

This is not much different from problems of erectile dysfunction that many able-bodied men experience, in which the cause can be either psychological or physical. Thinking, "Can I keep it up?" is almost a guarantee of not being able to do so. It is simply a case of performance anxiety. The ability to clear the mind during sexual intimacy is as important a psychological skill for everybody as it is for disabled. In any case, our desires ebb and flow with our body chemistry and the events of our lives at the time. No one is always ready for sex.

Psychogenic erection can rely on very subtle forms of touch and contact. Being subtle, these sensations might be overridden by bearing a partner's body weight or by body contact that pulls on hairs. A helpful strategy is to shift your attention to more subtle sensations that men with later disabilities might never have noticed prior to disability or might never have thought of as being sensual. These sensations, when allowed to rise above the noise, are in fact very powerful and gratifying. Sexuality educator Mitch Tepper notes:

> It's about getting in touch with subtle forms. I try to help people develop them with techniques such as breathing, focusing, and biofeedback.

Partners will need to work out techniques so that the disabled partner can still have the sensations that are pleasurable and maintain erection. Choose positions carefully, and emphasize the kinds of touch that are arousing.

An adolescent, injured at the stage of his peak period of testosterone levels (the male hormone) and his early sexual experimentation might imagine that he would have to maintain the degree of erectile rigidity he experienced as a teenager in order to be able to enter his partner. The inability to do so is thought of as a severe failure. According to this 36-year-old with spinal cord paraplegia:

> *I have since learned that all men reach a lesser degree of*
> *response as they age, which need not impair their capacity for*
> *intercourse. Age 18 is the point of optimal potency, but those of*
> *us injured at that time have no other point of reference.*

The "stuff" method is a way to share intercourse with a lesser erection. The flaccid penis is pushed into the vagina; this is more easily achieved in certain positions. Squeezing the base of the penis will direct more blood into the shaft and head, increasing erection. Keep pressure at the base—or use an erection ring designed for that purpose—to prolong erection and keep your movement gentle.

Always ask your doctor about the implications of any treatment or elective surgery you might be considering. You may well choose to surrender some sexual function in favor of reduced pain or some other benefit in order to extend your independence. Just be fully informed.

Methods to Induce Erection

There are a number of methods that reliably produce erections. Most men and their partners need to experiment to find the best solution. The invasive nature of some of these approaches is another reason to explore other sexual options rather than be overly reliant on penile intercourse.

Vacuum pumps have been used for erectile dysfunction over the last 20 years. A plastic tube with either a motorized or manual pump creates a vacuum that draws blood into the penis. An erection ring fits at the base of the penis, holding in blood to maintain the erection. The health of the skin on and around the penis needs special attention from regular users of the pump, particularly those who use catheters. Check regularly for irritation. Sexuality researcher Dr. Marca Sipski of the Kessler Institute for Rehabilitation in New Jersey says that:

> *Rings should not be used for more than 30 minutes. Gangrene*
> *of the penis has been shown to occur in men who have fallen*
> *asleep with the rings on.*

Prostaglandin—marketed under the name Caverject®—is a drug that is injected into the corpora cavernosa, the area of the penis that fills with blood and therefore produces erection. Men are trained in making the injections themselves prior to sex. The drug causes blood to flow to the corpora cavernosa, and the resulting pressure constricts the area, which allows the erection to last longer. Erection occurs in about 20 minutes and lasts generally no more than two hours, depending on the dosage. One needs to take great care with cleanliness and must avoid veins in the penis that could bleed excessively if violated by the needle.

There is a danger of overstimulation. Priapism is a condition in which blood held too long in the penis can begin to clot. In general, an erection that lasts more than four hours is worthy of concern. This is a serious enough event to require immediate medical attention. An overdose or the excessive use of injections can cause permanent damage.

The oral drugs Viagra, Cialis, and Levitra are relatively new treatments for erectile dysfunction. Viagra has some known potential side effects, such as transiently changing one's vision, it can pose health risks when taken with medications containing nitroglycerin, too high a dose can dangerously elevate the heart rate, it doesn't work for all men, it is expensive, and some insurers or HMOs do not pay for the drug.

Nevertheless, Dr. Michelle Gittler of Schwab Rehabilitation Hospital in Chicago says:

> *I can only tell you that my guys who rely on reflexogenic*
> *erections swear by Viagra.*

There are also permanent, surgical solutions. Penile implants are available in various forms. One is a solid silicone rod that provides an immovable, semi-erect solution. Another is a flexible silicone rod so the penis can be adjusted downward for comfort away from sexual activity. A self-contained implant will become firm when it is squeezed or bent and return to a flaccid state after a period of time. Lastly, an inflatable prostheses—the most expensive option—allows manual control of the degree of erection as needed. There is some risk that the pump—also implanted under the skin—may leak or that pressure sores could form inside the penis.

Since these are surgical alternatives, there is always some risk from the invasive nature of their installation and the presence of a foreign object inside of the body. Discuss these options in detail with your urologist, and take the time to speak with others who have experienced them. Mitch Tepper comments on the dangers of implants:

> *There is some risk of erosion from the inside. The rod can*
> *stick through the end of the penis or back near the testicles.*
> *There is more risk of complication from implants than from*
> *any of the other options. Even if you take it out, there is dam-*
> *age to tissue, and it may be difficult to go back to using injec-*
> *tions or any other method. The ability to get the same*
> *erections as before surgery may be reduced.*[3]

A couple should discuss how these solutions will affect their sense of intimacy. Will the partner feel that the artificial erection—whether drug induced or an implant—has less to do with how appealing she is? On the other hand, a greater sense of security about their erection can allow men to focus more on the sensuality of the moment. The range of positions can also expand as there is less need to prevent the overriding sensations mentioned earlier, which can counteract erection. And, best of all, artificial erections last long enough that you can participate in intercourse for as long as you choose.

Birth Control

Disabled women need protection from pregnancy as much as able-bodied women do, though some special considerations need to be made, especially for those who have limited sensations in the genital area. Find a gynecologist familiar with your disability who can advise you on the fine points.

Menstruation is usually interrupted in women after a spinal disease or injury but usually returns within six months as the body recovers from its shock. Women who are close to menopause may find that their menses will not start again.

The pill is the most effective birth control method, but there is an increased risk for disabled women of thrombophlebitis—blood clotting as a result of poor circulation in the legs from not walking. Women who experience spasticity are less exposed to this problem, since muscle contractions assist in the movement of blood. Your gynecologist can perform a test for susceptibility to clotting.

Some professionals feel that the risk of clotting plus the inability to recognize problems because of limited sensation are cause enough for disabled women not to use the pill. Guidelines developed by Planned Parenthood of New York City specifically recommend against them. Others say that, with today's lower dosages, the risks are minimal and that, if clotting has not occurred within six months after disability, it is unlikely to occur with the pill. You must also consider interaction with other medications you might take.

Progestagen injections provide protection for 90 days with a very high success rate. Progestin subdermal implants are also highly effective and can remain in place for up to five years.

There is disagreement on the wisdom of using an IUD. Its placement and removal can cause autonomic dysreflexia, typically an issue only for women with spinal cord lesions above the sixth thoracic vertebra. Women who use anticoagulants should not use an IUD. Excessive blood flow could occur during menstruation. Talk with your gynecologist for more information.

Diaphragms and vaginal condoms are effective about 90% of the time. A diaphragm also needs to be checked carefully for position, particularly for women who press on their bladder to assist in manual voiding. Extended wearing of a diaphragm also increases risk of infection. Women who used a diaphragm prior to injury should be refitted to account for weight change and reduced muscle tone.

A vaginal condom requires the use of a spermicidal foam or jelly. People who use a Foley catheter and leave the catheter in place during sex need to take care that the condom is not torn by the catheter.

Sponges and caps are moderately effective and available without a prescription. Like the IUD, diaphragm, and condom, they require sufficient hand function to insert and position. Sponges are more effective in women who have not already given birth.

Natural methods of birth control involving timing and abstinence are statistically the most unreliable. Some women opt for sterilization, having already had their children or knowing they choose not to be mothers. This is very effective but entails some surgical risk.

Pregnancy and Parenthood

Can disabled women conceive and have babies? Yes, in most cases.

Can disabled men make babies? Increasingly the answer is, "Yes."

Until recently, not many paraplegic men were producing children. But now men with spinal cord lesions are increasingly able to make babies. The question of childbearing seems to come up more with regard to spinal cord impairment, thus its emphasis in the following discussion.

The Baylor College of Medicine study on women with disabilities found that the medical profession is not serving women well with regard to pregnancy. Providers and the women themselves often operate under the false belief that such women should avoid pregnancy. Recent 10-year studies have found that women with SCIs are giving birth more often, yet:

> *Very few clinicians have experience managing pregnancy, labor, and delivery in women with SCI. Unfounded assumptions of poor outcomes may influence clinicians to behave as though risks are greater than they actually are. If the chance of a positive pregnancy outcome is considered slim, or threat to the mother's life too high, clinicians may encourage women who want to have their babies to have unnecessary or undesired therapeutic abortions.*[5]

This paraplegic woman reports being given incorrect medical advice:

> *I was 13 when I broke my back. (I'm a complete paraplegic.) I*
> *remember being told by my blushing 60-year-old doctor that*
> *I could have children, but only by caesarian section. I have*
> *since found out that that is totally untrue.*

Women in the Baylor study reported having trouble finding obstetricians or midwives willing to assist them in what were considered high-risk pregnancies. The Baylor report says that their own study and previous findings confirm:

> *Normal labor and delivery are possible, even routine, and*
> *generally pose little or no added risk to the mother or baby.*[5]

Physicians and midwives do need to understand issues faced by women with disabilities, including autonomic dysreflexia, urinary tract infections, skin breakdown, spasticity, and the effect on a fetus of medications they might be using.

Before you start trying to have a child, address health and emotional considerations. You'll probably wonder what it's like to be a parent with a disability. If you are a woman, you'll want to consider the consequences on your own health of becoming pregnant.

If you are disabled by a genetic condition, you will want to fully understand the odds and consequences of passing such a condition on to a child. This certainly does not mean you should choose not to bear children if there is a chance of passing on a disability. People with disabilities have historically been told that they should not be parents—much less be sexually active—because it would be wrong to bear a child with a disability. This attitude is widely viewed by people with disabilities as discriminatory. You have the right to bear children, and such testing for genetically passed disability is available to you for your own information. The decision is yours.

Can You Parent?

People with disabilities are raising children with great success, adapting creatively to childrearing just as they do to their mobility needs. Children are highly resilient by their nature and naturally adapt to your parenting style.

Slings, seat belts, and Velcro come in very handy for securing a child in your lap. Adjustable-height tables make it easy to lift your child from a lower position, then raise the child to a higher level for changing diapers and so on. For parents with limited hand use, buttons and snaps on children's clothing can be replaced with Velcro, and loops can be placed on shoes to help pull them on. A modest degree of family support or paid help might be necessary during early stages when physical demands are greater.

There are some potentially challenging cultural aspects to parenting with a disability. Once your child is in school, relationships with other parents and the community are a source of important support, information, and local advocacy. But other parents might not support your need for access to their home, or schools might plan events you cannot attend for lack of access. Some people might even imagine that the child takes care of the parent with a disability, an assumption that is insulting to parents with a disability, who work as hard as others on behalf of their children.

Through the Looking Glass is a group in Oakland, California, operating on a five-year grant from the National Resource Center for Parents with Disabilities. At an October 1997 conference, a task force met to review a recent national survey of 1,200 parents with disabilities conducted by Berkeley Planning Associates in Berkeley, California.[15] Here are some of the results:

- Thirty-six percent of disabled parents reported that their medical providers' lack of disability expertise caused problems in prenatal and birthing services.
- Thirty-one percent reported medical providers' attitudes caused barriers.
- Disabled parents reported needing assistance in recreation with their children (43%), traveling outside the home with their children (40%), chasing or retrieving children (39%), and lifting or carrying children (33%).
- Transportation affected more aspects of parenting with a disability than any other issue; 79% reported transportation as a problem that interfered with or prevented routine as well as critical parent-child activities.
- Cost was the most frequently identified barrier to childcare (30%), followed by lack of transportation (20%).
- Forty-eight percent reported that adaptive parenting equipment was too expensive; 32% reported that adaptive equipment was unavailable or not yet designed.
- Fifty-seven percent reported using personal assistance services for help with parenting; 54% reported that services were not available when needed; 46% reported that services were unreliable.
- Forty-three percent reported difficulty finding housing.
- Thirty-two percent reported facing discrimination.
- Fourteen percent reported pressure to have a tubal ligation; 13% reported being urged to have an abortion.

The Children

Children of disabled parents tend to be more independent, learning to do appropriate tasks for themselves that are strenuous for the parent. For example, very young children can develop the ability to climb onto a wheelchair and maintain their balance. These children also tend to develop a deeper compassion for all people, drawing a lesson from the perspective they gain through their parents about not falling into assumptions about who people are based on their appearance.

Don't be surprised if you find a lack of support for your decision to have a child. Unenlightened elements of society still imagine that a parent with a disability would put a child at risk by not being able to respond to an emergency or chase a child into a place where a wheelchair cannot go. Your family, friends, church members, or colleagues may withhold their support. In *Spinal Network*, a woman with mild cerebral palsy is quoted as recalling:

> *I was told quite bluntly by many that I had no right to have a child. I was told I was selfish; I was repeatedly told that I could not hold, care for, or look after the baby.*[16]

Children of disabled parents don't know the difference. To them, a wheelchair is totally normal. They know that their parents function fully and love fully—doing all they can to provide a healthy upbringing.

> *Donnie Herman—son of Paul, who is paraplegic, and Anne, who is quadriplegic—was asked at the age of 10 if he would like to see his parents cured. "Cured of what?" he answered.*

Getting Pregnant: Male Ejaculation

The question of the man's ability to produce a usable ejaculate is the obvious key to a couple's ability to bear children. Among those with SCIs, women are usually capable of conceiving, carrying the fetus, and giving birth. The challenge rests with the man with an SCI.

Depending on the type and level of impact on the spinal cord, a disabled man may or may not be capable of ejaculation. The response from the head of the penis travels to a given portion of the spinal cord—between T10 and T12—independent of nerves traveling to the brain. It is a completely reflexive process.

Semen and sperm are two separate substances, combined at the very moment of ejaculation, which is initiated as a biochemical and nervous system response. Three discrete steps take place:

1. Emission is the step in which sperm and other fluids are secreted from the Cowper's and prostate glands, the seminal vesicles, and from the testicles. These fluids assist the motility—the portion that is actively swimming—of the sperm, lubricate the movement of ejaculate through the urethra and out the penis, and include the sperm itself.

2. In the second stage, the bladder neck is closed to prevent semen from backing into the bladder during ejaculation. Disabled men with impaired nerve function might experience retrograde ejaculation, in which semen flows back into the bladder. The acid environment of the bladder and urine is a threat to semen, though, if urine is collected and sterilized, it can be possible to harvest semen from urine for artificial insemination.

3. Ejaculation is the forcible expulsion of the ejaculate, and the third step of the process. This occurs via the second to the fourth sacral segments. Complete injury in this area will usually preclude ejaculation.

For men with an SCI, there is less frequency of pregnancy. In a study at the Miami Project to Cure Paralysis, only 10% of men with an SCI who were able to ejaculate during intercourse succeeded in impregnating their mates.[17] In men injured at a younger age, the maturation of their testicles may have been hampered. In others, it is possible that irreversible structural atrophy can occur as a result of their disability. Such changes are more likely to occur within six months of injury, if at all. There is a suspicion on the part of researchers that there might be hormonal abnormalities in spinal cord-injured men that affect sperm production.

A severe bladder infection can cause sterility. An infection can spread from the bladder to other genital passages and compromise reproductive capabilities. Marijuana smoking also has damaging effects on sperm. One cycle of sperm production takes three months, during which time you would want to recover from any present infection, take extra care with your bladder program, drink sufficient fluids, and abstain from any damaging substances.

Assuming there is no physiologic damage, there are products that can help produce an ejaculate. A vibrator can stimulate ejaculation. A product from MMG Healthcare uses a specific frequency and amplitude of vibration to induce ejaculation; the FertiCare vibrator. The manufacturer reports a high success rate of ejaculates. Overstimulation with a vibrator, however, can be a risk to tissues if used excessively. For example, FertiCare and MMG recommend sessions of three minutes with a pause of one minute, repeated up to five times.

With electro-ejaculation, a probe is inserted through the anus to directly stimulate the nerves that elicit the ejaculation response. Men with sensation may require anesthesia for the procedure. The duration and voltage must be carefully monitored to avoid burns. Those with higher spinal cord lesions might be at risk of autonomic dysreflexia. Ejaculation may not occur on the first attempt.

The issue is not limited to simply gaining ejaculate; it is also about the quality of the product. Spinal cord–injured men have been found to have a normal number of sperm; however, the sperm have lower survival rates and less capacity to make the swim all the way to the uterus and the egg. An average male has a sperm motility of 60%. In a study conducted by Nancy Brackett et al of the Miami Project to Cure Paralysis, spinal cord–injured men have been found to have rates ranging from 23.5% to 30.9%.[18]

Temperature is thought to be a factor in potency. Consider the shape of the male genitalia, in which the scrotum hangs freely to allow the testicles to have plenty of air surrounding them for a cooling effect. Since disabled men sit most of the time, the testicles stay warmer. It has been postulated that this temperature difference compromises semen quality.

This view, however, is not without its detractors. Nancy Brackett reports:

> A cohort of men with SCI who walk and did not use a wheelchair for locomotion (i.e., they walked with crutches) had semen quality as impaired as that of men who used wheelchairs. Based on these studies, there appears to be no strong evidence to suggest that elevated scrotal temperature in men with SCI is a major contributor to their poor semen quality.[18]

Other factors suspected of affecting sperm motility, as discussed in the 1996 Brackett study,[18] include:

- Methods of bladder management. Men using intermittent catheterization had better motility.
- Infrequency of ejaculation. Intervals of less than one week but greater than 12 weeks resulted in ejaculates with lower sperm concentration or motility.
- Hormonal changes. Although men with SCI have been found to have the same levels of testosterone—the male hormone—as uninjured men, some study subjects had elevated levels of follicle-simulating hormone and were found to have no sperm in their semen.

The quality of semen is apparently affected by the method of collection. In another study led by Nancy Brackett, the percentage of motile sperm was greater for study subjects who used vibratory stimulation as compared to electro-ejaculation, although the sperm counts were comparable.[19] They found that there is a larger component of retrograde ejaculate with electro-ejaculation—sperm that had been exposed to the destructive acid environment of the bladder. This seems to account for the difference.

The potency problem can be solved by collecting and then freezing ejaculate, preparing it for artificial insemination at a later time. Not all frozen sperm recover the ability to swim, so this process involves gaining several samples and then combining them with a fresh ejaculate before inseminating the woman. In another study led by Osvaldo Padron at the University of Miami in 1994, freezing sperm of spinal cord–injured men was no more destructive than for able-bodied men.[20]

In some cases, taking hormones can help produce more sperm to aid this process. There may be supplements you can take to improve quality of sperm.

Getting Pregnant: Other Approaches

There are a number of methods for becoming pregnant—that is, when the traditional approach isn't working. They range in cost and complexity. Typically, you would start with the least expensive and least invasive methods.

Some couples are willing to invest almost any amount of time, expense, physical stress, and emotion to have a child of their own. It can be a considerable drain. A single advanced procedure can cost as much as $15,000 per try, whereas using vibration and at-home insemination is very inexpensive. Most who succeed say that, having had their child, it was well worth whatever they went through. Yet the success rate is not high, so there is the risk of being left exhausted and depressed—and broke! You and your partner need to fully explore your feelings about having your own biologic child and weigh what you discover against current medical options to decide what is best for you.

When the man is able to produce an ejaculate—by any of the methods mentioned earlier—sperm are collected and then the woman is inseminated by injecting the ejaculate with a needleless syringe. When a procedure such as electro-ejaculation is performed in an office or clinic, the insemination will also be performed there. A couple can also increase the odds of success by the use of drugs that stimulate the production of more than one egg per cycle and by using standard methods to identify the woman's peak ovulation.

When normal ejaculation occurs, the sperm is sent into the cervix at approximately 30 miles per hour. With the injection method, sperm have to be helped along with gravity by having the woman lie on her back and elevate her pelvis for a period of time after injection.

Modern science offers several options for uniting a sperm and an egg. A couple can consider:

- Intrauterine insemination. Sperm are collected and analyzed for quality and quantity. The specimen is washed and concentrated in preparation for insemination. The woman is monitored for her cycles, and, just before ovulation, a hormone is given to induce it. On the day of insemination, a fresh ejaculate is obtained, the concentrated specimen is added to it, and then it is injected directly into the uterus.

- Intratubal insemination. This method is recommended when there are two eggs in the same fallopian tube, which is where insemination normally takes place. With intratubal insemination, the ejaculate is delivered via a catheter while the physician watches with ultrasound, and the sperm are placed as close to the ovum as possible to increase the chance of success.

- In vitro fertilization-embryo transfer. Widely known as the test-tube baby procedure, the goal here is to generate as many healthy eggs as possible in order to harvest them before ovulation and perform the insemination outside of the body. In 24 hours, it is possible to observe if fertilization has taken place and then replace the embryos into the uterus. This procedure has shown only a 12% to 17% success rate.

- Gamete intrafallopian transfer. Eggs are harvested as in IVF, but, rather than being combined outside in a dish, the eggs and sperm are placed back into the fallopian tubes via a catheter. The process proceeds naturally within the woman's body with a 36% success rate.

- Zygote intrafallopian transfer. Insemination is performed in a dish to produce viable embryos, and then the embryos are placed into the fallopian tubes rather than the uterus. This procedure has a 37% success rate.

- Intracytoplasmic sperm injection. It is now possible to extract sperm from an ejaculate or directly from either the testicles or the epididymis—a very long, convoluted tube in which sperm mature and are stored until ejaculation. These sperm are then injected into an egg using the vitro fertilization, gamete intrafallopian transfer, or zygote intrafallopian transfer process. Only a few motile sperm are required for the process.

Pregnancy

Pregnancy involves major changes to the body and metabolism. Some of the possible effects for any woman include anemia, thrombophlebitis, swelling in the legs, blood pressure changes, carpal tunnel syndrome, infections, constipation, morning sickness, and so on. Any of these effects is minimized by being in good health at the beginning of the pregnancy and making a commitment to the best prenatal and postnatal care.

A pregnant woman using a wheelchair faces additional issues. As you gain weight, there will be increased ischial pressure and added risk of skin breakdown. Be certain to have a proper and well-maintained wheelchair cushion. A different product might be necessary during the later stage of the pregnancy. You will need to do pressure relief push-ups or change your posture more often to prevent sores, so some upper-body exercise for added arm strength might be in order. As you gain weight, you might even need a wider wheelchair, especially if you are being pinched in the hips, where there is risk of skin breakdown. Take measures to ensure the health of your skin, keeping it very clean, optimizing your diet for healthy tissue and circulation.

Any medications you take for bladder control, stool softening, control of spasms, or other implications of your disability need to be completely reviewed with your doctor at the earliest possible stage of your pregnancy. Bladder infections during pregnancy present a risk to the fetus. Certain antibiotics used to treat infections can be even more dangerous to the baby. Some women use Valium to control spasms. There are cases of babies who have had to endure Valium withdrawal after birth.

Miscarriage rates are no different for disabled women than for the general population. Spinal cord–injured women are at no increased risk of having children with birth defects. Birth weights are typically within normal ranges. Women with multiple sclerosis or muscular dystrophy may pass on genetic tendencies to these disabilities.

You might not sense the early signs of labor if you have spinal injury above T10 and could miss the opportunity to prepare for delivery before your water breaks. Normal vaginal delivery is possible in most cases, but, if you are without use of abdominal muscles, the doctor might need to assist in lieu of your inability to push down. Forceps, a vacuum extraction unit, or an episiotomy—in which incisions are made to enlarge the vaginal opening—might be necessary. Cesarean delivery—which recent studies have found is performed more than is necessary—may be necessary in some cases, but no more often than for nondisabled women.

Some doctors recommend beginning cervical checks at 26 weeks, since there is some statistical evidence of increased risk of premature delivery by spinal cord–injured women. They might even recommend hospitalization after 32 weeks to monitor the pregnancy as closely as possible. There is risk of dysreflexia during delivery for women injured above T6, a fact of which your obstetrician should be aware.

Disabled women can breastfeed. This is a reflexive response initiated by the baby's sucking. Some women injured above T6 experience a decrease in milk production after a time due to lack of nipple sensation.

For a woman using a wheelchair, pregnancy has its extra challenges. For this couple, it raised questions about having another child:

> My husband thinks having one child is perfect and doesn't
> even want to consider a second. I truly believe it is for the
> most part because he doesn't want me to have to go through
> the ordeal of pregnancy again. It was hard on me, but in a
> way I think it was just as hard on him to see me lose a little
> bit of my mobility. He thinks our son is wonderful but doesn't
> see a need to risk a second pregnancy. I am still torn on
> the subject.

Pregnancy is a demanding experience for any woman. When you provide for special needs while working with an obstetrician or midwife who understands those needs, you have the best chance of a manageable pregnancy in which you maintain good health.

Adoption

Only some couples unable to have a child of their own can afford the new high-tech approaches to producing a birth. Financially and emotionally, the cost gets too high. Couples may also choose not to have invasive hormonal or surgical treatments. Adoption is a possibility, but this is not an easy option either.

Most children available for adoption are from an ethnic-minority background. In the U.S., most parents looking for children to adopt are Caucasian and—like other prospective parents—prefer to find a child of the same race as their own. The competition is pretty stiff, since able-bodied parents tend to be given the advantage by agencies. Another portion of the children have health problems or were abused. It is harder to find homes for these children. They are a challenge for any parents to raise, but all the more so for a disabled parent, depending on the parents' capacities and resources. But, for someone with a disability who feels a passionate calling to share his or her love as a parent, these issues can be resolved.

Finding Your Own Way

Yes, there are a lot of adjustments to make, and some issues are complicated in the already treacherous milieu of love, sex, and babies. But, just as there are roadblocks, there are discoveries unique to sex with a disability if you have the patience and the adaptability to find them. If you can overcome the initial obstacle of being discouraged by all the cultural messages of youth and body image and the overemphasis on intercourse as sex, possibilities will expand. Your sexual nature is a gift of your existence, and no disability—no matter how severe—disqualifies you from the capacity for intimacy and sensuality.

References

1. Nosek MA. *National Study of Women with Physical Disabilities, Final Report*. Houston: Baylor College of Medicine, Center for Research on Women with Physical Disabilities, Department of Physical Medicine and Rehabilitation; 1997:3.
2. Sipski ML, Alexander CJ. Sexual activities, response and satisfaction in women pre- and post-spinal cord injury. *Arch Phys Med Rehabil* 1993;74(10):1025-9
3. Tepper M. Love bites. *New Mobility*. 1996;June:22.
4. Hale G, ed. *The Sourcebook for the Disabled*. New York: Paddington Press; 1979.
5. Rintala DH, Howland CA, Nosek MA, et al. Dating issues for women with physical disabilities. *Sexuality Disabil* 1997;15(4):219-42.
6. Kroll K, Levy Klein E. *Enabling Romance: a Guide to Love, Sex, and Relationships for the Disabled (and the People who Care About Them)*. Bethesda: Woodbine House; 1995.
7. Frankel A. Sexual problems in rehabilitation. *J Rehabil* 1967;33(5):19-20.
8. Alexander CJ, Sipski ML, Findley TW. Sexual activities, desire, and satisfaction in males pre- and post-spinal cord injury. *Arch Sexual Behav* 1993;22(3):217-28.
9. Sipski ML, Alexander CJ. *Sexuality Reborn*. VHS. West Orange, NJ: Kessler Medical Rehabilitation Research and Education Center; 1993.
10. Fisher HE. *The Anatomy of Love: a Natural History of Mating, Marriage, and Why We Stray*. New York: Fawcett Books; 1995:26.
11. *Sexuality & Body Image*. VHS. Minneapolis: University of Minnesota; 1994.
12. Robinson K. Caregiver and spouse: should the twain ever meet? *New Mobility*. 1998;Feb:12.
13. Travis R. Making love like a woman. *New Mobility* 1997;Feb:39.

14. Sipski ML, Alexander CJ, Rosen RC. Orgasm in women with spinal cord injuries: a laboratory-based assessment. *Arch Phys Med Rehabil* 1995;76:1097-102.

15. Toms-Barker L, Maralani V. *Challenges and Strategies of Disabled Parents— Findings from a National Survey of Parents with Disabilities.* Berkeley: Berkeley Planning Associates; 1997.

16. Maddox S. *Spinal Network.* Malibu: Miramar Publications; 1994:354.

17. Brackett NL, Lynne CM, Weizman MS, Bloch WE, Abae M. Endocrine profiles and semen quality of spinal cord injured men. *J Urol* 1994;151:117.

18. Brackett NL, Nash MS, Lynne CM. Male fertility following spinal cord injury: facts and fiction. *Phys Therap* 1996;76 (11):1221-31.

19. Brackett NL, Padron RP, Lynne CM. Semen quality of spinal cord injured men is better when obtained by vibratory stimulation versus electroejaculation. *J Urol* 1997;157:152-6.

20. Padron OF, Brackett NL, Weizman MS, Lynne CM. Semen of spinal cord injured men freezes reliably. *J Androl* 1994;15(13):266-9.

Chapter 6

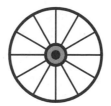

Spinal Cord Research

Recently, there has been dramatic progress in central nervous system (CNS) research. Researchers have begun to unlock the complexities of what happens when the brain and spinal cord are injured and what obstructs their ability to regenerate and recover function. Researchers are working on a remarkably wide variety of fronts to figure out how to promote the growth of CNS tissues and to get nerve pathways communicating again.

Many of the current lines of research might translate into increased function for thousands of people with disabilities. It is likely that research into conditions such as muscular dystrophy or multiple sclerosis will provide insights on spinal cord injury (SCI). What researchers discover about spinal cord trauma may well impact treatment of other conditions involving nerve cell damage. The advanced technologies now available to scientists have allowed them to make discoveries never before possible in shorter time frames than ever before imagined. Given the recent pace of discovery, it follows naturally that we can look forward to more insight into the CNS and what might be done to support it, making recovery reliable following insult. Plenty of researchers say with certainty that it is just a matter of time, and money.

CNS research is also about much more than functional recovery of ambulation—walking. Scientists are exploring issues that relate primarily to quality of life with disability—pain management, sexual function, bowel and bladder management, exercise physiology, and aging with disability among them. Even memory and life perspective are becoming better understood in the modern wave of neuroscience.

The Dream of the Cure

The very notion of walking again following paralysis is very potent, deep in the modern psyche, and used unsparingly in the media as a surefire device for tugging on emotional heartstrings. Not that many years ago, doctors thought it was inconceivable to solve the puzzle of how to repair spinal cord damage or brain cell damage:

> *At the time of my injury in 1973, my doctor told me plainly*
> *that the spinal cord simply does not recover, and it never will.*

However, the fantasy of walking again may yet come true. Significant advances in molecular and cellular biology have expanded the potential to understand and influence the human nervous system. There is considerable optimism with regard to repairing chronically injured spinal cords.

Spinal cord research is not just about getting the spinal cord to grow, but about mapping the structure of the body and its systems, methods of treatment and rehabilitation, and genetic advances that overlap into many other areas of medical research. Walking gets all the emphasis in the media when, in fact, there are many other benefits to be gained from CNS research.

Walking also depends on whether we are talking about acute or chronic injury and degree of completeness. Many people with acute, incomplete SCI who get treated quickly have a chance of walking out of the hospital.

Setting aside whether a given person or group of people will walk again, the real value of this research work is that some people with disabilities will be able to function at higher levels of independence and activity than they can at this moment. Life will change significantly for those who now suffer too much pain or whose time is so occupied with managing their disability that they cannot commit themselves to a career or to travel, for instance. Some people can barely leave their homes or find themselves trapped in an extended care facility. Such people are much more interested in increasing their freedom and independence in any way possible than they are in walking.

Ambivalence Toward Cure Research

The disability community includes people who have expressed concern— if not outright resentment—about the degree of emphasis on a quest for a cure. They resent being thought of as "broken" and resist the notion that they should happily change to fit the popular image of what it means to be "whole." Some see the quest for cure as prejudicial, as if a person with a disability is assumed to be incapable of living a meaningful life.

But the more widespread attitude appears to be one of balance. When you are injured, you get on with your life, which includes disability, while welcoming the potential for developments in research that can contribute to your quality of life:

> *I think many of the anti-cure people focus too much on the semantics of the word "cure." How about "fix" instead? I have a spinal cord injury, which cannot be "cured" since I am not "sick." It is not a disease. But while I live a full life now and don't sit around whining about a cure, I fully realize that I could function better if my spinal cord was "fixed." I spend a lot of time managing my spinal cord injury—time that in the past I could use on my career, my relationships, my personal activities, etc.*

> *So, hey, I don't care what they call it; I am all for science and medicine attempting to allow my bladder, my bowels, my reproductive system, or my legs to function the way they were designed to.*

Cure research can be a source of emotional support and hope for families, albeit with the attending danger of expectations that might not be fulfilled. Physicians tend to be extremely cautious discussing research with their patients for fear of building up unrealistic hopes. Many people find that their treating doctors are less informed on the status of research than they are themselves. Still, it's possible to be hopeful while taking what you get:

> *Regarding an SCI cure, my wife and I look forward to the day when I'll walk again. We don't spend our time thinking about it but are definitely heartened by the optimistic research.*

Others seem to use the potential for cure as an excuse not to face their disabilities, to allow themselves to be cared for, and to surrender to the fears and challenges that must be faced in adapting to their disability. According to an active disabled person:

> *I know folks who have my illness and live for a cure. They don't use assistive devices and spend most of their time in bed, because "a cure is around the corner."*

Christopher Reeve's Impact

The story of Christopher Reeve (not "Reeves") embodies the modern story of our cultural relationship to cure. Soon after his C2 SCI in a horseback riding accident in 1995, Reeve began to explore the research milieu and committed himself to supporting—in fact, dramatically accelerating—its efforts. In the early years, he made dramatic statements about his intention to walk before reaching the age of 50. At times, he stated a short number of years until the cure. These kinds of comments enraged some in the disability community, who felt that Reeve was winding back the years of advocacy work, the goal of which was to shift the view of disability from the "medical model" to the "independence model."

There were, in fact, protests where Reeve would make public appearances, and the effect of this was only to put a barrier between him and the leaders of the disability community who could have worked with him productively as he made the same adjustments that anybody else with a significant disability needed to make—both functionally and psychologically. In this way, the disability community missed the chance to influence the direction that Reeve would wield his considerable charisma and public visibility.

In fact, Reeve, his wife Dana, and those close to them were committed to quality-of-life issues with disability from the very start. Says close friend and former Reeve Foundation director Michael Manganiello, in an article in *SCI Life* following Reeve's death:

> *There were quality of life issues the minute we got him*
> *home. Chris slept in the dining room for the first year, with*
> *Dana on the floor next to him because the house wasn't*
> *accessible.*

The Christopher & Dana Reeve Foundation, as of 2002, includes the Christopher & Dana Reeve Paralysis Resource Center, which provides direct support to people with disabilities through its resource center, makes grants to a wide array of organizations that have to do with programs only for living well with paralysis, publishes a resource book and a series of DVDs on the same array of issues found in this book, and aggressively advocates for disability rights in the US Congress.

Quite a puzzle: A Spinal Cord Overview

The brain and spinal cord make up the CNS. The peripheral nervous system (PNS) carries motor impulse messages from the CNS to our muscles and sensory messages to the spinal cord, which carries them back to the brain.

When injured, the PNS recovers, the CNS does not. Why the difference? The PNS and CNS systems are distinguished by two essential qualities.

■   A different biochemical makeup. The PNS has a biologic environment that supports the process of regeneration, whereas the CNS doesn't have the right biochemistry for growth. The CNS has been found to contain factors that actually inhibit regeneration.

■   A different physical structure. Peripheral nerves have a system of sheaths that help direct a damaged nerve back to its "connection" as it regenerates. Central nerves have no such guiding channels. The small amount of regrowth that does occur after an injury has no idea where to go.

To understand the challenge of the immensely intricate research puzzle, we must know something about the way the spinal cord is built. Simplistically, it consists of long nerve axons surrounded by a protective coating called myelin. We need to know what happens to this system when it is injured and what would stimulate growth in a way that will restore function.

What Happens in SCI?

The spinal cord is composed of millions of fine nerve fibers called axons, which carry motor impulses to neurons that in turn pass the information to the peripheral nerves and onward to muscles. Sensory messages move in the opposite direction, from nerve endings throughout the body, through the cord, and back to the brain. These nerves are like telephone cables—dense bunches of thin "wires" down which electrical signals travel (Figure 6-1).

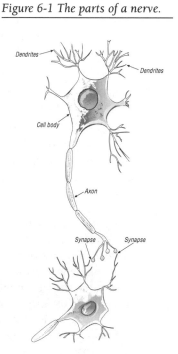

Figure 6-1 The parts of a nerve.

The spinal cord itself is made of up of gray matter, which carries both motor and sensory signals, and white matter, made up of myelinated nerves that carry signals from the gray matter between neurons. The spinal cord itself is made up of mostly long axons, which carry signals down to "cell bodies," which transfer these signals to and from the neurons that communicate with muscles and the body's largest organ—the skin and its sensory nerves.

Sometimes, in response to trauma, the body does manage to accomplish a degree of axonal regrowth on its own. Small amounts of nerve repair and remyelination have been observed. Central nerves have been known to sprout, sending out new shoots looking for a connection, but the odds are not good of linking up to a useful receptor without some help. The body really can't do this repair by itself.

As soon as a spinal cord is injured, a complex chain of events begins. The cord starts to hemorrhage, bleeding from the inside out. The cord—a soft, gelatinous material—is denied the basic nutrients and fuel it needs to function and maintain itself. The contents of the nerve, its axoplasm, leak out the end, immediately shortening the broken end of the nerve and putting distance between it and its former connection. The portion of the axon that is away from the neuronal cell body dies, while the cell body and remainder of its axon survive.

Soon after trauma, the body attempts to clean up the mess in a chemical onslaught that causes further secondary damage. As Melinda Kelley, PhD, former Associate Director of Research at the Paralyzed Veterans of America, describes it:

> Special cells called microphages and microglia help "eat" the debris and digest it. They also produce chemicals that detract from the regenerative process while they are in the area.

As damaged cells get digested by the body, some healthy ones get eaten too, spreading the extent of the injury. The body tries vainly to repair itself but, in reality, causes more harm.

The body has an intelligence of its own, a miraculous system of programmed responses to its own conditions. One such process called apoptosis is a sort of cell suicide. When cells discover they are no longer needed by the body, they destroy themselves. Spinal cord and brain trauma trick cells into believing they have completed their work and apoptosis begins, further increasing the degree of secondary damage. Spinal cord researcher Dennis Choi, MD, PhD, of Washington University in St. Louis has been addressing the question of apoptosis:

> A great deal is currently being learned that which is translating into specific strategies for inhibiting apoptosis. Overall, I would describe this research as still in early stages (cell and animal model testing). There are some theoretical concerns with the strategy of inhibiting apoptosis, that will have to be answered by further experiments. For example, the spinal cord may be better off if some badly damaged cells undergo apoptosis, rather than hanging on and getting in the way of recovery.

Within a week, nerve cells begin to degenerate, and whatever regenerative efforts the body had been trying come to a stop. Following injury, the glial scar—a physical and chemical barrier—forms, which obstructs neuronal growth. It is a chemical barrier due to growth inhibitors. The issue of glial scarring has been controversial, but current science appears to recognize it as a meaningful factor in the CNS injury puzzle.

Axons are surrounded by a protective material called myelin. When an axon is damaged and retreats, the myelin that surrounds it is also affected. As described by Dr. Wise Young of the W.M. Keck Center for Collaborative Neuroscience at Rutgers, the State University of New Jersey:

> Myelin is made by cells called oligodendroglia. Injury damages both axons and oligodendroglia. Each oligodendroglia myelinates as many as 20 to 30 axons. So, when oligodendroglia are damaged, they die and many axons may become demyelinated. Remyelination occurs, but many axons that survive the injury are either demyelinated or poorly myelinated.

Remyelination is a substantial part of the spinal cord cure puzzle, since a regenerated axon will not work without a restored myelin layer to protect it. In an incomplete SCI, it is not unusual for some axons to remain intact, yet be unable to pass impulses because of disruptions to their myelin. Nerve regrowth may not be the entire challenge here. Restoring myelin could mean a degree of renewed function for some spinal cord-injured persons. The majority of SCIs are incomplete injuries.

The degree of axonal death just after the injury is further exacerbated by a loss of circulation to the area. Blood supply through a system of very fine, microscopic capillaries is disrupted. Traumatized tissues are damaged by this loss of blood, but so are nearby healthy nerve tissues that have not been directly impacted but, nonetheless, need a constant supply of nutrients.

Blood and all of its nutrients and factors must be present to foster regeneration. For a true recovery, a permanent vascular system must be reestablished. This extremely delicate network of capillaries must integrate with existing tissues and maintain the flow of metabolic materials into and out of the new tissues.

The first successes in axonal regeneration—although exciting—produced disappointingly small amounts of growth. Recent efforts have been more encouraging in getting axons to grow over longer distances and are beginning to produce promising functional improvement.

The PNS has Schwann cells that promote growth and remyelination, but these are not present in the CNS. The central system has cells called oligodendrocytes, which produce myelin; however, they are unable to produce enough to compensate for the degree of damage involved here.

There are just not enough nerve growth factors present in the CNS to respond to trauma. The body apparently has figured that, once born, it no longer needs the capacity to grow central nerve tissue. Even worse, there are "inhibitors" that have been identified as getting in the way of the body's attempt to regenerate.

But there's more. Getting a nerve to grow with proper insulation is useless unless the nerve can get to the right destination. Remember that the CNS doesn't have the guiding channels found in the peripheral system. The axon has to reach the correct location. In animal studies, there have been cases of regeneration with no functional improvement whatsoever.

But it is not clear that specific nerves must make exact connections. The body might be able to retrain itself to use new connections, in whatever manner it needs to proceed. The receptor sites needing an axonal path to the brain might also have the ability reach out and grab a new axon, rather than having to guide an axon to the site itself. All of this is very preliminary.

In some cases, the spinal cord becomes attached to surrounding tissues. This is known as tethering and can restrict the flow of spinal fluids—which surround the cord—past the injury site. Pain and loss of function can result.

Surgery to untether the spinal cord is already being performed. Of 40 people operated on at the University of Miami and whose outcomes were reported by the Miami Project to Cure Paralysis, 79% showed improved motor function, and 62% had reduction in chronic pain.[1] For some people, untethering surgery might be necessary as part of a spinal cord regeneration therapy.

Suppose we get axons to grow—possibly as many as five million are needed—by supplying the growth factors and obstructing the inhibitors. We ensure that they are protected by myelin. We provide a continuing supply of blood and nutrients to the area and get the scarring out of the way to allow growth. We get the axonal end to grow long enough and direct it to the right location—or train the body to reroute its messages—and form working neurons and synapses to get the message out to the muscles. Can we walk now?

That depends. Now we need to ask to what degree atrophied muscles have the capacity to receive impulses and start to produce muscle fiber capable of sufficient contraction. In other words, will the muscles work, and how strong can they become? To carry the weight of the upper body and to work continuously without early fatigue is a tall order. After only months of atrophy from disuse, the degree of lost muscle strength is considerable. After years of disuse, who knows?

Whether muscles can work again depends on whether or not there is damage to "lower motor neurons," a particular type of cell in the nervous system that carries messages directly to muscles. Even if the brain-to-muscle communication is interrupted, the muscles can still be receiving enough signal for muscle cells to be maintained. Without lower motor neuron signals, muscle cells die. Ironically, spasticity (often seen as a disadvantage) preserves considerable muscle tone. People with spasticity will have less work to do rebuilding muscle if the cord is regenerated. There is also no question that spastic muscles have functioning motor neurons.

Many people with neurologic conditions develop contractures, in which muscles, tendons, and ligaments are permanently shortened. Even if the spinal cord can be completely cured, there are considerable issues of rehabilitation involved in getting someone into the right posture, building muscle, and re-teaching them the process of walking. Once the nervous system gets talking again, there is a major process of rehabilitation left to face.

When people don't walk for a number of years, their bones lose density, that is, they develop osteoporosis. This loss of bone density is another key question: whether the bones will be able to support the considerable weight of the body and tolerate the impact of walking.

Walking, as we've said, is not even the whole picture. What does all of this—nerve regeneration, myelin sheathing, establishment of blood supply, removal of scarring, nerve connections, muscle rebuilding, and bone strength—have to do with sexual function, bowel and bladder control, pain, and many other side issues related to various disabilities? Researchers gain insight into all of these areas when they perform research in basic science.

So this—extremely simplistically—is the puzzle that researchers face. One can understand the fascination of the challenge. With the availability of modern microscopes, laboratories, and computers, scientists can now study and engineer at the molecular level. They can see the processes, they can control them to some degree in the body, or they can reproduce certain aspects in the laboratory. They can attempt to reproduce some of the pieces through genetic engineering. How remarkable!

From this description, it could seem all but impossible to achieve a cure, but the progress made to date, if anything, answers what seemed completely impossible only a matter of years ago. The more researchers unearth the detailed physiology of what goes on with damage to the CNS, the closer we get to putting the impossible behind us, where therapies for acute—and even chronic—injury are a matter of course.

The Research Effort

There is a huge array of research projects geared toward disability-oriented research. It would take many encyclopedia-sized books to list them and even begin to describe their work—much less how the research fits together. Particular studies and researchers will be mentioned here to give you a sense of the variety of studies, the immense complexity, the excitement of the progress, and the skill and dedication of the researchers. However, for each project or person mentioned, there are dozens who deserve equal billing.

SCI Research Beginnings

The first attempt to understand SCI took place early in the 20th century, when a Spanish neuroanatomist named Santiago Ramon y Cajal conducted experiments with dogs and cats. He showed that the brain and spinal cord are made up of specialized cells, different from the rest of the body's nervous system. He was the first explorer who mapped the structure of neurons and axons that make up the system and is revered today by anatomists as a pioneer. He observed that, when cut, CNS axons made a brief effort to regrow and then stopped. His work is the source of the long-standing belief that nothing could be done to regenerate CNS nerves.

In the early 1980s, a Montreal Institute of Neurology team led by Dr. Albert Aguayo became the first to demonstrate that spinal cord axons could grow more than the slight distance that had been observed by Cajal. Suddenly, the accepted dogma that spinal cords could not regenerate had to be reconsidered. But this demonstration was still a long way from getting damaged axons to grow enough to bring about a "cure."

Dr. Wise Young, formerly at New York University and now the Director of the Neuroscience Center at Rutgers, State University of New Jersey, has been interested in spinal cord regeneration since well before it caught on in the neuroscience community. Early on, his attempts to get spinal cord research on the agenda at the Society for Neuroscience conferences met with little enthusiasm. But then Dr. Aguayo and his colleagues made the breakthrough that demonstrated that spinal cord axons could indeed grow. A few years later, Dr. Martin Schwab of the Brain Research Institute at the University of Zurich in Switzerland identified a growth inhibitor and began work on counteracting the inhibitor. Suddenly CNS research caught on, and Wise Young has been in the thick of it ever since.

Nerve Regeneration: Something Is in the Way

The first assumptions about the inability of axons to regenerate were that something was missing. Then, in 1988, Dr. Schwab discovered that something is in the way. His team found a protein that inhibits CNS regrowth after a trauma. The team has been experimenting with ways to turn off this protein to allow axons to regenerate. In 1990, they discovered an antibody called IN-1 that appeared to block the protein. The team observed about 11 millimeters of growth in the spinal cord of a rat. This was a major step in the research.[2]

But the inhibitor protein discovered by Schwab's team is apparently not the only one that exists. James Salzer, MD, PhD, at New York University discovered another inhibitor protein—a myelin-associated glycoprotein (MAG)—in the late 1980s. Actually, it was another researcher who found that the protein prevented axonal growth, and yet another who found that the IN-1 antibody had impact on it. At this early stage, it is hard to know if other molecules in Schwab's test rats also had an effect on the experiment. Such is the complexity of this research and an example of how collaborative the process needs to be.

The inhibiting proteins reside in the myelin—the fatty tissue surrounding nerve axons—in very small quantities. It is very difficult for scientists to purify and analyze the proteins in order to generate enough to be used for research. Scientists must refine the molecules with absolute precision to develop a usable treatment. It is painstaking work and an example of why this research takes so long. The difficulties of getting a quantity of usable protein for research also limits multiple laboratories from being able to participate in the work. There is not enough to go around.

Another approach to turning off the inhibitors is being explored with cellular adhesion molecules (CAMs). CAMs reside on the membrane surface of nerve cells. They foster communication between the nerve cells. For instance, CAMs help nerve cells to recognize an axon so that they know where to go and do their job of creating myelin. CAMs also help override the inhibitors and, so, play a similar role to that of the IN-1 antibody.

A CAM known as L1 has been shown to play a role in the regeneration of axons. Another Swiss researcher, Melitta Schachner, showed that L1 stimulates growth and does so in the presence of the inhibiting protein discovered by Schwab. L1 is known to be present in the developing brain and spinal cord but goes away after birth. L1 that is found in rats is 99% similar to that found in humans, making animal studies more reliable as indicators of what might happen in humans.

L1 is found on Schwann cells—which produce myelin in the peripheral system but not on oligodendrocytes—which create myelin in the CNS. This makes Schwann cells of great interest because they not only might remyelinate the spinal cord, but could promote regrowth of the axons. And, since IN-1 is so difficult to produce, L1 might prove to be a more practical solution, if only because it is easier to synthesize.

Factors like IN-1 and L1 can clear a path by overriding inhibiting proteins, but something more is needed to really get things growing. Dr. Naomi Kleitman, Director of Education at the Miami Project to Cure Paralysis, says:

> *Whether a nerve cell can regenerate is more a question of environment than the absolute ability of a cell in one or another part of the nervous system to be able to grow.*

The job for researchers is to create that right environment for regeneration to take place.

Growth Factors

Neurotrophins feed nerves and, so, stimulate growth. The brain and spinal cord already produce these growth factors but not in sufficient quantity to repair a trauma. There is quite a list of growth factors being studied by researchers. Nerve growth factor (NGF) was discovered in 1951 by Italian researcher Rita Levi-Montalcini and Viktor Hamburger of Washington University in St. Louis. Others include basic fibroblast growth factor (bFGF), brain-derived neurotrophic factor (BDNF), and glial cell line-derived neurotrophic factor (GDNF). Among many others, these growth factors are commonly referred to in research literature. According to Wise Young:

> *It is really important that we try and compare all of them. We currently do not know enough about the regenerating axons in the spinal cord to predict which one will work the best. It is likely that many of the factors play multiple roles in different tissue and at different times during development.*

Dr. Kleitman talks about the presence of up to 50 growth promoters present in the PNS.

> *Any nerve cell will respond to these if it has the proper receptor for it. We know that central nerves can respond to these as well as peripheral nerves in many cases. During the course of the life of a nerve cell, it might be receptive to a given growth factor at one point and a different one at another time.*

The one that has shown the most promise and has earned the most research attention is called NT3. In 1994, Dr. Schwab and his team used NT3 along with the inhibitor antibody, IN-1. They got nerve fibers to grow the entire length of a rat's spinal column—another groundbreaking step.

In the July 15, 1997, issue of *The Journal of Neuroscience*, researchers at the University of California, San Diego, reported an early success in axonal regrowth using gene therapy. They managed to get injured rats' own cells to produce growth factor right at the injury site. They used normal skin cells from the rats and altered them genetically to get them to produce NT3. When grafted back into the animals, these new cells secreted NT3, which produced axonal regrowth. Some rats recovered a degree of walking ability.[3]

Another good piece of news in the study is that the cells continued to produce NT3 for several months. This means that the cells were able to produce enough NT3 to be effective, yet were not what researchers call immortal cells. Such cells can cause cancer, since they continue to reproduce and ultimately spread where they are not wanted. Wise Young summarizes his optimism about future progress:

> The story is now becoming clear. There are facilitory and inhibitory proteins. In the presence of facilitory proteins, the inhibitory proteins do not prevent axonal growth. We are achieving a much better understanding of these proteins. It is a very exciting time in regeneration research.

Schwann Cells

When nerve axons die, so does their myelin. So, if axons are regenerated, the myelin must also be regenerated. In the PNS, Schwann cells promote growth of myelin and regeneration of injured nerve axons. In the CNS, oligodendrocytes perform the job of myelin production. However, says Dr. Kleitman:

> Oligodendrocytes have an additional inhibitor that is not present in Schwann cells. They seem not to be very aggressive remyelinators. For some reason, Schwann cells are really aggressive about doing what they want to do.

Oligodendrocytes in the CNS also have a tendency to cross over between axons, whereas Schwann cells have the ability to myelinate along the length of a single axon.

Since Schwann cells are not naturally present in the spinal cord, researchers are particularly interested in bringing them into the CNS and using them there as a possible tool for spinal cord repair. It is already well proven that Schwann cells are also able to regenerate myelin in the CNS for both sensory and motor nerves. The challenge remains to find how to create the conditions in which Schwann cells can accomplish this regeneration in a compromised spinal cord.

Schwann cells have the ability to create a connective framework that holds cells in place as they regenerate. This framework is a latticework of proteins called an extracellular matrix. The extracellular matrix looks like a blanket that wraps around the axon and the Schwann cells. This matrix—different in some respects from the extracellular matrix found in the CNS—is a key characteristic of Schwann cells and has growth-promoting features of its own. Its major component is a protein called laminin, which is also a promoter of growth. Kleitman states:

> *Not all cells like it. Laminin is just one kind of protein that some cells like to grow on at certain points in their lifetime.*

Schwann cells contribute to the regeneration of the nerve as well as the myelination and, so, perform a double duty. They help the nerve to grow and provide a myelin sheath in a controlled fashion along the nerve, and the matrix generates a structure that keeps the whole thing in place. Kleitman explains:

> *That is why these cells (Schwann) are so potent, because they basically bring their whole manufacturing system with them.*

At the Miami Project, researchers are working with Schwann cell "bridges." The bridges are based on work from Brown University, which produced a hollow polymer tube that can be wrapped around nerves. (Remember that the scale is microscopic.) According to Kleitman:

> *We took six million Schwann cells, mixed them up with a commercially available extracellular matrix mixture, and stuck it inside one of these hollow polymers. What happened was that the Schwann cells all lined up and created a nice little pathway that you can attach between severed ends of a spinal cord.*

This little pathway serves as a guide for nerve growth between two damaged axonal ends.

Schwann cells alone will not be the magic solution. Dr. Mary Bartlett Bunge of the Miami Project led a study in which Schwann cells were engineered to produce the growth factor BDNF. In the first set of studies, the researchers completely transected a spinal cord and laid down a trail of half a million Schwann cells. They found a lot more growth with BDNF and Schwann cells in combination than with Schwann cells alone.[4] Dr. Kleitman observes:

> *Almost everybody you talk to is going to talk about what combination of factors and cells we'll need to use.*

The following questions still remain about Schwann cells:

- Can enough cells be placed and controlled to bring about optimal repair?
- There are a number of different kinds of nerve tissues to be repaired in the spinal cord. Can Schwann cells affect them all?
- Can Schwann cells penetrate to the areas of the cord where regeneration is needed?

At this stage, getting nerves to grow in the spinal cord is not really the problem. Now it is a matter of getting enough of them to grow long enough and establish functional connections. Dr. Young estimates that about 10% of connections are sufficient to support substantial functional recovery in rats and humans. Since most people still have some connections remaining across the injury site, regeneration only needs to make up the difference.

Getting the Growth Factors There

Regeneration of the spinal cord is not just a matter of giving someone a pill or an injection. Growth factors must be integrated into the complex, continuous metabolic processes in the body. Growth factors must get to the right place, interact with other very specific molecules, and be replenished as they are used. Rather than just putting growth factor into the body, researchers are finding ways of getting the body to produce the growth factor itself.

A University of California, San Diego, team is using fibroblasts. These are cells in the skin that can produce substances that affect nerve growth. Fibroblasts have certain advantages. As Wise Young explains:

> Fibroblasts represent a very important candidate for delivery
> of growth factors to the injury site. Among other features,
> they can be isolated from the individual receiving the cells and
> then genetically modified in culture. This is the best way to
> prevent rejection of the transplanted cells when they are put
> back into the body. I believe that fibroblasts will be a major
> vehicle for delivery of factors to the spinal cord.

Making the Right Connections

Dr. Samuel Kuwada of the University of Michigan is performing a "molecular genetic analysis of axon guidance in the spinal cord." Neurons make connections with their appropriate target cells by relying on specific molecules that direct axons. Scientists believe that identifying and understanding these guidance molecules may help direct regenerating axons to the right place. The University of Michigan researchers use zebrafish embryos to help them generate molecules called netrins. Netrins appear to play a role in making connections during embryonic spinal cord development.

Dr. Marc Tessier-Lavigne is also exploring netrins at the University of California, San Francisco. His team's work suggests that a couple of different netrin molecules are found in the adult CNS. Their research abstract states:

> Netrins seem to attract some classes of axons and repel others. The work being proposed here seeks to pinpoint the receptors on axons that mediate the biological effects of the netrins. Candidate receptors have been identified in the past year, and their functions in development and regeneration of connections are beginning to be evaluated.

Pattern Generators

Then again, maybe the exact nerve pathways don't have to be recreated. Another avenue of research has studied exactly what the pathways are that produce the unique combination of impulses that make walking possible. There is some early evidence that the body has the capacity to reroute its messages, like a telephone operator plugging into a different line. The human body has some remarkable adaptive abilities, and part of the solution to the puzzle may involve letting the body do its own thing by simply removing the impediments and then giving it the building blocks it needs. These are known as pattern generation studies.

Walking apparently doesn't rely entirely on messages from the brain. Part of the process of walking happens below the level of the injury—impulses traveling between muscles and the spinal cord without having to make it past the injury and back to the brain. It is not clear to what degree this might be the case in humans, but Miami Project researchers have studied a person with a 17-year history of incomplete cervical injury who began exhibiting involuntary stepping-like movements in his legs. This study strongly suggests that there is a "central pattern generator," a group of nerve cells that synchronize muscle activity during alternating stepping of the legs.

This discovery—accelerated by Christopher Reeve's demonstration that continued activity can result in restoration of sensory and motor function, even years after injury—has fostered an entirely new avenue of research and rehabilitation: activity-based therapy. Spearheaded by neurologist Dr. John McDonald—who worked directly with Reeve—at Washington University and The Rehabilitation Institute of St. Louis, physical therapy gyms are now commonly equipped with a treadmill over which an injured person can be suspended in order to simulate walking. Functional electric stimulation (FES) bikes are another means of simulating motion in the legs for this purpose.

In this way, the pattern generators are encouraged to get involved. According to McDonald, this process even fosters the regrowth of spinal cord axons, creating functional connections. Activity-based rehab is the most notable and exciting recent addition to the milieu of CNS research.

Mapping the Spinal Cord

Recent computerized tools like CT (computed tomography) and MRI (magnetic resonance imaging) scans have fostered a revolution in medical care and research. SCI scientists are getting a highly detailed, three-dimensional look at the spinal cord thanks to these technologies.

Projects are underway that are designed to map the cord, including work at Purdue University and at Washington University in St. Louis, Missouri. At Purdue University, researchers are gathering information produced from 3-D images and making this material available as a database through computer networks that researchers can access. Dr. William Snider of Washington University believes that mapping the cord is critical to the process of achieving regeneration. He says:

> We think understanding how axons first find their targets in developing spinal cords applies to the situation after injury. A regenerating axon will likely have to retrace the same incredibly complex path to reform working connections.

A map of the spinal cord will also be a valuable diagnostic tool in the emergency room. The extent of injury will be much clearer to doctors, thanks to the ability to see a three-dimensional image of the injured cord. Researchers also benefit from being able to better witness the effect of their therapies.

Preserving and Restoring Muscles

We've already discussed the need for lower motor neurons to be present for muscles to retain the ability for recovery in the case of a spinal cord regeneration. Research is also addressing the question of producing sufficient muscle mass for walking.

To determine whether muscle tissues could contract if the cord were repaired, physicians might perform certain simple diagnostic tests for the needed lower motor neuron activity. They would use reflex testing-tapping with that little hammer that we have all seen as a stereotype of a doctor's checkup—or they might use an electrical stimulation device to see if muscles respond to a direct impulse. This would be evidence that muscle cells have not died and, so, would imply that lower motor neurons are in place.

If muscles are to be preserved and possibly restored in the future, at the time of injury, the lower motor neuron nerves need to be preserved or replaced before substantial muscle death occurs. According to Wise Young: "Neuronal replacement was considered science fiction until recently. The big discovery occurred rather quietly in the 1980s."

You can accommodate a degree of motor neuron death. Explains Young:

> *Muscles probably follow the same 10% rule that applies to the central nervous system, in which only 10% of the axons in the spinal cord are necessary and sufficient to support substantial function. Individual muscle cells can increase their bulk many times. A weightlifter, for example, can increase a muscle width by five to 10 times. This results more from expansion of individual muscle cells than from the production of more muscle cells.*

In other words, there can be a degree of muscle cell death from lost gray matter in the spinal cord where motor neurons reside, and it can still be possible to build enough muscle strength for functional use.

Embryonic Stem Cells

Embryonic stem cells have become very familiar in American culture, the subject of a dramatic political and cultural debate about the ethics of using them for research and whether federal money should pay for such activities.

Here is the science. Cells from a human fetus or embryo have the ability to form themselves into any of the roughly 200 types of human cells. This type of cell is referred to as "pluripotent." If we can harness and direct the capacity of stem cells to become any other kind of cell, then we can solve a huge range of medical conditions, not the least being regeneration of brain and spinal cord cells. People with Alzheimer's disease, Parkinson's, Huntington's disease, diabetes, leukemia, epilepsy, and other conditions are believed to be in a position to gain from stem cell research as well. There have already been early successes with Parkinson's disease.

When stem cells are inserted into another body, they are not seen as invaders, so rejection is less likely to occur. They integrate well with existing tissue. Several researchers have reported that they can induce these stem cells to differentiate into motor neurons. This suggests that it is possible to replace lost motor neurons in the spinal cord.

The missing growth factor needed for axonal growth is present in embryonic cells. These cells play a role in fetal development of the spinal cord, but "turn off" after we are born. Therefore, another avenue of research has been to transplant fetal cells directly into the spinal cord in the hope of switching back on the nerve growth capacity. Researchers choose embryonic cells rather than adult stem cells, which they do not believe have the same therapeutic potential.

The Politics and Ethics of Embryonic Stem Cells

Use of embryonic tissue is a delicate ethical and political issue. One of President Bill Clinton's first acts of office in 1993 was to remove the five-year-old moratorium on embryonic cell research that had been imposed during the Reagan/Bush era. The only fetal cells that had been allowed to be used were those from spontaneous abortion (miscarriage). Spontaneous abortions are often the result of conditions that render the tissue unusable. Research is therefore limited to efforts in laboratories in the US that are able to find sufficient nonfederal funding and those outside of the US.

When President George W. Bush took office in 2000, one of his first acts was to strike federal support for embryonic stem cell research, limiting monies to only the "lines" that were already in existence—64 of them, as the public was told. Many researchers have stated that a small percentage of the 64 lines are actually of value in the laboratory.

In the fall election of 2004, the voters of the state of California approved $80 billion dollars to be raised with a bond issue for stem cell research in the state. The following May, San Francisco was approved as the city to be host to the California Institute for Regenerative Medicine. The bond issue continues to be challenged in the courts. Meanwhile, the University of California has established the Human Embryonic Stem Cell Research Center (www.escells.ucsf.edu)

The primary ethical concern is around the question of whether an embryonic cell is equivalent to a human life. These cells are the product of an egg and a sperm creating a viable embryo, capable—in the right conditions—of growing into a person able to survive outside the womb. A significant number of people—principally based on religious beliefs—object to what they consider the destruction of life. Or worse, they view it as a form of enslavement, producing life in order to destroy it in the name of research. The potential benefits, in their view, do not override the essential ethical wrongness of using these cells for medical research.

A large number of human embryos are being generated—and stored—in fertility clinics, a product of new technologies that allow a woman's eggs to be removed from the ovaries, inseminated outside of the womb, and then placed into the womb to be carried to term. Necessarily, in the process, an excess number of embryos are generated to increase the odds that one will survive implantation into the uterus. From the many couples for whom this process succeeds, a considerable number of remaining embryos are destined for destruction. Supporters of embryonic stem cell research feel that it is, in fact, unethical to dispose of viable embryos that could be used to achieve potentially historic gains in medical therapies for such a wide range of human conditions.

At this writing, the 2008 presidential campaign is under way. Should a Democrat gain the office, we will likely see the release of federal funds for embryonic stem cell research. As long as this issue has the rhetorical power it does, we will see it swing back and forth depending on who holds majorities in the White House and the Congress.

In the hope of circumventing these complex ethical questions, there are efforts at hand to genetically produce cells with the same features as embryonic cells. If these efforts succeed, actual viable embryos will no longer be necessary for the therapy.

One solution to take the ethical controversy out of stem cell research is the development of somatic cell nuclear transfer (SCNT). SCNT uses a patient's own cells and an unfertilized human egg to make embryonic stem cells that match the patient's genetic makeup. The SCNT process does not use or harm an embryo or fetus. It is sometimes referred to as "therapeutic cloning" because it matches the DNA of the donor. This differs, however, from "reproductive cloning," in which the goal is to bring to life another being with the same DNA. SCNT is a process only for producing stem cells capable of differentiating into tissues that can be transplanted as a therapy without risking rejection. Some people object to SCNT, feeling that using a woman's egg toes the same ethical boundary as using an embryo.

In November of 2007, the journal *Nature* reported two dramatic advances that were widely reported in the international media and considered major steps forward that could potentially defuse the entire ethical debate over stem cell research. Shinya Yamanaka of the University of Kyoto in Japan and his team had "reprogrammed" human skin cells into essentially believing they were embryonic stem cells. They called them "induced pluripotent" cells. A team at the Oregon Health Sciences University had also succeeded in cloning the embryos of a monkey, the first time that this had been achieved successfully with a primate. However, neither of these research studies had been put to the full scientific test of whether they produce truly pluripotent stem cells that will supplant the need for the use of human embryos.

Other Transplantations

Researchers are experimenting with many kind of cells, from both human donors and animals. Cells are studied for the various features we have seen—a capacity to stimulate growth, to resist or suppress inhibitors, to multiply and go to the right place, and so on. The variety of possible sources for cells is huge.

In a study by Dr. Geoffrey Raisman, at the National Institute for Medical Research in London, cells were taken from inside the nose. These olfactory ensheathing cells succeeded in stimulating the recovery of a small SCI in rats. These cells are of interest because they are easy to collect and are continuously produced in the body, providing a generous supply. They are also the only type of cell in the CNS capable of regenerating themselves. There is also hope that they can act as a chaperone, helping newly generated axons to cross that difficult boundary between the peripheral and central nervous systems. This is the point where axonal growth often stops and is one reason why growth has not reliably led to functional improvement.

Controversial Treatments

In Tijuana, Mexico, a group of neurosurgeons is working with embryonic cells from the blue shark. Although they report improvements in the 16 human subjects with whom they have worked, they have not documented their research in a detailed fashion, making American researchers uncomfortable. Rather than conducting a carefully documented research study, the team at the Mexican clinic is interested in offering what they believe is a useful cure and are able to do so without the constraints placed on physicians in the United States by the Food and Drug Administration (FDA). Anyone considering participating in such undocumented research should go to every possible extreme to understand the work and its risks before considering an unregulated procedure.

Another controversial treatment for SCI is called omentum transposition. The omentum is a band of tissue in the abdomen of mammals that seals off abdominal injuries. A surgical procedure partially detaches the omentum, reconnecting it at the injury site. Removing it seems not to have a negative effect on the abdomen. The theory is that the omentum—which is rich in blood vessels—may supply the damaged nerve cells with vital oxygen and, possibly, may secrete chemicals that stimulate nerve growth.

Initial animal trials seem to show some functional improvement if the operation is completed within three hours of injury. Little or no improvement is shown when the procedure is done six to eight hours after injury.

Scarring at the cord, as well as abdominal complications, have been observed as a result of omental transplant. Clinical trials for people who have had a chronic SCI had been scheduled and were then canceled. This research has not been scientifically documented, so there is considerable skepticism regarding its value.

Methylprednisolone

Although the search goes on for an ultimate solution to regenerating the spinal cord, there have already been early accomplishments that help reduce the extent of damage to the cord at the time of injury. Methylprednisolone is a steroid that has been found to reduce the inflammatory process that occurs after injury.

A milestone in practical treatment occurred in May 1990. The results of the National Acute Spinal Cord Injury Study showed that methylprednisolone was found to reduce the extent of spinal cord trauma when given within eight hours of injury. Improvements of up to 20% have been measured, compared to people who were given no drug. The use of methylprednisolone with spinal cord trauma is now standard in emergency centers and in the toolkits of ambulance and EMT personnel throughout the United States.

The effect of methylprednisolone is significant, according to Wise Young:

> For someone with incomplete spinal cord injury and treated with methylprednisolone, the likelihood of the person walking out of the hospital is high. For example, athletes Dennis Byrd and Reggie Brown both walked out of the hospital. While people should not develop unrealistic expectations, they should also not become unduly pessimistic.

Methylprednisolone is an anti-inflammatory agent in common use for other purposes, such as a treatment for flare-ups of multiple sclerosis, lupus, severe asthma, and other conditions. The use of methylprednisolone has been the first time that treatment of any kind has been found to have an effect on the spinal cord.

Methylprednisolone might also play a role in regeneration. Future spinal cord treatment might itself be inflammatory, so the tissue would need protection. Dr. Kleitman of the Miami Project points out:

> Chances are good there would be some injury to the cord from putting cells in. If I were undergoing that, I would want [methylprednisolone] at the time of surgery.

The Multicenter Animal Spinal Cord Injury Study

The Multicenter Animal Spinal Cord Injury Study (MASCIS) was funded by the United States government's National Institutes of Health. MASCIS is following up on the initial work with methylprednisolone and other pharmaceuticals. These drugs have shown potential. The task now is to determine dosage, extent of follow-up therapy, and so on. This is a huge job, requiring thousands of experiments, well beyond the capacity of any one laboratory. Linda Noble, PhD, was a member of the MASCIS team. She says that the project is a very important development:

> It forced us to develop the best experimental model, putting it in all of the participating labs, and then following very specific guidelines for experimental design. This has never been done before in spinal cord research.

Such research is very slow and for good reason. According to Dr. Noble, the issue is reproducibility. What is done in one lab must be capable of duplication in another to prove consistent results. The only way to do this, and to find out the specific behavior of a drug or a therapy, is to closely control the conditions. She says:

> It's a very precise cookbook of instructions. It's very demanding on technicians and very time consuming. Because the process is so meticulous, it is fairly slow.

Established at a time when spinal cord research was uncoordinated and marginally supported, MASCIS represents an important step in making the research more efficient and a newfound cooperation among laboratories and scientists, making it possible for answers to be found that an individual lab could never have pursued on its own. This project is an important evolutionary step in the history of the research effort.

One of the greatest results of the MASCIS project was the development of the MASCIS Impactor, a device that accurately reproduces specific SCI in rodents. For research to be reproducible across various laboratories, there had to be a reliable and consistent means of creating the exact basis for the injury in laboratory rodents.

Hypothermia

Another method being explored to limit secondary damage at the time of injury is to lower the body temperature by two or three degrees, intentionally inducing hypothermia. This reduces the release of free radicals and glutamates, which destroy healthy cells not affected by the trauma. This treatment is counter to common sense, which would dictate that the body needs optimal circulation in order to respond to injury and recover. However, in the case of spinal cord trauma, it appears that interrupting the destructive process of secondary damage is of greater value. W. Dalton Dietrich, PhD, scientific director of the Miami Project, says:

> If you can cool the body by a few degrees and then, on top of that, provide a neuroprotective agent (such as methylpred-nisolone) or growth factor, you may see further dramatic improvements in the treatment of persons with acute SCI.[5]

Large-scale controlled studies have not yet been performed on this question.

4-Aminopyridine (4-AP)

The first effort to have an effect on the chronically injured spinal cord—well after the trauma—involved a drug called 4-aminopyridine or 4-AP, sometimes referred to as fampridine. Animal studies have shown that some nerve axons that survive a spinal cord trauma nonetheless fail to conduct an impulse past the injury site because of damaged myelin, the insulation of our spinal nerves. 4-AP appears to improve the function of demyelinated nerves. It does not actually restore myelin but, instead, helps existing axons with otherwise complete connections to relay impulses.

Dr. Andrew Blight of the University of North Carolina discovered the effects of 4-AP on the spinal cord. It was initially used as a treatment for multiple sclerosis and in the laboratory to study neurons and axons. The loss of myelin surrounding nerve axons allows potassium to intrude, among other effects, interfering with the passage of nerve impulses. 4-AP is a "potassium channel blocker," which limits potassium from interfering with conduction in demyelinated nerves, allowing these otherwise healthy axons to pass on an impulse. Since the greater portion of SCIs are incomplete—and presumably there are myelin-deprived but undamaged axons present—this could be a hopeful therapy for some people with CNS disorders.

Clinical trials performed in Canada in 1995 showed improvements in both motor and sensory functions following injections of 4-AP. Some of the subjects were more than a year post-injury. The degree of improvement varied. A man in Canada was able to consummate his marriage as a result of 4-AP treatment, yet other trial participants showed no reaction whatsoever. According to Dr. Blight:

> One third of the people with incomplete SCIs have experienced an improvement in quality of life in a variety of ways. In some

*people with significant preservation of motor function, the types
of benefits include reduced pain, spasticity, and muscle stiffness;
increased or more normal sensation; and some improvement in
motor functions, such as hand grip or walking efficiency. There
are also consistent indications of improvements in bladder control and male sexual functions.*[6]

Researchers were surprised to observe the reduced pain and spasticity.
If anything, they were concerned that pain and spasticity would increase,
since 4-AP amplifies nerve signals. All responses were temporary, yet scientists also found that benefits sometimes lasted for as long as four days, even
though the drug was no longer present in the blood. Further research is
exploring how it is that 4-AP continues to operate in the system.

4-AP works by increasing the excitability of axons, allowing them to
better pass on the voltage of a nerve impulse. It also increases the amount
of neurotransmitter at the synapse of the neuron, helping the impulse to
transmit itself better across the nervous system.

The search continues for a therapy that will permanently restore
myelin, either by stimulating the body to remyelinate its own axons or by
implanting new cells that would take hold and reproduce. That discovery
would cancel the need for the effects offered by 4-AP. In the meantime,
human clinical trials of 4-AP are underway at the time of this writing.

Since there is some progress in the use of transplanted cells to remyelinate axons, physicians need to know whether there are intact axons present
that would respond to such treatment. Toward this end, 4-AP could serve a
diagnostic role because, if someone responds to the drug, it means there are
intact but demyelinated axons present.

There is no question that recovery from an SCI will involve many different factors, as described by, Marco Saroni, a research fundraiser with
quadriplegia:

> *It's obvious that a cure is going to be complicated. There will
> be pharmaceuticals like growth factors, inhibitors. There will
> be surgery techniques, medical supplies, drug delivery, and a
> huge rehab effort. All of that is happening in parallel.*

Acorda Therapeutics

Acorda Therapeutics, the first commercial venture established specifically to
develop a spinal cord therapy, was established in 1995 by Dr. Ron Cohen.
After working at another biotechnology firm, Cohen took a sabbatical to
investigate what area of the industry would be exciting and had business
potential. He found about 20 different fundraising entities for spinal cord

research that were spreading their money around to various universities and research labs, with no coordination of the effort.

The academic laboratories are designed to make discoveries, not to develop them into something useful. A commercial entity is needed to conduct more extensive animal studies, conduct toxicity studies to make sure the therapy is not harmful, and then figure out how to make a pure medicinal grade product. Only then can you proceed with human trials.

At that time, no major pharmaceutical companies were showing interest in spinal cord therapy. They considered the market too small and were not convinced that the research would be fruitful. Another factor in deciding to pursue spinal cord research was the superb animal models developed by Wise Young and his team. Acorda's capacity to test as many as 3,000 animals per year owes its thanks in part to Wise Young's animal model.

Cohen gathered together the key players to discuss the issue and found them frustrated with the lack of organization and cooperation among the various funding groups and research labs. These scientists understood that research is of no value unless there is some way for its findings to be approved by the FDA, manufactured, distributed, and sold. These are tasks that happen in the commercial realm, so the spinal cord research community supported Cohen's efforts to establish Acorda.

Acorda is privately financed but has also received some institutional support. In 2008 the company became publicly traded. Acorda provides funds to its laboratory contractors and is poised to license therapies from the laboratories as they become available. Licensing will provide royalties to the universities where the labs are located, helping them to continue their work. Meanwhile, Acorda gets the right to produce and market the therapy. The first product Acorda intends to market is the drug 4-AP, which helps existing myelin-compromised axons pass on a nerve impulse. The Canadian Spinal Research Organization gained the patent rights for 4-AP and, in 1995, licensed them to Acorda. What makes the product unique is the "delivery method," a means of having it enter the bloodstream at a specific pace.

Acorda has reached FDA Phase III testing on 4-AP, including a disappointing result that shifted their protocol away from SCI to multiple sclerosis, in which results in controlled testing phases were more positive. The SCI community will nonetheless have access to the drug once it passes its final FDA testing, as doctors will be free to prescribe it as they see fit.

Who's Paying for the Research?

Spinal cord research has not been the kind of popular cause that attracts large amounts of money. Muscular dystrophy has the emotional image of disabled children, a well-known celebrity in Jerry Lewis, and a huge annual telethon to promote the Muscular Dystrophy Association's fundraising. AIDS has the fearsome quality of an epidemic and the political and cultural intrigue of our society's struggle with the acceptance of homosexuals. Cancer and heart disease happen on such a large scale at such extreme cost that large contributions by government and individuals seem modest in comparison.

The government has not been making the optimal investment in SCI research through the National Institutes of Health, instead, placing their emphasis on cancer and AIDS research. Lobbying efforts by the disability community have been focused on matters of employment, transportation, accessibility, and civil rights rather than on spending for cure research. The overall budget for SCI research is very small compared to what is spent on cancer research. When you compare it to the $9.7 billion that SCI is said to cost our economy each year—as estimated by the United States Centers for Disease Control and Prevention—it is mere pocket change.

Spinal cord research is now getting more money but, many would say, far from enough. The task of fundraising remains left to a variety of groups that raise money any which way they can, from individual memberships, corporate donations and endowments, to parties, golf tournaments, and the like.

The Organizations

Since the 1970s, a variety of groups have formed and reformed for the purpose of advancing SCI research. One of the first, begun by the wife of a spinal-injured man, was the Bermuda Conferences on Spinal Cord Injury Research, which has given an award every other year since 1972.

In the late 1970s, the Paralyzed Veterans of America, the Spinal Cord Society, the Paralysis Cure Research—formed by spinal-injured people—and the Help Them Walk Again Foundation were active. The Help Them Walk Again Foundation organized one of the first scientific meetings on SCI in 1979. The Spinal Cord Society funded much early research and earned national attention when its computerized walking demonstrations using functional electrical stimulation (FES) were featured on the television show *60 Minutes*.

When Christopher Reeve acquired high-level quadriplegia, requiring full-time ventilation for breathing, he began using his public fame and passionate organizing skills to campaign aggressively for CNS research. He joined forces with the American Paralysis Association, which soon transformed into the Christopher Reeve Foundation with the result of higher levels of fundraising and political advocacy. With Reeve's early death in 2004—and then, tragically, the loss of his wife Dana to cancer two years later—the Foundation has continued, and in fact grown. Now the Christopher and Dana Reeve Paralysis Foundation—reflecting Dana's very significant role—funds research, advocates, and provides resources for quality of life through their Paralysis Resource Center.

What was once a shifting mélange of groups has now consolidated into a few key entities that have grown and become more stable. Even more, where once they tended to be isolated and competitive, they are now cooperating and coordinating their efforts. The Reeve Foundation has formed the International Research Consortium on Spinal Cord Injury, the mission of which is "to promote structural repair and functional recovery in the acutely and chronically injured spinal cord." The consortium includes representatives from The Miami Project to Cure Paralysis, the Salk Institute, the University of Cambridge, and the University of Zurich.

Variety of Studies Being Conducted

There is a dizzying array of research projects being conducted under the auspices of these groups. Each season the Reeve Foundation, the Miami Project, and others all publish newsletters. The newsletter pages are graced with the faces of scientists next to their microscopes or banks of mysterious electronic devices, with summaries of their projects in very detailed terms. This is not reading for the average nonscientist, but it sure gets across the scale of talent at work. A few random examples:

- Dr. Robert H. Brown of Massachusetts General Hospital is working on a "non-viral vector for the targeted delivery of neuroprotective proteins to spinal cord motor neurons." The intent is to limit cell death from free radicals immediately after injury.
- Ron McKay, PhD, of the National Institute of Neurological Disorders and Stroke has been following up on a discovery made in the early 1990s. Stem cells in the brain and spinal cord have a unique ability to multiply and mature, giving added hope to the possibility of transplantation of cells.
- Jack Diamond, PhD, of McMaster University in Ontario, Canada, is exploring the "functional consequences of primary afferent intraspinal sprouting." Injured nerves often send out fresh sprouts that can't find a useful connection. This research attempts to find a use for the degree of regeneration that already takes place in the injured spinal cord.

- L.J. Stensaas of the University of Utah has studied the spinal cord of the newt. He found that astrocytes—cells normally found in nerves that provide nutrients—play a role in removing degenerating nerve axons and then act as a base for growth of new fibers.
- Dr. Amy MacDermott of Columbia University is looking into the "selective excitotoxic death of GABAergic dorsal horn neurons." Some people with SCIs become extremely sensitive to touch, which is often painful. Dr. MacDermott feels that there is a chemical process that overstimulates sensory nerves, and she hopes to develop a pharmaceutical treatment to minimize pain from this cause.
- Dr. James Guest, when completing his doctoral dissertation at the Miami Project, demonstrated that human Schwann cells support regeneration and myelination in adult rat spinal cords.
- Jian Zhou, PhD, of the University of Texas at Dallas addresses the "structural analysis of neurotrophin receptor signaling in neurons." This work intends to better describe the process of how signals are delivered through nerves by neurotrophins, which also support the nourishment and growth of nerves.

Reading these newsletters can leave you wondering how all these detailed studies fit together. They don't. There is intentional overlap, and various solutions are being explored for any given piece of the puzzle. One finding might shed light on another, or certain projects may suddenly add up to a solution that hadn't been considered (just as the discovery of penicillin was an "accident").

There seems to be more cause than ever to hope for some answers that will make a difference in the daily life of people with CNS disabilities. Hundreds of brilliant, highly educated, and highly trained people are working hard, and it is difficult to imagine that they won't make a difference in our life on wheels.

Who Else Benefits from SCI Research?

There has been a great deal of emphasis on spinal cord research here, but SCI research will benefit people with other disabilities, such as spinal muscular atrophy, stroke, traumatic brain injury, multiple sclerosis, Guillan-Barré syndrome, myasthenia gravis, and Alzheimer's and Parkinson's diseases. Elderly people with severe osteoarthritis can suffer the degradation of the spinal column itself, which can ultimately impact the cord. There are dozens of vascular, neurodegenerative, and congenital diseases that impact the spinal cord. Spinal cord tumors can occur in cases of metastasized breast or prostate cancer. People affected by all these conditions can benefit from this research.

When combined, people with these conditions far outnumber those with traumatic SCI. But SCI happens more commonly to young people, whereas these other conditions often appear later in life. Older people with other conditions will become wheelchair users. But their survival is often short, for example, once a cancer has spread, whereas a young person with a spinal injury is likely to live a normal life span. That difference in longevity makes the long-term costs of SCI greater, cold as that might sound. The fact is that there are plenty of forms of human suffering, all with their advocates and scientists clamoring for money from the same corporate and government sources. The fact that young people are being injured with a lifetime ahead of them is part of what justifies the amount of work done on spinal cord research. Fortunately, many others will get the chance to benefit.

Neurotechnology

The first "cure" effort to get wide public exposure involved simulating walking by using electrical impulses to make muscles contract. In 1970, scientists at the Rancho Los Amigos Hospital near Los Angeles and another group in what was then Yugoslavia got a person with paraplegia standing up with this approach, known as functional neuromuscular stimulation (FNS). In 1973, a test subject at the University of Virginia walked 40 feet, and a Vienna project got two people walking as far as 100 meters using crutches. In the United States, Dr. Jerold Petrofsky was a key player at Wright State University in Ohio and now leads the Petrofsky Institute, where FNS is featured.

FNS is a subset of FES, which is used in many other applications in which electrical impulse devices are used in places other than the muscles. A heart pacemaker is an example of FES, using electrical stimulation to balance the beating of the heart. FES is used for pain management and hearing enhancement and as an aid to male ejaculation, muscle strengthening, wound healing, and scoliosis correction. These uses are already accepted practice, and many other applications are either at the basic research level or as far advanced as clinical trials.

As with much "cure" research, FNS for standing and gait control has been overdramatized by the media. As a walking device, it is still at a very early stage, and its use is limited to a narrow population of qualified, potential users. Even with the increasingly small size of electrodes and the superfast processing speed of computer chips, walking with this technology is

not at all like using healthy muscles. It is very exhausting, although participants in trials have shown improvements with hard work and regular therapy and practice.

Yet, researchers have accomplished a great deal, including subjects
who have been able to walk up and down stairs using only the handrail.
Some have gotten far enough to use it for brief walking tasks such as walking down the aisle at their own wedding. Several current projects are
designed to achieve hands-free standing.

This is all meaningful progress, but FNS for walking still has a way to
go before it is a valid alternative to wheeling. Researchers at the Ontario
Neurotrauma Foundation are speculating that FES-assisted walking could
have secondary health benefits. Their study, initiated in April 2005, is com-
paring the incidence of urinary tract infections, pressure sores, and spasticity in people doing walking compared with those doing aerobic exercise and
resistance training. The study will be completed in April 2009.

How Muscles Walk

How a muscle is normally stimulated in the body is a very complex sequence
of events. Muscle stimulation is not simply a matter of how much electricity to send to which part of a muscle. This is a very detailed matter of how
the impulse intensity rises and drops and the maintenance of the impulse
during a contraction.

The body, it turns out, does not simply send a continuous stream of
electricity to the muscle but, rather, a stream of pulses. A continuous current quickly exhausts a muscle. Muscles also have different roles to play.
Some are for posture, and some are for movement, each displaying very different electrical profiles. Matching the natural pattern of stimulation is one
of the key challenges of FNS for walking, so that such a system can be used
productively without over-stimulation of the muscles. The system must
mimic the body's miraculous design, which makes the most efficient use of
its muscles to minimize fatigue.

Walking involves thousands of simultaneous signals going back and
forth between muscles and the brain, a tremendously intricate coordination
of sensations and contractions. The most sophisticated systems presently
use only 50 electrodes, though that number is sure to grow. At present, the
only possible stimulus is to make the muscle contract—the users get no
sensory feedback to know where their muscles are.

Electronics is one half of the system; the other half is bracing. In the
past, some people were fitted with heavy leg braces, which only added to the
weight that they had to balance, lift, and propel using crutches. This load
made more work for the electronics, too, so part of the effort has been to

develop lightweight bracing. The development of the reciprocating gait orthotic has been helpful thanks to its more lightweight design.

People who have been research subjects with early systems have been concerned with appearance. Most people don't want to go out in public all wired up and braced in a way that attracts unwanted attention. Lightweight braces and small power and control devices that can be worn under the clothes are being developed to make FNS more practical and desirable.

Locating the Electrodes

There are several methods of stimulating the muscles. Some designs use tight-fitting, stretchable pants that contain the electrodes. This is the most discrete method, but placing electrodes on the surface of the skin is the least effective way of getting the signal to the muscle. The signal has to pass through layers of skin and fat. This approach has the disadvantage of stimulating muscles in groups, with much less individual control. There is also some risk of irritating or burning the skin with the stronger current it takes to reach through the skin to the muscles.

The alternative to electrodes on the skin is to implant electrodes directly into the body, so they can contract specific muscles. Electrodes are either sewn to the surface of the muscle or a cuff design is wrapped around the tissue. Another type is implanted deep into the muscle and can be inserted by a modified hypodermic needle without the use of a surgical incision. Implants bring with them the risk of infection and can break or slip out of position.

Implantable electrodes have become remarkably small, can operate without attachment of actual wires through the skin, and can even have their batteries recharged from the outside using a remote device. The BION® Microstimulator was developed at the Alfred E. Mann Foundation at the University of Southern California and was still in clinical trials as of 2008. As described by Jennifer French, a neurotechnology advocate—and user:

> [The microstimulator] is specifically designed to coordinate
> the movement of arms and legs, and other bodily functions,
> for persons with neuromuscular ailments. It is programmable
> and contains sensors and a transceiver to coordinate with a
> pocket-sized computerized controller.

Parastep®

In 1997, the FDA approved the Parastep System, produced by Sigmedics of Northfield, Illinois (www.sigmedics.com) and originally developed at the University of Illinois Medical School and the Michael Reese Hospital and

Medical Center in Chicago. The user of Parastep operates controls on a walker, with buttons for sitting, standing, movement of the left and right legs, and intensity of the contractions. The Parastep System uses 12 externally applied electrodes. A small number of people are using the system with Lofstrand crutches—the type with the forearm loop. They use more of a swing-through gait, rather than the individual stepping that would be seen using a walker.

Parastep users like John Targowski, a student at the University of Michigan, report a variety of benefits. John values the increased muscle bulk from electrically stimulated contractions:

> *I like to keep the size of my leg muscles in good proportion to my upper body. Although other paraplegics might take some offense, I really don't like the typical appearance of huge arms and chests attached to stick legs. Secondly, I am an optimist and a future thinker. Soon, spinal injury will be curable or, at the very least, treatable. When this time comes, I want the bones, muscles, and tendons in my legs to be ready.*

Not a Cure Yet

FES/FNS is sometimes promoted as a replacement for a wheelchair. It is a limited option, requires a lot of effort to use it, and still has a lot of development work left to increase its usefulness. It also should not be thought of just in terms of walking. Standing, in and of itself, is valuable for preventing bone loss and to promote circulation. For many people, it is a great psychological boost to be able to stand. Some systems are geared toward assisting in transfers from a bed, wheelchair, bath, commode, chair, or sofa. Others use FES for increasing muscle tone alone, which wards off atrophy. This can mean wearing shorts without self-consciousness in public or protection from pressure sores thanks to the cushioning value of muscle tissue. Again, just as with spinal cord regeneration research, you should not be excessively caught up in the image of walking again.

Getting a Grip

In 1997, NeuroControl Corporation gained FDA approval for its Freehand™ System, an implantable FNS device to provide a grasping and pinch grip for people with C5/C6 quadriplegia. Implantation of the device involved a surgical procedure, significant rehabilitation, and a 12-week period of increased impairment until the benefits were fully realized. Because of the limited size of the market for this device, and a degree of reluctance on the part of the surgeons to implant an electrical device, NeuroControl has taken itself out of the spinal cord market.

A company in Israel, NESS, offers the H200, an external device that aids grip. It is of value for people with quadriplegia—who would need assistance putting it on and removing it—and for people with stroke or traumatic brain injury (www.nessltd.com).

FES Breathing

People with trauma at high levels in the spinal cord are unable to breathe on their own. This happens because the phrenic nerve, which causes the diaphragm muscles to contract, does not receive the automatic nerve impulses that it needs to work properly. Therefore, the diaphragm does not contract, and the lungs are not pulled down to create the vacuum that draws in air.

Phrenic nerve stimulation is an FES method to assist breathing by creating impulses in the phrenic nerve. Some people are able to be partly or entirely freed of a ventilator thanks to the implant. Christopher Reeve had been using the approach, first experimented with in 1964.

Think About It

Cybernetics Neurotechnology has been performing studies using an implant in the human brain, which can allow a person to literally "think" an activity to happen. As of 2007, users have been able to control the movement of a cursor on a computer screen using Cybernetics' BrainGate Neural Interface System. A sensor is planted in the motor cortex of the brain. It analyzes brain signals that the user can learn to control. The goal is for a user with quadriplegia to be able to access environmental controls, use the telephone, and control lights and television, and so on. The company also intends to explore the potential for the BrainGate system to control muscles. They are performing clinical trials for persons with SCI, muscular dystrophy, "locked-in syndrome," and stroke (www.cyberkinetics.com).

Who Are the Researchers?

The days of the lone scientist who makes a historic discovery are pretty much over. Hidden knowledge that could be found that way has been found already. Dr. Ron Cohen of Acorda Therapeutics says:

> There is a huge public misconception of the Louis Pasteur
> type of scientist alone in his lab who finds a vaccine and then

*finds a child to try it on and saves the child's life. There was a
time when that was the only way it could be done, when there
were no large pharmaceutical companies. We only heard
about the famous ones who succeeded, but, for every one of
those, there might have been hundreds who came up with
what turned out to be quack remedies that might have even
killed people.*

Times have changed, indeed. Researchers are now trained in years of
intensive study and clinical internship. People are increasingly specialized
in pursuits such as molecular biology, genetic engineering, or microsurgery.
Such specialization naturally requires people to work in teams, each applying focused knowledge according to her or his appropriate role in the
process. Research today is necessarily a collaborative process.

Researchers also have access to a tremendous amount of previous
experience and information, now all the more accessible via the Internet
and dedicated medical information services like Medline. Computers have
expanded the precision and capabilities of testing and measurement equipment many thousand-fold, making it possible to see into worlds that were
previously closed to the microscope. Calculations done in a moment by a
computer would have taken months—or years—by hand.

Researchers now operate under much more stringent regulatory and
ethical standards. Compared to the history of medical research, wanton
experimentation is all but completely ended. Researchers go to great
extremes to verify the value of human trials before they proceed. The FDA
demands that they offer extensive proof of their studies before permission
is given for human trials. There will always be risk with experiments, but,
when the initial groundwork is done well, the likelihood of life-threatening reactions to testing are very low. These, at least, are the standards you
should apply to any research project that you might consider participating
in as a subject.

Living by the Grant

Researchers rely heavily on grant money from many sources, public or private. If they conduct work that proves fruitless or unverifiable, they run the
risk of not being able to acquire additional funding. Remember, learning
from what doesn't work is different than having a failed experiment. The
test is not always whether they produce a usable therapy, but whether they
gain valuable information toward that end. Either way, researchers are very
motivated to work in a highly organized fashion. It affects their ability to
keep working by means of qualifying for grant money.

The only way that these labs can exist is to pursue funding from different sources, with many projects going at once. It is not unusual for several donors to contribute to the same research, though, when future licensing or other commercial interests are involved, such funding is carefully defined according to who would be entitled to possible commercial fruits of the work.

Commercial funding, such as that by Acorda, inevitably overlaps government money. The government does not mind investing in research that might result in a commercial product. It helps the economy, so Washington does not regard this as a conflict of interest. Says Acorda founder Ron Cohen:

> But when it comes to overlapping with another company, the lab will not take funding for the same project because the companies won't agree to that.

Paralyzed Veterans of America's Melinda Kelley says that:

> Most people don't know that the National Institutes of Health fund most of the biomedical research in this country—at least that done at academic institutions and medical centers. It is not the case that labs are usually funded by companies.

The Motivated Scientist

Researchers are often the unheralded heroes, working on extensive studies that are highly detailed, challenging, and time consuming. Some of them could probably be out in offices and hospitals treating patients and making much more money, but they chose the course where they feel they can make the most difference. They seem to be more interested in taking pride in their work than in following the money, which they have to beg for through the grueling process of grant writing and approval. Their motive is compassion; results are their reward. Dr. Noble says:

> I was a physical therapist, and, when I was an intern, I chose spinal cord injury as my specialty and spent a lot of time with these patients. I was very frustrated by the situation they were in, that they didn't get answers. I decided the best thing for me was to work in the area of spinal cord research.

Dr. Richard Borgens of the Center for Paralysis Research at Purdue University studied limb regeneration in salamanders as a graduate student. He won an award for the work from the National Paraplegic Foundation and encountered a room full of chair users at the award ceremony. He found himself uncomfortable as a person who could walk among so many wheelchair riders, having never even seen a person with quadriplegia. The human character of his work became clear, and he says:

> People with spinal cord injuries gave me an important profes-
> sional start—and I still strive to repay the debt.

What About the Animals?

Not all research can be performed on cells in dishes or simulated on a computer. Some tests require a working biologic system that parallels human beings, such as that in rats and dogs. Spinal cord research is not just about how to get a nerve to grow, as we've already seen. It is about the immensely complex system of chain reactions that occur in the real environment of living physiology. It is about the response of the body to a substance you might place into the system by any of a number of methods. It is about finding out that there are other factors at play that might not appear until you try what seems like a viable approach. This living research can only be studied in animals.

According to the American Academy of Neurology (AAN), less than 1% of research animals are dogs or cats. Ninety percent of research animals are rodents, such as rats and mice. AAN points out that more than 10 million unwanted animals are put to death each year in animal shelters, and only 1% of that total is released for research. In fact, most research animals are carefully bred for their purpose. AAN also points out that animal subjects have produced benefits for the veterinary community as well, benefiting animals as well as humans.[7]

Although some animal rights activists might draw comparisons to human experimentation in Nazi Germany, remember that such atrocities were performed with no concern for the experience of the subjects, often without the use of anesthetics, watching suffering of the deepest kind in order to "learn" from it. In the present, highly regulated setting of medical research, government inspectors make unannounced visits to determine the conditions of animal research. Besides, says the AAN:

> Treating research animals humanely is not only the right
> thing to do, it is a matter of self-interest. Scientists know that
> mistreatment can distort test results and ruin years of
> painstaking, costly work.

Using animals for research is widely supported by physicians, 97% of whom responded to an American Medical Association study with support for their continued use. The AAN says that "medical progress is simply not possible without animal research, and millions of people will pay the price if it is curtailed." They are concerned that animal rights activists will com-promise promising research into Parkinson's and Alzheimer's disease, trau-matic brain injury, meningitis, spinal cord paralysis, stroke, epilepsy, and many others. The AAN says that animals are used "with the dignity, gentle-ness, and respect to which they are entitled."

There was a time when research was sometimes carried out indis-criminately without concern for the suffering of the subject animals, but that time is past. There are very strict guidelines that laboratories must follow, and those that do not conform risk being forced out of operation. Dr. Noble notes:

> You have to be very careful about how the experiments are done and that you make sure you have people working in your lab who understand that they are working with living creatures entitled to as much care as you would give to a human patient. That's exactly how we work. Being a good sci-entist means that your use of animals is kept to a minimum. It's very clearly thought out. The quality of care that spinal cord injured rats get is superb. We basically run an intensive care unit. We are monitoring our animals all the time. My goal is to help the human population and I can't do it any other way.

You might find that the issue of using animals in research raises con-flicts for you, as you attempt to balance your desire for less pain and greater independence in your own life with an ethical and moral position regarding the treatment of all living creatures. This person with an SCI sympathizes with what animals were undergoing but doesn't want research to stop:

> I eat meat and wear leather, so I feel it would be hypocritical for me to take a stand against animal research. I also feel that if animal research ever results in a cure for SCI (or any other disease), or helps relieve human suffering in any way, I will thank and honor the animals that were used to bring this about.

Being a Research Subject

Before any research can be approved for use, clinical studies must be per-formed. At first, animal subjects are used, but ultimately human trials will be necessary. You might well be a candidate to participate in studies of ther-apies before they are approved for public use. This is a complex and very critical decision to make, one that demands that you be informed and think carefully about the risks that might be involved.

By their nature, research studies entail a degree of risk. The very point is to observe the effects—positive or negative—of the tests. The reason to participate in such a study is to help scientists develop useful therapies, not to get treatment before it is publicly available. There is no guarantee that the tests will be beneficial for you. The motive of most test subjects is the benefit of future persons who will use the therapy if it proves of value. That might include you.

Clinical Trials

As therapies and technologies evolve in laboratories and universities across the world, they eventually must go through a period of human clinical trials. Once the relative safety and potential efficacy of a therapy are established in animal models, then trials must be performed with a small—and later, a larger—group of humans.

There have been a great many clinical studies performed to evaluate the effects of exercise, pain management, spasticity control, and many other areas. In the coming years, more human trials will assess the regeneration of CNS tissue; some of the studies will involve invasive techniques such as surgery or injection of substances into the brain or spinal cord. Some trials will be specifically for those people with acute (recent) disabilities; others will be for people with chronic (long-term) disabilities.

The goals of these controlled studies are to:

- Determine the appropriate dosage of medications
- Observe side effects or the possibility of death
- Discover differences between results in humans and animals
- Prove the value of the therapy
- Decide whether or not to make the treatment widely available and for whom

A clinical trial is a carefully designed plan, prepared by doctors and scientists. The government's FDA might participate in the development of a clinical trial, as might a commercial entity interested in being the producer of the drug. This is a very precise project, defining specific criteria and methods.

It used to be that any researchers could go out and try the next "miracle cure" on anybody they could convince to go along. Doctors were under no restrictions in their experiments, and there were plenty of "snake oil salesmen" out pitching the latest elixir to cure any and all ailments. Even Coca-Cola was first promoted as a curative.

People sometimes died in the process of this uncontrolled approach. Today, the standards are very high. Scientists who do not work within a very prescribed process risk wasting years of work if their data are not found to have been responsibly and consistently collected. More to the point, the scientists conducting the study will be just as concerned with your well-being as with their reputations and legal liability.

Most trials employ a Data and Safety Monitoring Board, which reviews the study as it progresses. The Board members have the power to end the study at any point if they find that the therapy is not effective or is causing harm rather than helping.

The hospital, clinic, company, or university conducting the study will also have an Institutional Review Board that has seen and approved the study protocol in advance. The Board members receive regular reports and also have the power to suspend a study.

The U.S. government keeps track of clinical trials—those currently enrolling participants and those that are complete—at www.clinicaltrials .gov. The Christopher and Dana Reeve Foundation formed the North American Clinical Trials Network in 2004 to create the infrastructure for the increasing number of clinical trials that they see coming on the horizon. According to Foundation:

> *A number of fundamental scientific questions remain unanswered, both about the immense natural variability of spinal cord injury and how best to measure therapeutic efficacy. Such questions require large studies, involving multiple centers using the same examination criteria and treatment protocols.*

The International Campaign for Cures of Spinal Cord Injury Paralysis has published a comprehensive guide to clinical trials for SCI (www. campaignforcure.org).

Withdrawal

If you decide to participate in a clinical trial, you have the right to withdraw from a study at any time, but it may be possible that abruptly ending a therapy could itself be dangerous. You must understand that, when you agree to participate, you must follow the instructions absolutely and report any effects to your supervising physician. If you are considering withdrawing, discuss this with the doctor whose job it is to be your consultant, helping you to make the final decision. He or she should then advise you of the safest way to end the therapy and/or resume your previous treatment.

Placebos

Many studies involve use of a placebo, an inert substance given to some subjects rather than the actual drug being tested. This is to reveal whether some of the results observed might be because a subject believes she has been given a beneficial drug. It is now increasingly understood that attitude and belief can have a real impact on the physical—the so-called mind-body connection.

It is important to compare people who are getting the drug to people who are not receiving the drug to understand what real impact the actual drug is having. In some studies, you might consistently receive either the active drug or the placebo. In others, you might be getting one or the other at any one time.

It is not possible to request that you be given the active form of the drug. It would alter the results of the study if you knew which you were getting. Again, your reason for participating is to assist research, not just to gain early access to an unproved treatment.

You might be asked to cease taking a drug that has already been pre-scribed for you. Drugs interact with each other in the body, and the needs of the trial might require that you end your current treatment. You must balance the possible risks of going off of your present therapy against the potential benefits of your participation.

Blinded Studies

Clinical trials are generally either single-blind or double-blind. If you are in a single-blind study, you do not know whether you are getting the active drug or the placebo, but your doctor does. In a double-blind study, neither you nor the doctor knows. However, other investigators involved in the study have that information. If you were to have a severe reaction to treatment, it would always be possible to find out what you actually received.

Phases

Clinical trials are performed in three phases:

■ Phase I. This study is sometimes referred to as a "safety study." Its main purpose is to test the safety and effective dosage of a drug. This is the time of greater risk because less is known about reaction to the drug. High doses might be given to measure side effects of the drug. Only a few persons participate at this stage of drug testing.

■   Phase II. More people are included in the study, now that there is some sense of what the appropriate dosage should be. Now it is possible to begin to observe the effectiveness of the treatment. Several rounds of Phase II studies might be performed before the team feels ready for Phase III.

■   Phase III. Many more subjects are studied, often at a number of participating institutions. This is the time to validate the discoveries of the first two phases and to prepare statistical data to use in the process of gaining FDA approval for the potential commercial introduction of the therapy.

Money

Some trials pay their subjects for their participation, and some don't. There might be certain procedures that you would need to pay for, and you should check with your health insurer to see if they would be covered. There could be travel and accommodation expenses during periods in which you might need to stay near a medical center for initial tests and observation if you live away from where the study is centered. Or, your usual doctor might be able to participate and conduct some of the procedures.

On the other hand, you might benefit from additional coverage due to your participation in the study. You could be seen more regularly by doctors and, in effect, be getting more aggressive care of your condition at no extra expense.

You should not pay a fee to participate in a clinical study. These are always performed with funding from public, charitable, or commercial sources. The group conducting the study should not be in a position to profit from the actual study. They might, however, profit from future licensing or sale of the drug if it attains FDA approval.

Risks and Benefits of Participating

Some risks of participating in a clinical trial include:

■   Adverse reactions to the drug
■   Possible harm from receiving a placebo rather than active treatment
■   Physical discomforts from tests
■   Disruption in your personal schedule to be present for tests and examinations

Some benefits of participating in a clinical trial include:

■   Possible improvement in your condition

- More frequent monitoring by doctors during the study
- Improved coverage of expenses
- Personal gratification for your role in assisting the study

Questions to Ask

You have the right to ask any questions you have about the study and your role in it. You should seriously reconsider your willingness to participate in any study in which your questions are not fully and patiently answered. Among the things you should know are:

- If you live a distance from the study center, how long will you need to be available to the researchers and at what stages of the study?
- What kinds of tests will you be asked to submit to during the study?
- How long is the study expected to last?
- Is there a possibility that you will be receiving a placebo?
- Will your usual doctor participate or be informed about your role in the study?
- Who will know that you are participating in the study? Is your participation anonymous or simply confidential?
- What risks are already known about the substance or therapy being studied?
- What are the potential benefits the study hopes to demonstrate?
- Are there any results already known about the drug, good or bad?
- How many others are participating in the study?
- Will you need to go off of your present drug therapy?
- What, if any, portions of the study will you need to pay for?
- Who will pay for treatment if you should experience an adverse reaction?
- Who is financing the study?
- What forms will you be asked to sign, and what legal obligations do all the parties agree to?

Inclusion Still the Priority

For the foreseeable future, we will remain a human community with a significant population of people who have physical disabilities of various sorts. Regardless of the modern miracles that continue to be pursued by science, everybody is entitled to full inclusion according to their true capabilities. We need to support research that can improve quality of life but not at the price of continuing to cast people with disabilities in the role of damaged goods. Maybe some people will walk again, maybe not. Either way, we mustn't let any hope we place in research prevent us from continuing the progress disability advocates have made in removing social and physical obstacles that now prevent too many people from living to their full potential.

References

1. *The Project: News from the Miami Project to Cure Paralysis* 1998;11(1-Spring):6.
2. Maddox S. *The Quest for Cure: Restoring Function after Spinal Cord Injury.* Paralyzed Veterans of America; 1993:95-6.
3. Gallo G, Lefcort FB, Letourneau PC. The trkA receptor mediates growth cone turning toward a localized source of nerve growth factor. *J Neurosci* 1997;17(14):5445-54.
4. Kleitman N, Bunge RP. The Schwann cell: morphology and development. In: Waxman SG, Kocsis J, Stys P, eds. *The Axon.* New York: Rockefeller University Press; 1995:97-115.
5. *The Project: News from the Miami Project to Cure Paralysis.* 1997;10(3-Winter):7.
6. Blight A. Development of 4-AP for chronic spinal cord injury. *CSRO Quarterly* 1997;8(2). Available at: http://www.csro.com./CSROmag-v8i2.htm. Accessed on: March 10, 2008.
7. *Sensitive but Sensible: the Absolute Importance of Animal Research for Neurologic Disease.* St. Paul: American Academy of Neurology. Available at: http://www.aan.com/globals/axon/assets/2344.pdf. Accessed on: March 10, 2008.

Chapter 7

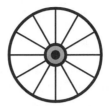

Home Access

A home should be flexible enough to handle everyone's needs, without people finding themselves trapped by obstacles or unnecessarily dependent. *Building for a Lifetime*, by Margaret Wylde, Adrian Baron-Robbins, and Sam Clark, documents the results of research conducted at the Institute for Technology Development under a grant from the National Institute for Disability Rehabilitation and Research.[1] It details the concept of the Lifespan home, which not only accommodates people with disabilities, but considers the needs of all family members at all stages of life and health, including children and elderly people.

The authors describe four fundamental needs that homes provide:

- Privacy. A space of your own and a chance to be left alone.
- Belonging. The ability to share spaces with friends and family, to be able to join in preparing meals and social activities.
- Control. The ability to go where you want and do what you want.
- Safety and security. The ability to move efficiently through the house, open doors, and escape in an emergency.

In the Lifespan model, you evaluate your home, keeping in mind these four aspects and looking for the highest possible quality of life for everyone, rather than simply thinking in terms of getting in the front door and using a bathroom. Each person finds his or her own priorities. This woman moved into an accessible apartment in New York City:

> *My apartment was built for a wheelchair user. The kitchen*
> *has a roll-under sink. The bathroom door is very wide and*
> *opens out. The bathroom is very large with a huge turning*
> *radius. The switches are lower and the outlets are higher, but*
> *that doesn't mean as much to me as being able to use the bath-*
> *room and wash the dishes. My balance is really good, so I*
> *don't rely so much on grab bars.*

You might resist making home modifications. The process can amplify negative emotions about your disability. Particularly if you have a progressive condition like multiple sclerosis or amyotrophic lateral sclerosis, planning for a future of additional disability can be upsetting. Louis Tenenbaum is a carpenter and building contractor in Maryland who specializes in access modifications. He describes his work with a client:

> *She fought me all along the way because she thought that mak-*
> *ing changes was giving in to her disability. But in the end, every*
> *one of the changes has increased her independence.*

Universal Design

The philosophy of Universal Design aims to increase independence for everyone in the home, while keeping the home attractive. When efforts began to remove architectural obstacles, terms like *barrier-free* or *handicapped-accessible* design were widely used. These are terms that tend to stigmatize a building, implying it has been somehow compromised or institutionalized. Increasingly, architects and product suppliers are developing alternatives that fit seamlessly into the overall design, with respect for aesthetics.

The late Ron Mace was an architect with a private practice and was director of the Center for Universal Design at North Carolina State University. He had polio as a child. Mace saw that making the world accessible benefits everyone. He saw that the existing terms did not promote integration and, in fact, generated resentment:

> *Universal Design says, why not change our thinking and*
> *design for everyone all of the time? Let's not call it "design for*
> *people with disabilities." Let's call it "good design."*

Proponents of this philosophy speak of a home where one can "age in place." As you and your family members get older and encounter any of the variety of physical changes humans encounter, your home can remain friendly and usable for everyone, or at least easier to adapt. And that includes guests with disabilities.

Most people eventually experience a disability of some sort, even if only for a matter of weeks using a wheelchair or crutches. A broken leg or temporary disease could mean being physically limited for months or years. An entrance without steps and an accessible bathroom are suddenly useful at such times. The demographics of the United States are shifting dramatically toward an older population. As you age, you will increasingly value features of Universal Design in a home. You might be able to stay in your home longer, despite an illness that might otherwise mean moving to a residential care setting.

More and more, people with disabilities are out in the world, achieving higher education, pursuing careers, and raising families. These people will be buying homes and deserve a selection in the marketplace. It makes good business sense for builders and landlords to incorporate Universal Design principles:

> Here I have a big down payment and a pre-approved mort-
> gage, but, because I use a wheelchair, I have much, much less
> to choose from than anybody else in the housing market. It is
> extremely frustrating because the place where I will live is the
> key to the quality of life I want to make for myself. This
> severely restricted market is keeping me from my dreams, and
> I don't appreciate the idea that I should have to compromise.

Universal Design also makes monetary sense. The cost of later modifications is much higher than doing it right in the first place. Wide doors are easily available, and the construction details of water-safe, level, outside entrances have been refined and well proven.

On the other hand, modifying an existing home is likely to be very expensive. You might not be able to afford all of the work it would take to achieve full access. Tenenbaum notes that you often have to make tough choices:

> I worked with a woman where we decided that her best solu-
> tion was to build an additional room on the first floor, but [the
> design also] meant she wouldn't be able to go upstairs to yell
> at her kids about throwing their clothes on the floor. It's very
> hard, because we're being controlled by budget. Universal
> access is a goal, but we often have to compromise.

Universal Design also suggests building for adaptability, an approach referred to as *handicapped-adaptable*. With some foresight and simple measures during construction, future accessibility needs can be more easily met. For instance, make sure that walls in bathrooms are reinforced in advance for grab-bar installation. Ron Mace explained:

With adaptable design, they don't have to put the grab bars in.
You can just put them in where someone needs them. Or in the
kitchen, the builder puts the base cabinet under the sink, but
makes it removable. He just doesn't bolt it down. You take a
couple of screws out and put it in storage.

Building codes sometimes offer builders an alternative. They can make a certain percentage of units accessible, or they can make more units adaptable. Variations in a city depend on local policies and the choices made by housing developers.

Private Homes and Accessibility Codes

There is no national requirement for private, single-family homes to be made accessible. The building industry has resisted such provisions, fearing it will impose added costs on them, raise the selling price of the home—and slow down the permit-approval process, delaying the moment when they can sell the house and close their interest-accumulating temporary construction loan.

Current building methods do not lend themselves to easy accessibility. For example, the typical style of home building puts the main floor up at least several inches to prevent water from flowing in from the ground level, in theory at least. Some homes are raised to allow a "crawl space" for air to circulate under the home—again to remove moisture—or to make room for windows to allow light into a basement space.

When you consider accessibility codes in terms of how legislation would apply to private homes, the issue gets trickier. On one hand, some people hesitate to force accessibility on private homes:

This is coming from a wheelchair user who hates visiting
people in homes that are uncomfortable or difficult for me.
I would never tell someone that they must build their house to
suit me. Maybe I, in my wheelchair, can't deal with a sunken
living room, but that should not prevent someone from having
one, if that's what they want.

On the other hand, millions of people with disabilities have to live someplace and, in the present environment, have very little to choose from. You could be forced to leave a neighborhood you prefer or to have to spend extra money for adaptations just because there are no requirements for basic features of access.

But why not require that all new private homes be required to meet minimum standards of accessibility, rather than just public or apartment buildings? We don't accept that someone can just decide, "Oh, I don't feel like having my new house meet all of those expensive, fire-safety and structural-integrity requirements." The public interest is said to be best served by ensuring a minimum standard of safety for both the first residents and any future residents. Is it unreasonable to expect this of basic accessibility?

Finding existing homes that are either accessible (pretty difficult, in all honesty) or can be modified with the least expense is a challenge and typically takes more time than people in the market who don't need accessibility features (for now, at least!). Rental agents and landlords generally have poor knowledge of what makes something accessible, though it is really a matter of what you specifically need.

That said, you could get lucky, as did this chair user with a stroke who lives in an area where basements are a common feature of freestanding homes:

> *I ended up purchasing a house that did not have a basement.*
> *No one wants a house with no basement, except a guy in a*
> *chair. So I got a good price on it.*

Visitability

Access questions extend beyond your own home. Your life takes you to the homes of relatives and friends. People throw parties. Someone you love might need help because they are not well. The "visitability" of other homes is a significant factor in the quality of your life:

> *When I visit a home where I need a lift up the steps or have to*
> *control my liquid intake for lack of a bathroom I can use, my*
> *hosts are very apologetic. Consistently, people wish that they*
> *could provide a setting that works for me. Some will go out of*
> *their way, as a dear cousin of mine recently did by building a*
> *portable ramp for the garage entry.*

As of 2006, 14 states and 32 municipalities (get the latest from The University of Buffalo Center on Universal Design, www.ap.buffalo.edu/idea/visitability) have established a visitability ordinance that requires a minimum of one accessible outside entrance, doors and hallways wide enough for wheelchair passage, and one usable bathroom on the ground floor.

Will it Look Like a Hospital?

Many people fear that making their home accessible will make it look institutional and damage future resale value. Ramps, grab bars, lowered switches and raised outlets, or kitchen counters that leave space for leg room all raise the specter of not being able to sell the home when the time comes.

It is a fallacy that an accessible home must become unattractive to potential buyers. Remember, when you think in terms of Universal Design, you are making your home safe, comfortable, and convenient for everyone. Because the design quality of products—from grab bars to kitchen and storage systems—has improved, your home can remain attractive and not look like a hospital.

Building contractor Louis Tenenbaum puts it simply:

> *Beauty really is in the eye of the beholder. One person's institutional is another person's attractive. Personally, I think what's ugly is breaking a hip because the environment was unsafe.*

Adapting What's There

Most people with disabilities will be faced with adapting—and adapting to—an existing home or apartment. Wheelchair access is not what architects and builders are thinking about when they design and construct housing.

A rental landlord is not required by law to make a house or apartment accessible, but landlords are required to allow you to do it yourself. They also have the option of insisting that you return the house or apartment to its original state when you move out.

You will likely encounter issues in the public areas of an apartment complex, which are covered under the Americans with Disabilities Act (ADA). This chair user found that:

> *One complex had inadequate parking; they had the wheelchair sign up in a regular space and thought, "problem solved." The van I had at the time took up two spaces to be able to get in/out. Complaints ensued, informed them of ADA specs. They finally made only 2 wide parking spaces out of 20 spaces. I've found that approaching apartment managers diplomatically (presenting ADA info in a non-threatening way) instead of going in all fired up and angry making threats, complaining, accusing, etc. works a lot better and things can be negotiated. Most of the time.*

The degree of adaptation you can make depends on:

■ What you can afford
■ The existing design features of your home or property

■   What control you have over your home—that is, whether you own or rent your home

Start with measures that cost nothing, such as moving furniture around to make space and teaching your family to not leave items where they impede your path. You might move to another bedroom in the home, rearrange what goes in which kitchen cabinets, or remove the door to the bathroom in the master bedroom. It might even be necessary to accept not having access to certain parts of your home without assistance.

Next, there are measures that don't cost much money. Wooden ramps can be built easily; portable, folding metal ramps are available at reasonable cost. Doorknobs can be converted with inexpensive lever handles, and door hinges can be changed to a hinge type that pivots the door aside so the door's thickness no longer blocks your way. Grippers, reachers, and various other tools help to extend your reach and use what strength you have. Remote-control systems allow you to turn almost anything on or off in the home, as well as open doors or answer the telephone.

More expensive is the construction cost associated with major work, such as widening doors, pouring a concrete ramp and grading the land outside, replacing a bathtub with a roll-in shower, or adding a new room to the house. You might also consider taking down a wall that is not load bearing—perhaps between the dining room and den—to open up space for ease of movement. Depending on your income and where you live, tax credits might be available for some of these expenses. Some banks extend long-term loans with minimal down payments for disability-related construction. Your local center for independent living (CIL) might have access to modification funds.

If you are doing substantial work or buying significant new items such as major appliances, this is a chance to improve your home with quality construction and well-made products that will last, with a minimum of maintenance. Adapting a home for access can be a chance to increase the convenience of your home for everyone and, in the process, improve the home's long-term value.

Seeking Home-Modification Funds

There are some sources that will assist with home modifications. Federally funded Community Development Block Grant monies are available through various entities that administer home-modification programs, very possibly your local center for independent living. These funds are available only to people with qualified disabilities who have a household income below a certain level. Because this is a government program managed by a nonprofit, be prepared for the possibility of delays and complexity—though it is not impossible that you can get the support of people who really know how to make this program work well. The slow spot is typically in the process of inviting in multiple contractors for estimates.

Local charities or churches or a Rotary group could be a source of contributing not only money, but also materials and muscle, to make home modifications.

The US Department of Housing and Urban Development has programs that help provide accessible housing, including the Section 8 voucher system, in which you are given a certain amount of money each month to rent housing in certified units. These kinds of programs tend to be overburdened, involve being on long waiting lists, and require you to deal with the kind of bureaucratic complexity that lives up to the stereotype of a Federal agency.

Insurance companies also contribute to the expense of modification, particularly if you are covered by a long-term disability plan, fall under Workers' Compensation, or are a veteran. In all of the above cases, be sure to take the time to learn all of the requirements and boundaries involved, such as the surprise that this woman, spinal cord injured since childhood, encountered:

> *After jumping through hoop after hoop to get my approval, I was presented with a contract that stated that if these modifications were done, I would be required to live in that house as my primary residence for the next 10 years, otherwise I would owe the money spent on the modifications back to the insurance company. As a girl just starting out in life after college and my career, I don't know where I'll find myself in 10 weeks, let alone 10 years!*

Building Your Own

If you're fortunate enough to have the resources, you can build your home from scratch. You might work with a homebuilder who is putting up a new project—giving you the opportunity to make changes to one of the floor plans the builder has to offer. In this case, you will be limited to working within the broad structure of the existing design, but you will have considerable flexibility moving around walls that are not structural; selecting appliances, sinks, tubs, and so on; specifying placement of light switches and power outlets; and working to design the zero-step entrances you will need. You could even have an elevator put in for a second floor.

The deluxe approach is to design from scratch with an architect. Obviously, this takes a lot more time and money and involves a much greater number of decisions to make—not the least of which is the aesthetics and style of your home. You'll also need to find the piece of property where you'll build.

This is exactly what Rosemarie Rossetti, PhD, a wheelchair user since a tree fell on her while she was riding her bicycle in 1998, did. Paraplegic from the injury, Rosemarie has been writing, speaking, and consulting ever since. Not only are she and her husband Mark Leder building their own house from the ground up with an architect, but they have made it the centerpiece of The Universal Design Living Laboratory (www.udll.com) in Columbus, Ohio, where they live (Figure 7-1). The process is being documented for a public television broadcast, and the home will be made available for tours once it is complete.

Figure 7-1 Front elevation of Rosemarie Rossetti's Universal Design Home.

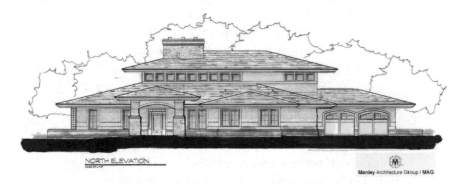

NORTH ELEVATION

Manley Architecture Group / MAG

Using Professionals

Doing construction in the home is quite stressful. The stereotype—often true—is that things take longer, cost more, and disrupt your life in ways you never imagined. Many people find themselves in conflict with the contractor or their spouse, arguing over scheduling, costs, design choices, or quality.

It is easy to underestimate what construction will cost, even if the task seems simple. Contractor Louis Tenenbaum observes:

> *We volunteer with a program at the local Center for Independent Living, where we help with consulting and evaluation. They had the impression that they could do a lot for $2,000 per house. That's just not true. $2,000 doesn't go very far.*

The right professional will give you good advice on the reality of the work—the costs and the actual tasks. Many builders are still not experienced with accessible design, beyond simple tasks like adding grab bars or using wider doors. However, there are contractors who make a specialty of accessible construction. It is worth some effort to find the most experienced people. You would be well advised to interview a number of builders, find out about their experience, invite them to evaluate your home, and ask for references.

There are efforts aplenty to help builders learn their way around Universal Design. The EasyLiving Home program offers certification. Contractors who demonstrate the ability to provide Easy Access, Easy Use, and Easy Passage get their seal of approval and participate in various co-marketing activities (www.easylivinghome.org/elh.htm). The National Association of Homebuilders has been gradually but surely overcoming its resistance to recognizing the value of supporting and disseminating information about accessible housing. Universal Design and aging-in-place information is available on their web site at www.nahb.org.

Some architects have also emphasized access in their practice, for doing modifications, new buildings, or both. Although it might cost more to pay an architect's fee, architects understand how to maintain the quality of your home's appearance and overall function—and, in the process, preserve, or even enhance, your home's value. Architects will also have worked with local contractors, so they can advise you on who does quality, reliable work. Ron Mace noted:

> It happens all the time that people build something ugly
> instead of something that is well integrated and looks
> good. They make terrible, brutal home modifications,
> sometimes at great expense, because they don't know
> what they can do.

Adapting a home is a multi-disciplinary process involving many players. Therapists have a contribution to make, because they understand how the physiology of your disability affects your interactions with the home. Home modification is a sub-specialty within the profession of occupational therapy.

The process also includes you. Observe the details of how you function in your present home. Note what is stressful, fatiguing, inconvenient, or awkward. Make notes to have with you when you start to discuss changes. No professional can automatically know about your specific needs and preferences. If you can clearly describe your needs from your everyday experience, you will get the most from their services.

Defining the Problems

Start by defining the problems. Take time to evaluate your home, consider how your disability needs to be accommodated, do research and reading, and invite in people with experience. Check with your local center for independent living, many of which offer evaluation services or even programs to help perform or finance changes. Tenenbaum finds that people often come to him with preconceived notions about what to do:

> *I find the most important thing is to avoid discussing solutions until we identify problems. For instance, the problem is "How do I get into my house?" not "How do I get in my front door or in my garage?" Or even "How do I build a ramp?"*

Considering Private and Public Space

Maintaining the separation between private and public space is important to your quality of life. The bedroom is a private space, whereas the entry foyer and den are public. A bathroom is a private space, but one bathroom might be where you have your private toiletries and adaptive equipment and the other bathroom would be for guests and, therefore, a more public space.

Some families whose homes have all of the bedrooms upstairs find themselves changing a downstairs room into a bedroom for a person who can't go up the stairs. Tri-level homes also pose problems of this sort. There may be only one level where you have access to a bathroom or the ability to freely come and go from the home.

Putting a bedroom on a lower level can violate the separation between public and private space. The normal flow of family life is disrupted by the loss of family space downstairs or by the movement of activities upstairs in which you can no longer join. Guests coming in may see a bed or medical equipment, perhaps in what used to be the living room. This kind of exposure can be uncomfortable for the whole family—especially the person with the disability.

If a formerly public space must be made private, try to relocate the public space somewhere that is still accessible. One family in a tri-level home made a bedroom of the ground-floor living room because it had the easiest access. The father—the chair user—opted to accept being assisted up a ramp around the side of the house to get to the new living room on the next level.

Too much privacy can mean isolation for the person with the disability. Even if the solution is to build a totally accessible addition to the house, keep in mind the need for everyone to share in the community of the family, and place the highest priority you can on maintaining independent accessibility.

Product Selection

Choose the best products you can, even if they are more expensive at first. Well-designed products will last longer, be easier to operate and simpler to maintain, and often be better looking. Well-designed products don't tax your strength, their operation is self-evident, and they provide you with auditory and visual cues that they are operating correctly.

Consider all features when choosing products. A door handle might be easy to turn but have a key lock that demands fine dexterity or pinching strength. A flat stove surface might make it easy to slide pots onto and off the heating element; it should also indicate, by some color, that it is on to prevent accidental burns.

Strength and Stamina

Keep both strength and stamina in mind as you consider adaptations you make in your home. Strength is how much force you can exert briefly. Stamina is your ability to continue performing an activity. For example, opening a door and making the bed by lifting the mattress are strength tasks. Making a door spring less tense or choosing a lighter mattress can preserve strength. Washing the dishes and doing container gardening are stamina activities. Locating a kitchen or gardening task so that you can sit comfortably affects how long you can work and how much strength and leverage you can apply, depending on your balance and physical capacity.

Wheelchair Width

If you are selecting a new wheelchair, you should account for the narrowest door or passageway that you will need to get through. A narrower chair doesn't necessarily mean narrower seat. Frame design and the type of wheels and hand rims also have an effect on overall width.

Your chair can be adjusted to optimize your access. The more camber you use—adding angle to the wheels to increase your base—the wider you are. If you have adjustable axles, you might also gain some clearance by bringing your wheels closer to your body. Obviously, your stability and comfort in the chair are the high priorities, but the fraction of an inch you might gain could make the difference between getting someplace independently or not.

Dimensions

There are published standards that detail exact dimensions—often expressed as a range—for wheelchair clearance and accommodation. In reality, the ideal measurements depend on your specific needs. Just because a home does not technically conform to accessibility guidelines does not mean there will necessarily be obstacles for you. You might not need every recommended access measure, so you might as well save your money. That said, keep the future in mind if you expect your disability to change in ways that limit you further.

For instance, a circular area five feet in diameter is typically recommended as the space necessary to fully turn around in your wheelchair. You might actually need more or less space. You might need more if you need to elevate your footrests and have a ventilator on a tray behind your chair, or you might need less if you are using a high-performance, lightweight, rigid frame manual chair in which your feet are under your knees. Front- and mid-wheel drive power chairs can turn in smaller spaces than can rear-wheel drive chairs.

Consider whether you even need to turn around. Going backward out of a small room like the bathroom might not be a large problem. On the other hand, having to wheel backward often, over a greater distance, could lead to stress in your neck and shoulders from having to crane around to see where you are going:

> *I once lived in an apartment with a small bathroom. I couldn't turn around, but I could close the door once I was inside and get to the toilet, the tub, and the sink. Because I am flexible enough to reach behind to open and close the door, and because I can wheel backward accurately, it was fine, although not ideal. Everything else about the place was just right, so I decided to accept it.*

By all means, acquire the published standards; they have much to offer. But consider them a guide, not law. Do your best to think in terms of principles—being able to move, reach what you need, be independent, and use your energy efficiently.

In fact, there are no legal requirements for accessibility measures in detached homes, and they are nominal for other forms of housing. Your legal concerns will have more to do with local building codes and permit approval.

Being Creative

To modify your home, you don't always have to call a professional contractor, pay top dollar for new products out of catalogs, or even restrict yourself to products that are designed solely for access. Keep your thinking—and your eyes—open to solutions in unexpected places. You might have a friend who just loves tinkering and solving problems. Give him a call. Those skills can come in very handy.

Your building contractor can use the same creative approach, as did a builder in Canada for this person with a spinal cord injury:

> While I was in the local auxiliary hospital, waiting for our home to be constructed, we phoned a company to see what it would cost to have a door opener installed. They wanted $2,000 plus traveling to come about 75 miles to install one. My contractor said, "That's ridiculous." He bought a garage door opener for $270, mounted it sideways above the patio doors with a rod and a chain so it pulled the doors open or closed instead of pushing them. Then he hooked the on/off switch to doorbell buttons inside and out, and I could go in and out whenever I wanted. It worked like a charm, and altogether it only cost $450.

Creative contracting solutions should be done with care. Automated equipment needs to be properly installed. Anyone adapting equipment needs to understand how it will withstand the stresses placed upon it and ensure that the structure holding it can support it. For example, a standard garage door opener is a fairly heavy item not designed to operate on its side. Improperly executed, a low-cost approach can lead to injury, as this woman with a mobility disability notes:

> It is usually cheaper in any situation to rig up something that was intended for another purpose. But when you call a supplier you are pretty much asking them about the installation of equipment specifically made for that purpose. A supplier has their reputation and liability to think of. If they jerry-rigged something and the door somehow closed on you or hurt you in some way—well, they would be the ones in trouble. If a door opener made for that purpose malfunctions, then you can go back to the manufacturer for satisfaction. If you are using something made for another purpose, the manufacturer is going to say, "Too bad."

Many creative ideas don't involve expensive or heavy equipment, only simple solutions. This contractor found a simple solution to the problem of keeping a door open while someone helped the chair rider up a ramp:

> One easy modification that comes to mind is a chain with a hook on a post at the edge of a porch where I built a ramp. It connected to an eye that I attached to the storm door. This allowed the gentleman caregiver to hook the door open when

he was pushing his wife in her wheelchair so that he did not have to hold the door with his knee or something. Though it is a small thing, it did make things easier for him. The low-tech way—that's what I love.

Typical Building Features

A number of building features impact the ease of access to your home. Doors, flooring, windows, electricity, and other features need to be considered for the ways in which they obstruct your independence or can be better designed.

Entrance

Ideally you would prefer to go in the front door like everyone else. For some people, this ability to enter your home can affect your sense of being an equal in the household. Having more than one choice of entry is better yet. The primary entrance is ideally close to the car and allows you to bring things into and out of the home as easily as possible. In an apartment complex, this might mean convenient access to an elevator from a parking garage.

Your goal is to achieve a "zero-step" entrance. Homebuilders often hesitate to build zero- step entrances because a primary concern is protecting the house from water. They also fear that they might not pass a final construction inspection required for handing the house over to the buyer and collecting their money. But the details of building zero-step entrances have been well established and well proven in many homes. With a proper seal at the door threshold, and a minimal slope away from the doorway, water will not find its way into the home. A protected doorway also helps keep the rain away from the door altogether.

A paved, reasonably level, smooth surface is best for approaches to doors, patios, decks, gardens, and parking areas. Widths of five feet are considered ideal. Consider whether the entrance should be protected with an overhang if you live in a rainy locale. Chair riders often need a little extra time to get a door open, so they will be exposed to the weather. An overhang also suggests the need for additional lighting so that you can find your keys, see the pavement when approaching the door, and see the doorknob well enough to operate it. A small shelf next to the door is an idea that would give you a place to put down a bag of groceries while you are unlocking the door.

If you can afford more-extensive changes to a private home, you might regrade the driveway to bring it up to the level of the house. This way, you can take advantage of the car to get up the slope so you won't have to push or drive your wheelchair uphill.

Construction details and planning information are available from a wide variety of sources, notably the University of North Carolina Center for Universal Design (www.design.ncsu.edu/cud) and the Center for Inclusive Design and Environmental Access of the School of Architecture and Planning University at Buffalo (www.ap.buffalo.edu/idea).

Ramps

A ramp is a common and generally affordable solution. Some people might simply lay down a piece of wood so a chair rider can be hauled up it in his chair, but that might not achieve independent—or safe—access.

The usual slope recommended for ramps is 1:12, which means that, for every one inch of vertical rise, there are 12 inches of horizontal run. This angle can be too steep for some chair riders, as well as for some people who walk, or in winter or rainy conditions. A gentler slope of 1:20 is likely to be usable by most people. Figure 7-2 shows the difference between a 1:12 and a 1:20 slope. At 1:12 or greater, most codes recommend or require handrails, so another advantage of less slope is less visual clutter from handrails—and lower construction costs.

Figure 7-2 Preferred and maximum ramp slopes.

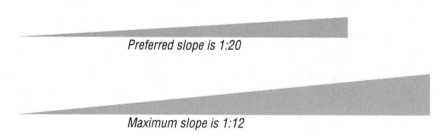

Preferred slope is 1:20

Maximum slope is 1:12

The angle you choose also depends on space. The less the angle of slope, the more distance the ramp will run. If there isn't much room, more slope might be the only solution. Some riders do have the strength to climb slopes even greater than 1:12. But, no matter how strong you are, when you have a bag of groceries in your lap, you can't climb as easily because you can't involve your upper body, since your load will prevent you from leaning forward as you push. And, of course, there is a point at which too much slope will be likely to cause the wheelchair to tip back altogether.

The ramp does not have to run in a continuous rise but can "switch back," making a turn and coming back in the opposite direction. Or you can use a dog-leg design that makes one 90° turn—an approach that can be used to run part of an exterior ramp along the side of the house, minimizing its visual impact. Such designs need a level landing at the turn. All ramps must have a level landing of five feet for every 30 inches of rise, providing manual wheelers a brief respite from pushing uphill or braking down, as well as the option to pause if desired. Tenenbaum emphasizes the need for a landing before a doorway:

> *The main thing is to have a landing at the top. People sometimes mistakenly run the slope right up to the door, with no curb or handrail.*

Managing a sloped surface while opening a door is very difficult. You will also want to provide enough level surface on the side of the opening edge of the door so you can be clear of the door when it swings open.

Ramps of concrete and asphalt are ideal surfaces that require little maintenance, but, for rises of more than one foot, these materials will usually not be practical. Too much concrete or asphalt can crack under its own weight. Wood or metal grating is used for ramp surfaces. If you are using metal grating, be certain that openings are not large enough to catch a crutch tip or a shoe heel. Take drainage into account so that the surface will stay dry and free of puddles.

Handrails are an important safety element of a ramp, just as they are for a stairway, and are usually advisable even with a gentle slope. Provide handrails on both sides. Some chair riders prefer to pull themselves up the ramp by grabbing the handrails, which is sometimes easier than pushing the wheels. Wood railings must be well finished so that there are no splinters. Other materials, such as metal, can solve this problem but might not be appropriate for winter climates. Rails should not be more than one and a half inches in diameter so that they can be gripped reliably. A round shape is best. Handrails should not be too close to the wall—one and a half inches is recommended. Handrails should extend one foot beyond the bottom and top of the ramp so that it is possible to have support as you approach the rise and until you reach secure, level ground. For exterior ramps, provide for nighttime lighting.

A ramp has a strong visual impact. Take into account the design of your home, and use compatible materials, colors, and patterns. You want to avoid communicating, "A disabled person lives here and we had to make our home ugly because of it." Rather, you want the design to communicate, "Our home is a place that welcomes everybody." Landscaping can better integrate the ramp into the design of the home.

A poorly designed and aggressively installed ramp can indeed affect the value of your home. Ron Mace observed:

> *The ramp is the cheapest thing you can do, but it has the disadvantage of being very obvious. It devalues the home in the view of Realtors. They usually discount the house because they feel that, in order to put it on the market, you're going to have to spend more money to take the ramp off. It's something that nobody else will want.*

You don't want to build a ramp in a way that will feed into these attitudes. Regrading is desirable, if possible, or you could install the ramp in a way that it is easily removed but still structurally sound. Alternatively, perhaps the ramp could go inside a garage; this can be the most convenient place if you will be driving and typically enter the home through the garage door. Putting the ramp in a garage also protects the ramp—and the person using it—from weather.

Temporary and Portable Ramps

Temporary ramps are often acquired or built. In some public settings, a removable ramp might just get left in place rather than building something more permanent. Inspect such a temporary ramp for stability:

> *I fell out of my wheelchair on a ramp at a funeral home. The ramp was removable, and, when my front wheels hit it, the whole ramp moved. I fell and my power wheelchair came down on top of me. I broke my elbow and scraped my knees.*

Portable ramps in various lengths are available for sale. Some are individual tracks that you set a proper distance apart to accommodate wheel position. This design makes them lighter overall and easier to transport, but either track can shift independently out of position. Other types are full width, some of which fold up to reduce their bulk for transporting. Check what weight these ramps can handle. If you are a large person in a power chair equipped with a recline system and a ventilator, you might find yourself having an experience similar to this man with his new, portable metal ramp:

> *We made it into the house all right, but, on the way out, the left ramp collapsed, nearly tipping me and my chair over, and almost ruining my wife's and my attendant's backs. When I phoned the dealer, the first thing they said was, "Were you in the wheelchair when the ramp collapsed?" I said, "Yes, I was." They replied, "I'm afraid your warranty is void then. If*

you look in the owner's manual you'll see that they are not
recommended for use while the wheelchair is occupied." I
looked and sure enough that's what it says.

Interior Ramps

Ramping inside the house is more problematic, since there is less available space. There is a tendency to keep the ramp from taking up too much precious floor space by making it shorter and steeper. But the steeper the ramp, the more likely you are to lose control going down, get stuck on your footrests at the bottom, not have the strength to push yourself up it, or tip over backward in the effort. If you are in peak condition, you might have no trouble, but, as you age—or when you become ill or tired—such a ramp could become more of an obstacle and risk. In general, building next to a wall is advised because it allows you to put a handrail on at least one side of the ramp.

The Ramp Project

In 1991, the Minnesota Center of Independent Living (MCIL) developed the Ramp Project, which has helped people build quality, appropriate, exterior ramps for very low cost. Their program is based on the use of volunteers who pitch in to help construct and move ramps. MCIL reports that many ramps have been reused in different locations thanks to their modular approach, which was reviewed and modified by a professional engineer.

The plans for these ramps—with specific structural details—are available from MCIL for a modest price. They offer a booklet that includes planning guidelines and also discusses issues such as permit approval and how to order materials.

MCIL has developed a modular ramp system that requires no footings. That means it is not necessary to dig down into the earth to set posts in stone or concrete below the frost line—the usual construction approach. Their design is stable and does not have problems with shifting.

Lifts

Lifts can be used as a way to get to an outside entry or up interior stairs. They have some disadvantages but can be a solution when nothing else works.

Many homes have a front porch with perhaps four or five steps, a driveway next to the house, and small front yard. There just is not space for a ramp. A mechanical lift would be the solution. Ron Mace said:

I recommend lifts when there isn't enough land or room to put
up a ramp. Besides, ramps in icy locations are not much good
half the year. In winter settings, even if there's space, it can
make sense to do a lift anyway.

A lift can cost as much, if not more, than constructing a ramp. Being mechanical, it can break down. Although landscaping can conceal the lift, and you can locate it in the least conspicuous place you can manage, lifts are bulky, and it is more difficult to integrate one into the appearance of your home. An exception is the Everhard lift, which is enclosed in a concrete pit underground.

It is important to take care of a lift: keep it lubricated, observe weight limits, and have the dealer make regularly scheduled maintenance checks. Lifts need more maintenance in winter environments.

For interior stairs, a vertical platform lift could be a solution for a short run of four or five steps but not for a full flight of stairs. Stairway lifts are available that consist of a seat that rides a rail along literally any stair configuration. One must have sufficient transfer and balance skills to use one safely—and another wheelchair to use at the top. Installation of a full elevator is a much more elaborate and expensive undertaking, but it is an option if you have the resources and space—which might mean giving up a precious walk-in closet, for instance. Elevators do not have to look commercial or institutional. For instance, the elevator door could be designed so that it looks like a normal interior door.

Doors

Doors are the most likely bottleneck to free movement through the home. A number of conditions could make a door an obstacle. A doorway should

- Have sufficient maneuvering space at the approach
- Be wide enough for a wheelchair to pass easily
- Have hardware that can be easily gripped or turned
- Require little force to open
- Have a low threshold

A door without one of these qualities could rob you of independence and threaten your safety if you need to use the door in an emergency.

When you are thinking of how to modify your home for maximum access, think of the functions of a door. Doors provide safety, privacy, acoustic control, climate control, and aesthetics. The function of safety should not be compromised. However, you can weigh other priorities. Any door that does not provide these functions might not be needed at all. If a door only gets closed when you sweep behind it, why not remove it altogether?

Doors are places where collisions are most likely to happen. Paint gets chipped, or chunks get taken out of door jambs or walls. Sometimes space is just tight, and, no matter how skilled a driver you are, for the number of times you'll go into and out of the door, odds are really high that you're going to make contact now and then. Thus this advice from a man with cerebral palsy:

> *Protect doorways with hard plastic trim. They're much easier*
> *to replace.*

Door Width

A door must be wide enough for you to fit through. Wider doorways also allow you to carry an occasional wide package on your lap and reduce the chance that you'll bump into the frame and damage it or the paint—or your hand! Bathroom doors are typically the narrowest in the house. Bedroom doors can be narrow or oriented to the hallway in such a way that you can't wheel straight through. Although making the door frame wider is not always an option, there are other possibilities to give you more clearance, such as using a different kind of hinge that takes the door out of the way or installing a pocket door.

Wider doors do not add to the cost of a new building. There are many benefits, according to Mace:

> *When you use wider doors, there's nothing different about*
> *them. They're just doors. Buy a wider door and you're put-*
> *ting in less wall. The wall actually costs more than the door.*
> *It's a direct tradeoff that doesn't cost anything. It doesn't look*
> *any different from any other door. I've never heard anybody*
> *complain about the look of a wider door. It's a lot easier on*
> *moving day. It increases circulation and air flow and*
> *increases views into the room. Deaf people get better*
> *sight lines.*

Door Types

Many people report that sliding glass doors are the easiest to operate, but they sometimes have difficulty getting over the metal channels at floor level. Sliding doors are best installed in a recess in the floor to make the surface flush, assuming that water infiltration would not be a problem. Sloped thresholds—or "mini-ramps"—can also be installed to help wheels over the frame. Some sliding-door designs use lower-profile channels.

A pocket door slides into and out of the cavity of the wall, so it takes up no space from the door frame. The door rides on easily gliding tracks that require little exertion to operate the door. When the door is open and fully tucked into the wall, there is usually a small hook on its edge, which you grab with your fingertip to pull the door in order to close it. This can be a dexterity problem for some people. A D-pull handle solves this but then will limit the ability of the pocket door to fully recess into the wall. If enough clear space is not left to pass through the doorway, you can cut a notch in the wall to recess the D-pull so that the door can open all the way (see Figure 7-3).

Figure 7-3 Detail of recessed D-pull on pocket door.

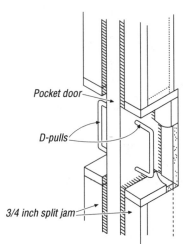

Installing a pocket door in a wall is a significant construction task—which might also involve redirecting electrical switches or outlets—and some people complain of difficulty with maintenance. If properly built, the door should glide easily and stay on the track. A less costly and simpler approach is to install a surface-mounted pocket door. Such a door can be attractively installed on the outside of the wall, with proper trim and hardware, and without the problem of having to cut a notch for a D-pull. The only drawback is the loss of some wall space (Figure 7-4).

Figure 7-4 A surface-mounted pocket door.

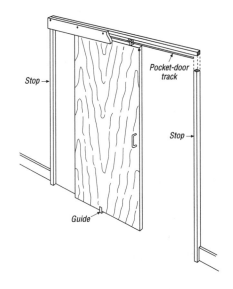

Closets typically use double-leaf or folding doors. These door types don't impose themselves as far into the room when they are opened. Two smaller doors can provide better access to a closet space. Folding doors are often inexpensive and not of high quality. They tend to jam, fall off their tracks, or require more dexterity to operate.

Door Hardware

Door hardware has a large effect on independence. A door with difficult-to-use hardware is also more likely to be damaged as it becomes necessary to push, kick, or use the wheelchair itself to get through it. Lever handles and D-pulls are the easiest to use. A hook latch or handle with a thumb latch require dexterity and strength.

Lever handles should be used on both sides of entry doors. Contractors or installers might think that a person with a disability will only open the door from the inside but be assisted when coming from the outside, which, of course, may not be true. A second door pull, placed closer to the hinges, can help you close a door you've passed through. The latch can be too far to reach once you are through, so the additional D-pull allows you to close the door without strain.

Lock hardware also can be inaccessible. Many people are unable to put a key in a lock, grasp it with their fingers, and twist it to turn the lock. Some people tend to install many locks for an increased sense of security, but, instead, these locks can serve to imprison and endanger someone who has difficulty operating them.

Keyless locks are now commonly available; a keypad is used to enter a code with gentle pressure from a fingertip. Generally, you choose the code, so you can change it occasionally for security reasons. You also can never lose your keys—though you can forget the code. Make sure the control is installed at a reachable height. Some of these products come as an integrated system that includes a doorbell, mailing slots, or intercom.

Often a small bathroom is rendered inaccessible simply because the door swings into the room. The door can't be closed because there is not room to wheel far enough into the room to clear the door. The door might also block your access to the tub, shower, toilet, or sink. This can be solved by reversing the swing of the door. You can remove the door and put the hinges on the other side of the frame so that the door swings out instead—which means you'll need to take extra care opening the door from the inside into the hallway where someone might be passing by.

The thickness of a standard-hung door occupies one or two inches of the space of the door frame when it is opened. There is a replacement hinge available that pivots so that the thickness of the door is effectively removed from the passageway when it is opened. These hinges are easily installed and inexpensive. Figure 7-5 shows how this type of hinge works.

You may be able to remove a bathroom door altogether. If privacy is an issue after removing a door, hanging a curtain in the doorway can often solve the problem:

> *I removed a bathroom door in one place where I lived. It was never a problem because the bathroom was accessed through the bedroom, so I could simply close the bedroom door for privacy. In another apartment where I lived, I simply never closed the bathroom door because the room itself was too small for the door to close while I was inside. If I had guests I simply told them to stay in the living room, and I turned up the music!*

Another common obstacle is a screen or storm door at the front door of a house. Having two exterior doors can be solved with automatic door closers or by enclosing the doorway area with a porch. Then you can deal with each door separately.

How easy is it to open the exterior door? Most doors in a home do not have a closer, which applies some spring resistance to the door when you open it. Apartment buildings, however, will likely have closers on the door to the apartment and certainly on the door at the street entrance. The spring tension needs to be adjusted so that it is not difficult for you to open and then pass through comfortably. It is also important that doors open fully to a 90° angle to the opening to provide a clear path that allows you to continue in a straight line. This also makes it easier to hold the door and use the handle to pull yourself through. There might be conflict with building management who want to keep the spring tension tighter at the street for security reasons so that the door will close faster. But it is management's responsibility to properly maintain the door to close securely without requiring greater spring tension to slam it closed.

Figure 7-5 An offset door hinge.

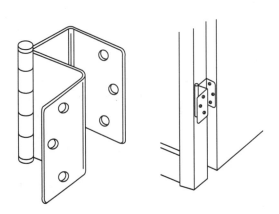

Floors

Flooring surface has a big effect on how easily and comfortably you are able to use a manual chair at home. Since many quadriplegic, elderly, or weak users switch to a manual chair while at home, floor surface has a significant impact on many people.

Most floors in a home are carpeted. A thick pile carpet on a soft under-mat is very difficult to wheel on and will fatigue you quickly. For power chairs, thicker carpet puts more demand on the motors and, so, uses up the batteries. It is more difficult to wheel in a straight line on thick carpeting, which forces you to constantly make adjustments with each wheel as you go. You will not coast very far either, which requires you to push the wheels many more times. Since you tend to repeatedly travel the same paths in your home, a thicker surface will develop visible tracks:

> Eventually, tracks start to show in the carpet because I usu-ally follow regular paths at home. They sort of disappear when you vacuum, but eventually they get pretty set in. It's just part of the wheelchair experience, I guess. They used to have a thicker pile carpet in the hallway of my apartment building, and friends who didn't come over very often used the tracks to help find my door!

Carpets with tight weaves provide better rollability. A pad underneath the carpet is not usually necessary but, if required, comes in thinner profiles. Some people have installed industrial-grade carpeting in their home, designed for public environments like offices.

Many homes use large rugs over a wood floor. Rugs are unfriendly to wheelchairs and can get twisted up in the front casters. A rug can be secured with Velcro. If you are placing a rug over carpeting, you will need only the half of the Velcro with the hooks, attached to the underside of the rug. Vel-cro strips in various widths with a sticky backing are available in rolls from office supply stores.

Hard floors are very easy to roll on. For wood floors, make sure no nails or screws are coming up from the surface that could threaten a tire. Look for wood splinters that could puncture a tire or get caught in the wheel—and then in your hand. Stone or ceramic tile can be very bouncy to wheel on. Deep spaces between tiles are usually the source of a bumpy ride, though the tiles themselves can be made with an uneven surface. The spaces between should not be too wide, and the grout that fills these spaces should be close to the top level of the tile for a smooth wheeling surface.

Floors need to be level. It doesn't take much slope for you to begin to roll downhill. Frankly, it is hard for builders to get all floors perfectly level, and a building inevitably settles a bit over time. If an existing house has noticeably sloping floors, however, check for problems with the foundation. If you are going to use a very heavy power chair, that is all the more reason to ensure the structural integrity of your building. If you are building something new, you should strongly emphasize this point with the building contractor.

Windows

Natural light contributes to quality of life in the home. Windows also help maintain contact with the outside world. You can look out to see what might have caused a sound or see who is asking for entry into your home. Using operable windows for ventilation is an efficient way to manage temperature and is the best way to get fresh air throughout the home and circulate impurities out of the air.

What if you are adapting an existing home? Even if adding or changing windows is beyond your budget, you can orient furniture—particularly the bed—so that there are views to the outside. You can add landscaping to make the view more appealing or trim branches to let in more light.

There are different types of windows:

- Casement windows open toward the outside by turning a crank. Casements are easier to open than other types and are more likely to open enough for an emergency escape. Handles can be found for the crank that are large and easier to grasp.
- Vertical sliding sash windows are common in homes. Because of their weight and the force required, opening them usually requires two hands and considerable upper-body strength and balance. The latch is usually at the top of the lower sash, often out of reach from the sitting position. Some products locate the latch at the sill.
- Horizontal sliding sash windows cannot unexpectedly close due to gravity and are easy to open. They usually are designed with a lip that runs the entire vertical edge of the moving window, offering variety in where to push or pull. They come with different kinds of latches, some of which are spring loaded, placed high, and require pinch force—a difficult-to-use design. A simple latch placed at the bottom that is easily lifted and stays in place is best and commonly found. Only one half of the total window width can be open; this might not leave sufficient room for escape in an emergency.

As with doors, remote window openers are available for many of these types of windows, depending on the brand and design.

Walls

Do not place rough textures on areas of wall that you are likely to touch, such as plastered surfaces that are laid on with a decorative texture or some wallpapers such as grasscloth. These surfaces are often rough enough to injure your hand if you slide your hand across the surface or need the wall for sudden support.

When turning a corner in a manual wheelchair, it is much easier to make the turn by placing your hand on a wall, rather than grasping one wheel while you push the other. The same is sometimes true for going through doors: placing a hand on the wall as you pull the door open can make it easier. Unfortunately, that means that, each time, you will leave a little bit of oil and dirt from your skin on the wall. This eventually starts to show as a dark area. Choose wall coverings that are easily cleaned and that don't show dirt as well. Glossy rather than matte-finish paints tend to be easier to clean. Small plastic shields can be attached to walls where they are commonly touched and can be replaced more easily than the paint or wall paper.

When a circulation path passes close to a wall, it is more likely to be bumped or scraped by a wheelchair, no matter how skilled the rider. Wainscoting with wood or with vinyl or plastic covers protects the underlying wall surface and can be attractive.

Furniture

Just because you are a wheelchair user doesn't mean that you will always stay in the chair. Many chair riders are able to easily transfer to furniture—and want to. It can be a real relief to get out of the chair.

Be conscious of the surface you choose to sit on. Just because it is soft, doesn't mean that it will provide appropriate support for the prevention of pressure sores. The foam in some upholstery is soft enough to compress almost all the way, resulting in focused pressure on your skin. You might supplement a chair or couch in the home with a foam pad, a piece of lamb's wool, or the cushion from your wheelchair. To facilitate cleaning, or to rearrange furniture for the great party you're throwing, chairs and sofas can be equipped with caster wheels. Include two that can be locked so they won't roll out from under you during a transfer.

Knee and foot clearance at tables are key issues. A central support for the table is more likely to be in the way of your feet when you sit on the side of the table, or a central base could be large and thick enough to block your front wheels from going as far forward as you need to sit close. Many dining room tables include a skirt around the edge that might be low enough to keep your knees from going under the table. Tables sometimes come with extra leaves to extend the end of the table. The extra leaves hang out over the edge and often allow that extra inch or two of clearance for your knees or feet. This explains why chair users so often find themselves sitting at the head of the table as a dinner guest:

> *I had my table put up on blocks so I could roll under it. Same thing with the table for my computer. I hired someone to make the changes for me, and it was a very simple solution.*

Stacking tables and folding chairs, such as director's chairs, can be kept aside for clearance and then used for company. Coffee tables that go in front of a couch are an obstruction, both to travel within the room and to your ability to transfer to the couch.

I have friends with two couches and a large table in between. If there are other guests while I'm there, I simply cannot get into the rest of the house. No room left to pass.

Lighting

When you are considering lighting, think about being able to reach and operate switches and being able to change bulbs. Typically, room light switches are located just inside the door. The placement of a switch might be too high or require a degree of dexterity beyond your ability. When you are unable to reach a switch, a noise-actuated switch can be installed that responds to a clap or a loud vocal sound. Unfortunately, these switches sometimes respond to sounds when you don't want them to, turning a light on as you sleep or leaving you in the dark prematurely. A more costly approach is to literally move the light switch down, cutting a new hole, and filling the old one.

Of the many types of light switches, rockers and push buttons take the least dexterity, involving no gripping or pinching. Thumb wheels, rotary knobs, and slide bars are generally more difficult. Figure 7-6 shows various types of controls ranked by the difficulty of operating them.

A remote-control unit is a reliable solution for people with limited hand dexterity. These systems usually involve no electrical rewiring; there is a small unit that you plug into the power line and then program the remote control to recognize it.

The design of a fixture might prevent you from changing a light bulb. Many lights require that you pinch a small set screw to remove a hood or globe to access the bulb. A lampshade might have been replaced too tightly by a friend or family member to be removed. Some attention to detail can make a big difference in independence. Multiple light sources, fixtures with

Figure 7-6 Electronic controls, from easiest (1) to most difficult (7).

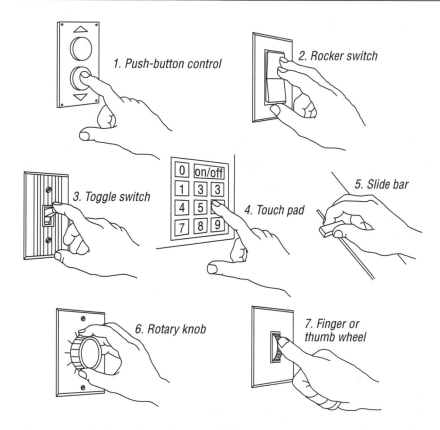

two bulbs, and a backup desk lamp help ensure you won't get left in the dark. Ceiling fixtures can be found equipped with retractable cables so that you can bring them down for a bulb change; grabber arms can be handy.

Outdoor lighting is important so that you can see the path and avoid any surprise obstructions. Motion detectors can turn a light on when it picks up the arrival of your vehicle or your approach from the sidewalk. Motion detectors then can turn the light off after a set period of time, which presumably leaves you enough time to get inside the house. Timers can be installed and programmed to turn the exterior lights on at a given time each day.

Electrical Wiring

It is critical that you have enough electrical power. If you are charging a power wheelchair, have a bed with motorized adjustments, use a ventilator or oxygen, have a remote-control system for lights and so on, these will place considerable demands on your power supply. The last thing you want to risk is overloading a circuit and shutting off a ventilator. Using plug taps, power strips, and extension cords so that you can plug more items into existing outlets than would otherwise be possible can quickly overload a circuit and present a real fire hazard. The issue is whether you have enough "amperage" in a given circuit for the amount of power you ask of it.

It might be necessary to add more power to your home or reroute existing power to where it is needed. Some outlets—such as in the basement or garage—might be underused and more valuable when routed to the bedroom, for instance. Running new wires through walls—if necessary—can be very costly and disruptive but is the first choice for aesthetics. An easier and less expensive approach is to use cable raceways that are surface mounted. They can be placed unobtrusively or covered by moldings.

In the bathroom, incorporate ground-fault circuit interrupters into outlets in the wall. These are widely available and found at any hardware store. An interrupter is not a major piece of equipment but will shut off power at the plug rather than at the main circuit if water gets in.

If you need it and can afford it, a battery backup system can be installed that will provide you with a number of hours of emergency power if the system goes out. A generator that runs on a small gasoline engine is another backup option. Call your local authority—city, township, and so on—and let the authority know if someone in your home is at risk if power is lost. In the event of a blackout, the local emergency plan should put a priority on protecting people whose lives might be threatened without electricity, though don't be surprised if the plan has not yet addressed disability emergency preparation. You might find yourself a local advocate on this issue.

Some local utility companies offer special rates for people with disabilities or have programs that allow you to spread out payments during winter months when the bill might be substantially higher. You should also ask if the companies have a registry or special number to call in the case of an emergency, in the event you need a high priority for having your power restored.

After you've checked that you have enough power and can protect yourself in the event of outages, you'll also want to look at other matters of safety and convenience.

Power receptacles low on the wall are often obscured behind furniture and can be difficult to reach. You can effectively raise power outlets with a power strip—several receptacles on a strip at the end of a two-foot cord. It gives you flexibility for where to position the power and often includes electrical protection from power spikes, which can injure sensitive electronic equipment, and usually includes a master switch that allows you to turn off several items with one push of a button.

Heating, Ventilation, and Cooling

Temperature control is very important for people with certain disabilities. With multiple sclerosis, excessive heat can encourage exacerbations. People with arthritis are sensitive to temperature variations, as are older persons, who generally need more heat. Some people with spinal cord injuries are unable to sweat, so they need to keep cool. People on fixed incomes have difficulty spending more money on heating, ventilation, and air conditioning, so they are faced with the tug between saving money and ensuring their safety. Some people address the need for more heat with space heaters, which are often inefficient, are expensive to run, and can be more likely to cause a home fire.

The placement of thermostats is important. Put the thermostat within reach for everyone and make sure it is not in direct sunlight. Zoned heating and air conditioning can be a valued feature. You might want to set a cooler temperature for a bedroom where a temperature-sensitive person sleeps or spends more time during the day. Some thermostat designs are more difficult to use; avoid designs that require pinch and hand strength or on which the numbers are too small to be easily seen. Programmable thermostats allow you to set temperature changes for different times of the day.

Think through emergency procedures for utilities and make sure that shutoff valves are accessible to every family member. For example, you can install a gas shutoff valve that can be turned easily by a long lever-type of handle, without great strength or tools. Also ensure that the path to shutoff valves remains accessible.

Before spending money on expensive heating and cooling equipment, take measures to control air movement and sunlight with passive energy methods:

- Be sure windows and doors are well insulated.
- Weather-strip around door and window frames.
- Make sure that doors to the outside have a good seal at the threshold.
- Spray an insulating foam into walls.
- Manage the sunlight: when you need heat, open shades and let the sun shine in; close shades when you're warm enough.
- Awnings or eaves of the correct depth will block the sun in summer and let it in during winter.

Fireplaces can remove heat. The heat of the fire travels up the chimney flue and creates a vacuum effect that actually draws warm air out of the house and out the top. Be sure not to leave the flue vent open when you need to keep heat in the house.

Telephones

The ability to communicate over distances is key for people with limited mobility. The phone can be the link to your social world, maintaining relationships through calls with friends and family. It can allow you to conduct business from home or function as an advocate—for yourself or others. A phone line for an Internet connection can be a link to a wider community, as in the case of this man with Friedrich's ataxia:

> The Internet has enhanced my life a great deal. I'm an amateur writer, and the World Wide Web has been a great research tool for my writing projects. I have been able to converse with some great people about many different things. By using a computer, I am more independent than I would be otherwise. The computer has been the impetus for some of the best things I feel I've ever done. I use a wheelchair, my hand/eye coordination and balance are very poor, but the computer allows me to function as a productive member of society.

Telephone jacks are best placed near electrical outlets, since computers, fax, and answering machines also need power. General advice is to have at least one phone jack in each room where you are likely to spend more than a few minutes at a time.

A telephone line is also a lifeline. A speaker phone with a speed-dial button might only require pressing one or two buttons, without having to pick up the handset, to make an emergency call. There are services that allow you to carry an alarm button that will make an automatic phone call to a healthcare facility or security agency. Some medical equipment can have similar features, in which a phone call is made if the machine experiences a shutdown that could be life threatening. Dedicated phone lines might be needed in these cases.

Many telephone companies have disability programs to provide special equipment. For example, AT&T gives people speakerphone headsets, or telephones are available with large, lighted buttons that are easy to press. They are free of charge once you and your physician fill out the application.

People with little arm movement can freely access the telephone via puff-and-sip control systems that allow them to choose from a preprogrammed list of numbers or dial a new one. Hands-free telephone access is possible.

Remote—or cordless—telephones are very helpful. It can take some time to get to a fixed telephone set—for instance, if you are not in your wheelchair when the phone rings—and you might miss calls. (You can let people who call you regularly know that you might need more time to answer, and, if you have voicemail, you will want to specify a sufficient number of rings before voicemail answers for you.) A remote phone goes where you go, which is especially helpful in the bathroom. These products have improved a great deal in recent years. The sound quality is good, multiple channels are available in case you get static, and 2.4 GHz phones can have a range of 1,000 feet or more.

Intercoms

Intercom systems allow easy communication or monitoring and are especially useful for people who have very restricted mobility or who must spend a share of each day in bed or on a breathing apparatus. Intercom systems can be helpful for monitoring guests at the front door. Commercial systems are now available for the home with video capability, so you can see who is there and can speak with them as well.

There are two types of intercom systems. One uses its own wiring, usually threaded through the wall cavities—an approach that provides the clearest sound. Wiring is best done during new construction but is possible to install in an existing home; surface conduits can be used.

The other type of intercom system uses carrier current. The intercom is integrated into electrical wiring, which carries the signal alongside the electricity. Components plug into outlets to transmit the signals. Some static is picked up from the shared wiring. These systems are generally less expensive than intercoms with their own wiring.

Home Control Systems

There are home control systems that allow you to:

■   Control the volume of televisions or sound systems
■   Adjust lights
■   Lock and unlock or open and close doors and windows
■   Control heating and ventilation
■   Control appliances of all kinds
■   Use telephone systems
■   Turn on your iPod

Some systems are designed specifically with disabilities in mind. When you shop for a system, assess the details of how it operates. Operation should be clear, intuitive, and not demand much memorizing of commands. Controls should be easy to operate without fine dexterity or the need to apply much force. The controls for a home control system can be integrated into a power wheelchair's control system, including puff-and-sip or head remotes. Some can be activated by voice control or blinking an eye.

Appliances you already own might not be compatible with some control products.

As with intercoms, there are hard-wired versions and carrier-current types of home control systems. The X-10 standard is an example of a carrier-current type of system. Modules are purchased that plug into power outlets, and then the appliances to be controlled. Such a system can be expanded over time, as your budget allows:

> *Everything is working fine with the X-10 protocol; I've never had a problem. It controls lights, electric devices, temperature (heating/air conditioning), built-in alarm system, and medic-alert, with scenarios that you can program. For instance, when I enter the bathroom, the lights fade in by themselves and fade out after a predetermined number of minutes. You can control everything by phone, with a remote, or by a touch-screen panel.*

Ron Mace liked the product because it met his criteria for Universal Design:

> *The X-10 product came out as a consumer product—not a disability access/adaptive technology product.*

The X-10 protocol continues to be available into the late 2000s, part of the increasingly wide and less-expensive array of environmental components available from a variety of suppliers of home control systems such as Smart Home USA (www.smarthomeusa.com) and Break Boundaries (www.breakboundaries.com).

Automated Door Openers

Door openers are a sort of subspecialty, produced by companies that focus only on this particular solution. They generally don't involve major construction. Examples are from Door Motion Technologies (www.doormotion.com) and Power Access (www.power-access.com).

Alarm and Warning Systems

A loss of mobility implies increased risk in the event of an emergency. Early warning is critical for a person with a disability.

Warning alarms include smoke, fire, and gas detectors. The alarm design should consider a variety of sensory needs. A buzzer or siren for warning might not be sufficient for those with hearing loss. Products are available with strobe lights that can waken sighted people from a deep sleep and, thus, also serve people with hearing disabilities.

Check alarm batteries often. Smoke and heat sensors need to be placed high up on a wall or on the ceiling, since heat rises. Provide some means for a person with a disability to turn off the alarm, even if that is with a broom handle kept nearby. Some homes and apartment complexes have systems that notify a security office or the police or fire station in the event of fire or emergency. Be sure that everyone in the household knows the codes for setting and defeating these systems.

It is a good idea to inform building management or neighbors that someone is in the household who might need assistance in an emergency. Local police and fire departments might also keep such lists. Find out what kind of emergency assistance programs exist in your community. Put a wheelchair symbol in your bedroom window to identify yourself, and develop an escape plan with your family, neighbors, or personal assistant.

Lift and Track Systems

For those people who are unable to perform their own transfers to and from the wheelchair onto and off of places like the bed, the toilet, or the tub, there are a variety of lift systems that ease their being assisted—or these people may even be able to perform the operation on their own. Typically a sling is positioned under the person to be lifted, which then attaches to the lift arm. There are manual lifts as well as battery-operated ones, and there are lifts capable of lifting bariatric weights. Options include a lift on a structure that can roll, so you can be taken anywhere in the house. Hoyer is known for making this type of lift—as well as a reasonably portable one that can travel with you for use in hotel rooms. They also provide customized track systems that can be installed on the ceiling to take you from room to room and specific locations. The SureHands system (www.sure hands.com) does not require an assistant for those people who are able to use their arms sufficiently. It is specifically designed to be easier to get into and out of yourself. SureHands can also be configured on a stand or a ceiling track system. Says this man with quadriplegia:

> After installing a Surehands ceiling lift to save attendants'
> backs and make things easier, I created a lift into a whirlpool
> tub, which I love. It transverses the toilet and bed also. My
> next project takes the bath lift to the outside to drop me in the
> pool and convertible, and bike, mower etc.

The Bathroom

The bathroom is often the space that is the greatest challenge to make accessible. In a 1993 US Census Bureau report, 4.5 million people with disabilities reported having difficulty bathing, and 2.1 million had trouble using the toilet. Millions of people are inconvenienced—even endangered—by inaccessible bathrooms. Any impediment to easy access to the bathroom can lead someone to delay their bowel or bladder program—which can have secondary health consequences. A bathroom that is easy to use protects your health (see Figure 7-7).

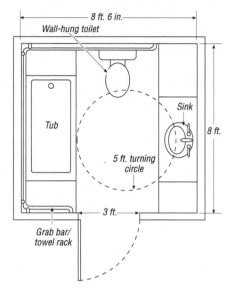

Figure 7-7 A small, wheelchair-accessible bathroom.

An existing home might have several bathrooms. They don't all have to be accessible. Ideally, there should be an accessible bathroom on each accessible floor of the home.

Creating a larger bathroom for access does not have to rob the rest of the home of space. Ron Mace explained:

> All we need to do in bathrooms is increase the size by about a foot to get enough maneuvering space for a wheelchair. If you plan it carefully, you're only adding about five square feet, and you can get that by just taking a few inches out of adjacent rooms. You hardly notice the difference, except that the bathroom is a bit more luxurious.

Builders of new apartments benefit from providing access:

> People who move into an apartment with a large bathroom don't even know it's for access. They just love it. It turns out to be a marketing plus.

Safety

The bathroom is a site of many household accidents. The US Consumer Product Safety Commission reports that more than 110,000 accidents occur in bathtubs and showers each year. Some chair users make several transfers each day from their chair to a toilet or bath. More than for any room in the house, you need to think of safety as much as simple access to the space.

For a chair user who is able to stand to use the shower or bath, a slippery surface can be extremely treacherous. Various floor materials respond differently to being wet. Some new ceramic tiles or rubber-based linoleum surfaces have better slip resistance. Keep the bathroom floor clear of small objects on which you could slip, and use cleaning products that do not leave a slippery film.

Toilets

Toilets are often too low for people with disabilities. This can be solved with a riser to elevate the seat, available in various heights. Some riser products lift out of the way to allow others to use the lower seat. You could also replace the toilet with a wall-mounted unit. A wall-mounted unit not only lets you install it at exactly the height you need, but also frees up floor space underneath, which increases the turning radius available to you by allowing additional clearance for your feet.

Individual chair users have their own unique needs and preferences for how they position themselves relative to the toilet. Some people get onto the toilet only occasionally; possibly only for their bowel program. Those who use catheters empty their bladder into a plastic container, which is then dumped into the toilet. Others wear a leg drainage bag and need to be able to get the drainage tube into the toilet to empty the bag.

The side of the toilet or bidet needs to be placed at the right distance from the wall. If the side of the toilet is too close, you risk bumping the wall during transfers. If it is too far away, you could fall between the wall and the toilet while reaching for the tissue dispenser or a grab bar.

Toilet paper holders or items that might extend from the surface of the wall need to be placed for easy reach from the toilet. They should not be too far away or behind the plane of the shoulder, making it necessary to reach behind oneself. Many people lean forward and drop their head as they transfer from the toilet to the wheelchair; make sure that nothing, such as towel rack or decorative artwork, is in the way of your head.

There needs to be sufficient clear space in front of and next to the toilet or bidet to get your chair in the optimal position for transfer. In public, far too many so-called accessible bathroom stalls are wide enough to enter but leave you sitting directly facing the bowl. This requires you to do a full 180° transfer—a treacherous feat for many chair users with no ability to stand at best. For safe transfers, it is generally necessary to be able to achieve a 90° angle to the toilet. Some people being assisted are best transferred from a position next to and parallel to the bowl.

Tubs and Showers

Getting into a bathtub is difficult for many people with disabilities. They cannot step or lift themselves over the edge of a tub or, once in, cannot lift themselves back out. Yet they yearn for the luxury of a good long soak, after having to typically settle for showers or, worse, sponge baths in bed.

One design that lets you down into the tub is a sort of balloon that is "inflated" with water. The balloon lowers you down into the bath when you release the water from inside it. You refill it from the tub tap to raise yourself back up. Some people also use sling lifts in the bathroom to make transfers onto a shower chair or down into the tub. A portable lift can do double duty in the bedroom and bathroom.

Sitting on the floor of a tub is a problem for people with posterior muscle atrophy. There are a few tubs designed with a foam base under a heavy, vinyl-like covering. Some people have found success with the proper density of foam that provides support but does not float. An air-floatation cushion could be used if it can be partially filled with water to keep it from being buoyant, which would make you unstable in the tub.

A tub becomes usable as a shower with a shower chair or tub seat. Some designs allow you to get into the chair outside of the tub and then pivot or slide into place. A hand-held shower head gives you or your personal assistant the ability to hold the shower head to rinse easily.

Antiscald controls allow you to set a maximum possible water temperature. Your inability to quickly move out of the path of the stream or your inability to sense dangerous temperature makes this a valuable device. These devices also control water pressure, which can affect water temperature when it fluctuates. You'll find these in some hotels.

Shower and tub controls are typically placed in the center of the wall over the spigot, which can be difficult to reach from a chair when you are outside the tub. Controls would ideally be located closer to the outside wall and lower down for easy access. Many people who prefer to sit in the tub would benefit from having controls on the side wall where they can be reached from inside the tub. In either case, a single, lever control is easiest, compared with knobs or handles that require a strong grip. Make certain that the contractor understands the reason for the location of controls because they—and building inspectors—are accustomed to seeing controls in the center and could unwittingly override this valuable access detail during the plan review and permit-approval process.

A range of bath and shower units are being developed for the convenience and comfort of those with disabilities. For example, the Freedom Bath® is a bathtub with a side wall that raises and lowers and includes a seat formed inside the tub (see Figure 7-8). You can transfer onto the seat at normal height, raise the wall, and fill it with water for your bath. There is no need to deal with the dramatic change in level to get to the bottom of a bathtub, but you can still be immersed for a good soak. It is the size of a normal bathtub.

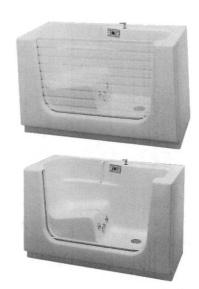

Figure 7-8 A side-entrance bathtub.

Some stall showers have a molded seat built in; others use a fold-down platform that lifts out of the way for use by people who stand. You might need to add a cushion to such a platform, in which case you need to be careful that the cushion would not slip and that you are very stable. Also note where the grab bar is located—sitting back against it might be uncomfortable, especially if it is cold metal. Be sure your need for upper-body balance and stability are being met. Prefabricated shower units are designed to roll into, accommodating rolling shower chairs designed for the purpose. Prefab units have only a small lip at the edge, rather than the three-inch or larger lip that is common to most stall showers. These units can be used in new construction or replace an existing bathtub.

Another solution is to build a wet room—a space, sometimes just the open corner of a large bathroom, that is tiled with a drain on the floor. Faucets, shower heads, and handholds are installed on the walls, also tiled. You wheel into the area in a rolling shower chair to wash.

Grab Bars in the Bathroom

Grab bars are essential, particularly around the shower, toilet, and bidet. A grab bar needs to be secured to a solid structure in the wall, typically horizontal reinforcement between vertical studs that can be drilled into. Builders are now encouraged to provide support structure in bathroom walls for the eventual addition of grab bars, but it is not yet a standard construction measure. When sufficient structure is not already present, it is sometimes necessary to break into the wall to add the structural backing:

I moved into a newly built apartment complex that used the handicapped-adaptable approach. In my smaller, second bath-room they couldn't put a grab bar in the bathtub because they hadn't reinforced the wall. There was nothing to attach it to, so they just put the grab bar vertically at the front of the tub. It's totally useless and just a waste of money.

Sometimes a brace can be added across studs on the surface of the wall, which can then carry a grab bar. But a brace near the bath or shower becomes a trap for water, which will eventually cause damage. Another approach is to sheathe the wall with 3/4-inch plywood, which creates a strong structural base for grab bars. The plywood sheathing is more costly than adding one or more studs but allows installation of support at any loca-tion you choose. Grab bars need to be able to carry as much as 300 pounds. A towel rack is not a grab bar and should never be used as one, even momen-tarily. It is not able to carry your body weight.

A mobile home might have some walls that are only made of particle board, fiberglass, or sheet metal. These materials are incapable of support-ing a grab bar, but it might be possible to add reinforcement behind these surfaces. There are grab bars available that clip onto the side of a bathtub or toilet and don't require structural support from a wall. Be very certain they are firmly installed, check the attachments regularly to keep them tight, and then test carefully in advance by applying force in several directions before relying on them for support.

Although there are standards that offer advice on specific grab-bar heights, optimal height and position for grab bars depend on your exact capabilities and size. A grab bar that is standard height might be too high for some people because of their height or because the muscles they would need to use are weak or unavailable. In your own home, you are not bound by code standards that apply in public settings, and you may set grab bars at the position and height that are optimal for you.

Some people benefit from supports immediately next to the toilet, functioning as armrests. For others, these can be obstructions during trans-fer from a wheelchair. Some products are hinged from the wall, so that they can be raised out of the way during a transfer and brought down for safety and stability while using the toilet.

In *Building for a Lifetime*, the authors suggest thinking more generi-cally in terms of handholds—places in the room where people might require support as they bend or lean in the course of their business. Hand-holds might indeed be grab bars but can include a shelf, countertop, or a ledge around the bathtub. This kind of thinking might mean you reinforce the support of the sink, for instance. The authors recommend using "a generous supply of handholds."[1]

The selection of access products for the bathroom has expanded. Major bathroom appliance manufacturers have been applying their skill to the design and appearance of accessible fixtures. Grab bars, for instance, are available in options beyond the once-standard stainless steel. They can now be found in a variety of colors and designs. An accessible bathroom is an enhancement to your home, and you should have no reservations about proceeding with such changes that both enhance safety and are aesthetically pleasing.

The Bathroom Sink

Many bathroom sinks are set in a cabinet top. The cabinet can often be removed from under the sink to allow room to get close to the sink, after making certain that the cabinet is not supporting the weight of the sink. Remember to cover the water pipes under the sink with insulation to ensure that you don't burn your legs.

The best sink faucets are single-lever types. Antiscald devices are useful here. Use a spout that extends far enough out so that it is easy to get your hands fully underneath the water, unobstructed by the back of the sink, and so that you are not forced to lean forward away from your chair back.

Choose a faucet with an easy-to-use control for closing the drain. The old-style rubber plug with a chain is easy to use.

Regulating Air Temperature

There are unique temperature-management issues in the bathroom. Warm water in the bath or shower generates heat and humidity. On the other hand, you tend to feel chilled when you open the shower curtain and let in the cooler air from the rest of the room or house. For people with temperature sensitivity, heat and cold can be managed with:

- A dedicated air conditioner
- An infrared heat lamp
- A wall-mounted heater
- An exhaust fan
- An operable window

Because of the amount of water in a bathroom, a space heater placed on the floor is dangerous and not recommended. In bathrooms, windows tend to be installed higher for privacy but may be important for ventilation and temperature management. Some window controls can be extended with a chain or a pulley system to allow them to be operated from a lower position.

The Kitchen

The kitchen is much more than a place to make food. It is a central gathering place and social center for the home. Access to the kitchen is crucial for participation as a full member of the household.

When looking at kitchen design, think in terms of the two-cook kitchen. Leave wider aisles, and create work spaces that allow knee clearance so that the wheelchair will not obstruct circulation in the space. Then the chair user can join in, rather than become an obstacle that prevents others from working with him in the kitchen.

To be able to cook from your wheels, you need a surface that is low enough for cutting vegetables and for other food-preparation tasks. Normal-height counters can still be reached easily to hold items not in use but are usually too high for a seated person to comfortably use for cooking preparation. At the least, you can set a cutting board on your lap, possibly with a piece of thin foam underneath to level and support it.

Ideally, provide a lowered work surface. The surface should be within reach of the sink and stove so that you won't have to be moving back and forth as you work. The surface should have knee clearance and unobstructed leg room. A cabinet could be removed and a height-adjustable surface installed, controlled either by a manual hand crank or a motor. Lower surfaces also let children get more involved in the cooking process, and elderly or temporarily injured family members can sit on a stool to work in the kitchen. Space underneath this counter might also accommodate a serving cart or recycling bins.

Lowered surfaces can also be created with pull-out counters installed into the kitchen cabinets. They are hidden when not in use and greatly expand counter area for all users. They are especially valuable near the stove, where foods can be cut and placed directly into pots. A pegboard with hooks or a countertop container allows you to keep commonly used utensils, like a spatula or spoons, within reach at all times rather than having to open and close drawers and cabinets. You should not have to struggle to operate anything in the kitchen or risk having something heavy, hot, or sharp fall in your lap because a sticky drawer forces awkward movement.

Kitchen Sink

Ideally, it should be possible to sit straight at the sink, saving you from the need to twist continually while washing vegetables or dishes. A shallow sink can both help provide better leg room and spare you from having to reach down into a deeper sink. If you are installing a garbage disposal, it is best placed to the side and rear to preserve leg room. A garbage disposal can help keep trips to the trash can to a minimum. Pipes and plumbing underneath the sink must always be insulated to protect your legs from burns.

Height-adjustable sinks are possible thanks to flexible drain pipes that allow the sink to move. Flexible pipes can be used underneath the drain while maintaining a trap—the U-shaped form that keeps water in the hose and prevents gases from rising back up through the drain into the house.

Use a single-lever handle on the sink. Use a spout that is high enough so that there is room underneath to place pots. The spout should also extend far enough forward for minimal reach and be able to rotate. People with the ability to grip can benefit further from a hand-held spout on a flexible hose, very commonly found in plumbing sections.

Appliances

In general, choose appliances that are easy to operate, with clearly readable controls that function intuitively. All appliance controls should be in the front, especially on the stove, so that you will never have to reach over a hot heating element.

With an electric stove, choose a stovetop that includes a warning light when a burner surface is turned on, to prevent accidental burns. A stove with raised heating elements presents a greater risk of a hot pot falling off the edge, since the pot has to be lifted to be moved. Ceramic stovetops allow pots to be more easily slid safely to a counter surface at the side. A disadvantage of the smooth ceramic stovetop is that there is less capacity to catch spilled liquids, increasing the risk of burns for someone who is seated near the stovetop.

Stovetop burners should be staggered so that it is not necessary to reach across one burner to access another. It should be evident which control affects which burner. An angled mirror above the cooktop will allow you to see inside pots from a sitting position.

Oven doors generally open downward, forcing you to either lean over the door or position yourself to the side, assuming there is space next to the appliance. Either way, you are not in the best position for balance, especially to handle heavy, hot items. A wall-mounted oven with a side-hinged door allows you to be closer but also increases the risk of a spill, unless there is counter space immediately adjacent where you can set a hot dish without having to drive the chair. A pull-out surface immediately underneath the oven is the ideal.

Microwave ovens are often installed up high, over a traditional stove. This location can be too high for some people, who need the microwave placed on a counter top or installed into cabinetry at a lower level. Microwaves come with various types of door latches, some of which require pressing a button while pulling. These are difficult for people with reduced gripping ability.

Dishwasher designs suffer from the same issue as an oven, with a door that pulls down, although there is not any risk of burns. A dishwasher needs to have sufficient clearance at the side so that dishes can be put in directly after being rinsed in the sink.

In refrigerators, put the heaviest items at chest height, where they are easiest to access. Side-by-side refrigerator/freezers put more freezer space within easy reach.

Kitchen Cabinets

In the traditional kitchen, a great portion of cabinet space is often inaccessible. Cabinets are too high, too low, or too deep to be fully accessible by someone sitting or older household members who also have difficulty reaching or stooping. Cabinets can be made more useful by any of several measures that improve visibility, accessibility of contents, or height.

- Use shallow cabinets that keep more items within reach and within view.
- Use windowed doors to save the need to search for items by opening many cabinets.
- Remove cabinet doors altogether, particularly on lower cabinets, where you have to move away from the door as you open it.
- Put the most-often used items on shelves that are easiest to reach.
- Use a grabber arm to get items on shelves that are out of reach (see Figure 7-9).
- Adjust cabinet shelves to a more convenient configuration.
- Store more items on the counter. A small stack of shelves can make good use of a countertop, or small cabinets with doors can be built in.
- Place a lazy Susan in a cabinet or on a countertop.
- Move overhead cabinets lower to bring them into easier reach.
- Install automated units that can be lowered to counter level.

Drawers bring objects within reach and view and into the light. The back half is as useful as the front, unlike a cabinet. Use roller tracks that glide easily, and do not overload the drawer with heavy items that will make the drawer harder to slide in and out. Provide handles that don't demand fine dexterity or strong grip. Cloth loops added to handles can help people with no grip open drawers. Be sure there is room for the wheelchair next to the drawer. It is not necessary to reach every shelf in every cabinet in your kitchen. Louis Tenenbaum observes:

> *My experience in the kitchen is that we use a whole lot fewer things than we have. What it's really about is spending the time to figure out what things you need to have close by. In many cases, the things you don't have close by, you use rarely. For stuff that you only use when you have company, wait until your guests arrive, and ask them to get it down.*

Kitchen Electrical Issues

Switches and power outlets are typically placed on walls at the back of counters. These are especially difficult to reach in corners of L-shaped or U-shaped layouts. Outlets can be relocated to the front of floor cabinets or just under the surface if there is an open space for leg room. A switch or outlet box can be placed underneath a surface where leg room has been provided, taking care to put it to the side so that it does not obstruct or potentially injure your legs. There is some risk at this location of a cord getting caught by an arm or your chair, or grabbed by a curious child and of an appliance being pulled off the counter. Many kitchens have false panels, particularly underneath the sink, where a hole could be cut and wiring extended to install an outlet.

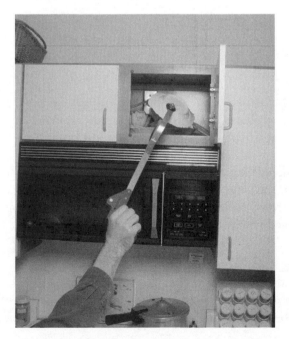

Figure 7-9 Using a grabber arm for a high cabinet.

Another option is to place power underneath overhead cabinets—which also keeps them beyond the reach of children. A cable raceway can run underneath the front edge of upper cabinets, providing a series of outlets along its length.

Most kitchens benefit from lighting placed underneath upper cabinets. These lights make counter tasks easier to see and also bring light switches within reach. Choose fixtures that will not create glare or shine directly in your eyes from the seated angle. Natural light is appealing in a kitchen, so provide window shade controls that can be reached from the seated position.

Kitchen Layouts

The most efficient layout for a kitchen is a U-shape, which puts more surface within reach without a user having to move. A drawback is that deeper spaces in the corners are more difficult to reach. The U-shape layout also makes it easier to provide room for you to fully turn around in your chair.

A kitchen with two longer parallel surfaces has its advantages, too. If the kitchen is properly arranged, you can be within reach of surfaces and facilities on either side of you and have a pull-out surface installed at a good height for cutting and food handling. It is critical to establish good relationships among all features of the kitchen and make the best use

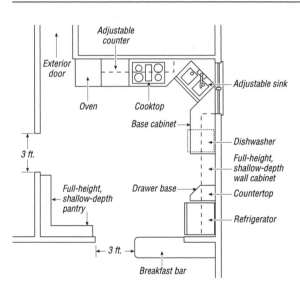

Figure 7-10 An L-shaped kitchen.

of accessories. This layout also allows you to enter or leave the working area from either end. Figure 7-10 shows an example of a good option for a kitchen layout.

If you need to make do in a kitchen with major appliances that are difficult to use, don't discount the value of your local appliance store. Toaster ovens, crock pots, waffle irons, griddles, rice cookers, and hot plates are lightweight, easily positioned, inexpensive, and energy efficient.

Bedrooms

The ideal bedroom is spacious enough to allow full turning radius, particularly next to the bed, where people often are forced to back out of a space close to a wall. Non-fitted bed linens and spreads can narrow the space even more and get tangled up in the wheels. Backing up is easy for many wheelers but awkward for others, in which case the wall or bedclothes can suffer from contact with the chair. Narrow spaces next to the bed can also make it very difficult to get to a telephone, typically kept on the bedside table.

The bedroom is a place where additional electrical power might be needed for adjustable beds, home control systems, medical equipment such as ventilators or oxygen machines, television, stereo, or computer systems. The trick in planning is to be able to reach all of these things. Once in bed, for instance, how do you turn off the lights? A bedside lamp with a chain switch (which might need to have a loop added to it for those who can't grip) could be the answer, though the lamp should have a heavy base so that it won't easily tip over. A more advanced solution is to put switches in the wall directly next to the bed.

Beside the bed, you might need room to have a lamp, a book to read before you go to sleep, medications, or remote-control units, especially if you use an environmental control system. It could be difficult to twist far enough around to reach a bedside table that is placed back against the same wall as the headboard. A bedside stand with wheels can be rolled forward after you are in bed.

Bedroom dressers and tables often have drawers that do not slide easily or use handles that require strength and agility in the fingertips. Better designs use ball-bearing tracks so that the drawer slides with little force and handles that are large enough to grip with all of your fingers. Even then, adding loops can help make drawers more accessible, such as for this woman with rheumatoid arthritis who also has a vision impairment:

> For the bedroom, we added brightly colored belts to drawer handles, so that I can loop my arm in them, to see inside. To make it more of a family thing, we put them on everyone's drawers, as this way I am not singled out and it actually made it easier for other family members to get into the drawers, too. Also, some of my blankets have loops at the top that I can loop my arm through to pull them up or down.

The ultimate bedroom is a master suite with an accessible bathroom and roll-in closet. These spaces could use pocket doors, which are easy to open and close and don't invade any space by swinging out.

A close relationship between bedroom and bathroom is highly desirable. Getting dressed is more effort for most chair users. A private route to and from the bathroom spares you the need to dress until you are fully prepared for the day. If you receive assistance, you are best served when the helper has easy access to the bathroom. A lift can be installed on a ceiling rail that travels from the bed directly into the bathroom, allowing you to go from your bed directly into the tub or shower.

The more time you spend in the bedroom, the more important it is to have an escape route. There might be a door to a deck or patio, but, at the least, there should be a window that is large enough to get out.

It might not be possible to have access to an upstairs bedroom. Depending on your resources, you could consider installing a stair lift, converting a space downstairs, or adding a new bedroom. If you add a bedroom, ensure full access to the rest of the house. Louis Tenenbaum describes seeing a plan for a bedroom addition:

> There was no way for the father—quadriplegic from a work injury, using a power wheelchair—to make the turn through the kitchen from this new master suite.

Storage and Utilities

There is now quite an industry in closet organization, with shops, catalogs, and consultants presenting products for optimal efficiency. The typical closet has a horizontal rod for hanging clothes, with a shelf above it. Both can be out of reach for a wheelchair user. Hanging rods must be lowered or a height-adjustable product must be installed. Sometimes this allows installation of another rod higher up that can be used by a standing person.

Apart from moving rods, you can gain storage space with an array of accessories. Stacking storage boxes, drawers, and shoe bins can make the most of existing closet space, while bringing more items within reach. Placing folded clothing in drawers or shelves can be easier on the arms, sparing you the need to extend your arm forward to lift clothing on hangers off of the rod.

Every home has a space for tools, wet boots, and brooms and where laundry gets done. In an apartment, these things get squeezed into a closet. If you have a utility room, consider the height of shelving, ability to access closets, and the type of washer and dryer. A small, stacking washer and dryer unit can be very hard for a wheelchair user to reach. Front-loading types are easiest to reach.

Outdoor Spaces

Access to the outdoors and any yard is an important consideration. Ramped sidewalks or ramps from rear patios and decks expand access to the outside for family barbecues, working in the garden, or just sitting in the sun. A sun porch added to the rear of the house or a screened-in balcony in an apartment offers greater opportunity for fresh air, protects from bugs and direct sunlight, and removes the need for a screened door at the entry, which complicates access.

Some surfaces are easier to wheel on than others. Thick grass, especially on damp ground, is difficult for wheeling, and grass can hide invisible depressions a wheel could sink into, tipping you over. If you intend to wheel on a lawn, keep the grass cut, and inspect the yard for depressions to be filled in. On unpaved surfaces, gravel and stones make an unfriendly surface, whereas crushed limestone or packed clay makes it more passable.

If you will be encountering substantial rough terrain, wider, knobby tires can help or you could use an all-terrain vehicle instead of a wheelchair. Clearance of footrests can make access difficult if footrests are too low, since there is a greater chance of the main wheels settling a bit in soft ground.

Finding a Home

You need to take responsibility for determining whether a home or apartment can work for you. Telling landlords or real estate agents that you require wheelchair access will usually not do the job. They could either exaggerate or minimize your needs. They don't know how you adapt or what is hard or easy for you to do. They may think that you must have a home formally designed for wheelchair access, according to general standards and codes.

You will have better luck getting what you need with newer construction. Depending on the state you live in and whether the developer gained any exceptions to accessibility codes, a certain portion of new apartment units or townhouses in a newly constructed complex are generally required to be accessible. This might mean "handicapped adaptable," an approach in which the unit is designed to be adapted in certain ways if it needs to accommodate a wheelchair user. For instance, the management would be prepared to install lever handles on the doors and plumbing, add grab bars, or switch the stove and oven unit for one with controls on the front.

Thanks to the recent history of access codes and the ADA, the building environment is much improved. Builders tend to be more aware of the standards and of product offerings that satisfy legal requirements. But there is a difference between the codes and what really works best. If you have the chance to influence the design of a home or apartment complex before construction, you might be able to offer some guidance to a builder who is interested:

> *I had a hard time finding accessible housing after I was injured. I finally met with a builder in my area who was planning a new apartment complex. Because of my contact with him, he made two apartments in the complex very wheelchair accessible (roll-in shower, etc.), and all apartments are accessible (wide doorways, level entrances). He would not have done so without my influence, not because he didn't care, but because he wasn't aware of the needs, or how easy and inexpensive it was to make the apartments accessible.*

This is unfortunately more the exception than the rule, particularly if you are buying, because of business and permit approvals. A builder might not be allowed to accept money for a housing unit until it is finished. Since you can't commit to the purchase in advance, builders can't risk making special accommodations, since they can't be certain you will actually buy it.

Developers are just beginning to witness direct demand for Universal Design in their new apartments and homes. Ron Mace described how some consumers are planning ahead:

> *We had a developer come to us who said that six clients had recently said they had heard about Universal Design. They wanted the developer to build houses that would last the rest of their lives. These were families without a person with a disability. They were baby boomers who saw their own parents have to leave their homes when they got older and couldn't climb the stairs or use the bathroom anymore.*

Mobile and Modular Homes

Some people have found a workable solution for accessibility in mobile and modular homes, which are usually limited to one floor. A mobile home is attached to a steel frame, which provides structural stability. It can be placed only in a mobile home park or other site zoned for mobile homes. A modular home is more akin to conventionally built homes. However, it is largely constructed indoors in a factory, transported to the site, and then placed onto an already constructed foundation—which is where the worst complications can occur if the foundation is not carefully laid. Modular homes can be located in most residential areas, depending on local zoning ordinances and building codes.

Mobile and modular homes are built with the outer shell providing the structure. Interior walls are generally not load bearing. Because of the construction of these homes, there is usually more flexibility in modifying interior design. Modifying an existing unit can also be much easier, since interior walls are less likely to be structural. Doors can be widened and walls moved without worrying about the ceiling falling in. A ramp added to a mobile home will usually need to be structurally freestanding, since the building is not designed to carry the additional load.

Beyond Physical Changes

You might need to train family members and friends about keeping a clear path for you around the house. People who walk tend to leave shoes, bags, or packages recently brought into the house in your path of circulation without realizing they are obstructing your way. You also need to train others to return chairs fully back under the table and out of your way. You often need to remind people a few times before it really sinks in. Most people will understand and adjust. Often, other people tend to think that because, as a chair user, you spend all day in a chair, you must be accustomed to it:

> *When I have guests to my home, I end up staying in my wheelchair more than I otherwise would. Part of the problem is that there is a lot of competition for my favorite recliner— definitely the most comfortable spot in the house! But the other issue is that people don't understand my preference to get out of the wheelchair.*

If you're not getting to move out of your chair enough, feel free to speak up and let others know your needs, saying something like, "I'd really like to get out of this chair and be more comfortable."

What else is involved in making a home usable aside from building ramps, enlarging doors, or buying the right stove? Louis Tenenbaum suggests:

> *I often think that to make all this work, these homes need reasonably priced, friendly, maintenance contracts. I think that is going to have to be a vital component of independent living.*

Independent Living

An accessible home makes for a much greater quality of life, yet true independent living needs the community surrounding that home to be accessible, too. What good is it to be able to come and go freely from a household where you are a true participant if you can't get around on the streets where you live, go to school, go to work, or go have fun?

The ramped curbs at intersections that are now so common did not exist until the 1960s, when the Independent Living Movement began in Berkeley, California—the location of the very first curb cuts. Ed Roberts, who was quadriplegic as the result of polio, fought his way to acceptance into the University of California and, along with other devoted advocacy pioneers, achieved the first curb cuts, sought accessible housing, provided needed services on campus for students, and established the first independent living center in Berkeley to provide these services. This began a movement resulting in independent living centers across the country, thanks to the availability of federal funds through the Rehabilitation Act of 1978. Your local independent living center may have specialists who can help you solve accessibility issues in your home and, possibly, even help find funding to pay for them.

Ed Roberts, by the way, eventually served as the Director of the California Department of Vocational Rehabilitation—which had attempted to deny him tuition funding to attend the University of California, Berkeley. Thanks to the successes of people like Roberts, your home is not just where you live, but is a base from which you can live a full life in your community and beyond as you explore the very wide range of possibilities for getting out there!

References

1.   Wylde M, Baron-Robbins A, Clark S. *Building for a Lifetime: the Design and Construction of Fully Accessible Homes*. Newtown, CT: Taunton Press; 1994.

Chapter 8

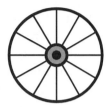

Getting Out There

Going Out

Even in the smallest towns, there are movie theaters, playhouses, sports events, restaurants, concerts, and other activities that you will want to attend. In larger cities, there might be the symphony, opera, museums, or tourist attractions.

The Americans with Disabilities Act (ADA) now requires all public facilities owned by private entities to be made accessible. Public facilities include restaurants and bars, theaters and stadiums, convention centers and lecture halls, shopping centers, retail stores, libraries, museums, zoos, amusement parks, schools, social service centers (including homeless shelters), and recreation facilities such as gymnasiums, health spas, and golf courses. The language of the law is that these facilities may not "refuse service or deny participation" in an activity. They must provide access under the reasonable accommodation provisions of the ADA or else establish alternative service. If you cannot enter a store, for instance, the store personnel are required to provide curb or home delivery service at no extra cost to you.

Most theaters, sports arenas, concert venues, and museums in the United States and Canada now provide substantial access. This is increasingly true in Europe where, for instance, the Louvre and Musee D'Orsay in Paris are fully and easily accessible. Some facilities will even offer you a discounted entrance fee. In some cases, you will need to go around to a side entrance, which should be clearly marked by an access symbol, but, in general, you have a good chance of getting in the front door and of being able to park nearby.

Seating in theaters and stadiums is more complex. There are a limited number of seats dedicated to wheelchair users, and those seats might or might not be well spaced throughout the facility. Often the accessible seating is toward the back of the theater or away from the lower levels of the stadium or arena. This limited choice of seating can be frustrating. It's wise to get tickets early, since those seats sometimes sell out faster than the rest of the venue. Recently built movie theaters have widely adopted "arena" style seating, in which there is literally only one row that is accessible in the middle of the theatre.

Typically, spaces are left open between or next to regular seats for a wheelchair user to park, but some riders prefer to get out of the chair to sit in an upholstered seat at a movie or concert. When that is the case, the question arises of where to park the wheelchair. If you want to sit closer to the screen at a movie, odds are you will have to allow your wheelchair to be parked elsewhere by a companion or a theater employee, particularly if it has a rigid frame. An unfolded wheelchair will be too much of an obstruction in the aisle, and even a folded chair is likely to violate fire codes, which require exit ways to be kept open. These restrictions might affect your choice of where to sit if you are uncomfortable being away from your chair or reliant on others to bring it to you in case of an emergency.

Many sports arenas have begun to install a system of seats that can be folded up and out of the way to allow a wheelchair to park in the remaining space. That method of construction gives you the option of staying in your chair or not and lets chair users have more options for where to sit throughout the arena. The arena can also sell more seats to able-bodied customers as the event begins to sell out, rather than having to leave spaces empty that could only have been used by a wheelchair rider.

A key problem arises around how many people you might want to have along at an event. If you want to make plans with a group of a dozen friends, you might have a lot of trouble getting that many seats together. Chair users want the freedom to make plans with a group like anyone else. On the other hand, the facility needs to preserve the accessible seating for those who need it, limiting its use by people who can walk. When you call for tickets to an event, be prepared to hear that you are only allowed one "attendant" to be with you in the disabled seating section. In some cases, this is a policy of the ticket-selling agency. If you call the arena or team offices, you might find someone willing to sell you the tickets you need.

The wheelchair seats are sometimes the best in the house. A platform might be set up at a large arena concert with the most unobstructed view in the place. It is also not unusual for a performance space to allow wheelchair users in first to avoid the crowd, which can mean you get the pick of the seats. As you attend events at local venues, you will learn their policies, how to get the best seats, when to arrive, and how to get around.

Public Transportation

Having control of where you go makes a big difference in how much you can accomplish. All of the therapy and adaptive devices in the world don't mean much if you can't get to a job, run a simple errand, or meet your spouse for coffee. Freedom to move and go where you want is also central to your sense of self.

Public transportation has come a long way. In major cities, buses are now widely equipped with lifts. There are seats on the bus that lift out of the way, revealing a clamp that holds onto a wheel. There is also a seat belt. The drivers are trained in the operation of the lift and how to assist wheelchair-using passengers. The quality of service varies:

> *I have had three experiences of getting on a bus and then having the lift fail to work to get me off. The bus had to be emptied. The driver was getting no response to his calls to the maintenance department, and I missed my appointments. I'm not inclined to trust the bus system, but realize that this is just one aspect of a huge set of problems with the bus system.*

When you use city buses regularly, you will encounter a variety of conditions and drivers:

> *I had a lot of trouble at first negotiating with bus drivers, but over time I've learned to assert myself. I was a real "people pleaser" before my accident and so I had to develop interpersonal tools to get what I need. Seventy percent of the drivers are wonderful, 28% get the job done adequately, but the other 2% still give me grief and I have to use a stick rather than a carrot.*

Cities such as New York, Washington, Portland, and San Francisco have rail systems and subways that provide varying degrees of accessibility. Northern California's BART (Bay Area Rapid Transit) system has accessible cars and stations but has had problems with the maintenance of the elevators from the street level. In 1998, a judge ordered BART to increase its efforts and spending to ensure that elevators are kept clean and operating and that the system in general remains accessible.

Most cities offer a paratransit service, with which you can make an appointment to be picked up and taken directly to your destination. Once you qualify through an application, the service is made available at modest cost. Unfortunately, the quality and reliability of paratransit services vary widely, with many people finding that they cannot rely on the service to be on time or even to show up in some cases. For transportation to a job, paratransit is not usually a good solution. If you want to get to a store or the park for a little sun, you can afford to be a little late or go the next day if the driver doesn't show up. Do some research. You might be lucky enough to be in a city with a well-run system.

There is little, if any, public transportation to choose from for many people outside of urban areas. Some will be able to rely on neighbors or family to get a ride and have this suffice for their transportation needs. However, greater access to public transit options might be enough to convince rural wheelchair users to move to a larger metropolitan area.

Inadequate transportation is more likely to be a problem for those with disabilities, finds the 2000 NOD/Harris Survey of Americans with Disabilities:

> *Inadequate transportation is considered a problem by*
> *three out of ten (30%) adults with disabilities. 16% report it*
> *as a "major problem," 13% a "minor problem," but only one*
> *out of ten (10%) adults without disabilities report a problem*
> *with inadequate transportation, a gap of 20 percentage*
> *points.*

Your Own Vehicle

For many wheelchair users, the ideal transportation is their own vehicle— car, van, or truck. Driver's training and lessons in how to load a wheelchair are often included in rehabilitation programs or offered on an outpatient basis.

You will develop your own method for loading a wheelchair in a car. Folding chair users who drive a two-door car generally put the chair in the back seat by sliding over to the passenger side, pulling the driver seat forward, and then pulling the folded chair in by rolling it in over the rocker panel. People using a rigid frame chair remove the wheels and lift the frame—with the back folded down against the seat—over their torso onto the passenger seat or back into the rear seat. Those driving a four-door vehicle generally enter from the passenger side, pulling the chair in after them and securing it with the seat belt. Folding and lifting a chair in and out of a car every day can be fatiguing in the long term, causing wear and tear on the arms and shoulders. Ultralight wheelchair frames might allow you to drive a sedan rather than a van.

Quadriplegics with enough balance but not the strength to throw their chairs around, or people who need to be able to drive from their wheelchair, have many option for adapted vehicles. A number of companies specialize in minivan conversion. They lower the floor so a ramp can be used instead of a mechanical lift (Figure 8-1), install a kneeling system to bring the van lower to the ground to reduce the ramp angle, and put in tie-down systems to keep the wheelchair secure during driving, whether or not you stay in the chair. The door, ramp or lift, and door locks are controlled by switches in the vehicle as well as by a remote control that you keep on your keychain.

Figure 8-1 The floor is lowered so a ramp can be used instead of a mechanical lift. A kneeling system is installed to bring the van lower to the ground to reduce the ramp angle and a tie-down systems is put in to keep the wheelchair secure during driving.

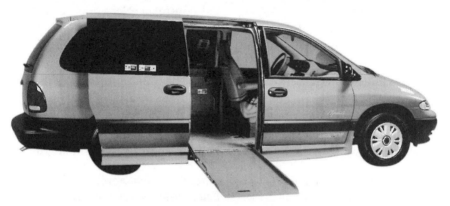

Hand Controls

Hand controls on vehicles can be electronic or manual. Electronic controls manipulate the brake cylinder or engine components, such as the fuel injectors, and are initiated by a joystick or other controller in the cabin (Figure 8-2). Manual controls are mechanical devices attached directly to the pedals, usually supported by the steering column.

Electronic controls are generally used by people with minimal upper arm capacity. Installation is complex, more training is required to operate them, and they are much more costly. Programming features set the sensitivity of a joystick or button and allow people with limited arm strength to control the transmission, accelerator, and brake.

Manual hand controls brake by pushing forward on whatever control lever is used. There are no gears or linkages for the brake—the control uses

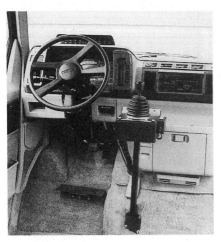

Figure 8-2 A joystick or other controller can be used in the cabin.

a strong rod attached directly to the brake pedal so that there can be no possibility of failure.

How manual controls press the accelerator varies. Some designs attach a rod directly to the pedal—particularly those designed for quick installation. Most designs use a system of gears or levers to decrease the amount of pressure your arm must exert to press the accelerator. Driving with a hand control is a lot of work for one side of the body, especially if you do a lot of stop-and-go driving.

There are three styles of manual-control accelerators. One is like a motorcycle control, which you rotate; the second is pulled toward the body; the third is pressed downward toward the floor to press the gas pedal. The first two styles are more likely to cause repetitive strain injuries because you have to maintain muscle effort to use them. The third type involves the least strain, since the weight of your arm and hand can be used to maintain speed with much less muscle exertion, although it requires sufficient clearance between the control and your lap for its downward movement. For any accelerator style, cruise control is recommended to reduce arm fatigue:

> *My first set of hand controls operated like a motorcycle. You would rotate the handle, which had a little extension where you could rest your palm to get more leverage. It was fine for many years, until I moved to San Francisco. I found I had to press harder to get up hills because my car's acceleration wasn't so great. I started to get tendinitis in my left elbow, so I switched to the type you press down on.*

There are no commercial hand control products for driving a vehicle with a manual transmission, although a few hardy souls have made their own creative adaptations to operate a clutch and gear shift while still keeping a hand on the steering wheel.

Parking

All states issue parking permits that allow you to park in designated spaces. They are typically extra wide to accommodate opening your door fully or to extend a lift or ramp. Parking spaces along a curb on a city street do not provide extra space, and you might not be able to use some of these spaces because your lift or ramp would have to open into traffic.

The permit is issued to the person with the disability, not to the vehicle. Anyone driving your vehicle or assisting you needs to understand that the privilege does not extend to them personally. You will get a hanging placard, which is typically designed to be placed on your rearview mirror when you park. You have the option of getting special license plates that designate you as a disabled driver. Even if you have the special plates, you will still need the hanging placard for the times when you are riding in another car or are traveling.

Permits generally allow you to park at any metered space without paying. You must still obey time restrictions, such as for rush hour or street cleaning, when you could receive a ticket or possibly be towed from the street for parking illegally. Don't count on any favors because you have a disability permit. Be sure you understand what privileges your state is providing you.

Disabled parking has essentially expanded into elderly parking, as well as parking for people with heart conditions, bad knees, or temporary injuries. Doctors only have to sign the application for someone to get a permit. Each state defines what conditions qualify, but these boundaries are rarely enforced. Certainly there are many people who are not chair riders who cannot easily or safely walk distances and are fully and fairly entitled to disabled parking privileges. At the same time, there are far more permits issued in many cities than there are reserved parking spots. The competition for spaces has become fierce, and, too often, a chair user who needs the wider space has no parking to choose from because spaces are increasingly being used by people who can walk. Walking permit holders should use a non-reserved parking spot—assuming it is an acceptable distance from their destination—and preserve the wider spaces for chair riders and vans rather than automatically using the blue spots simply because they have a permit. They still get to park for no charge with no time limits at meters.

Gasoline

You have the right to be assisted at service stations. It varies state by state, but, in general, you should get serviced at the self-serve pump—for the lower price—when there are two or more employees on the premises. If there is one person alone in a booth at a completely self-serve station, she is not obligated to come out to put gas in your vehicle. The trick is how to get attention. Here is another reason why those with special plates still need the blue placard—so you can wave it at someone to ask for help at the pump. Usually, you will find station owners and employees willing to help. They might even clean your windows and check your oil. If you are able to enter and exit your car without too much difficulty, you might find it easier to just get out and serve yourself.

Travel

Want to go someplace in the world? Depending on how much you want to deal with, you can go just about anywhere. Like any traveler, you'll need to get there, find a place to stay, and get around to see the sights.

Airlines

Flying as a chair rider is a bit of an art. The more experienced you are, the more you learn how the system works and the easier it is to avoid pitfalls. First, know that you have a right to travel by air. In 1986, the United States Congress passed the Air Carrier Access Act. Here are some of its provisions:

■ New aircraft ordered after April 5, 1990, must be accessible.

■ Planes with 30 or more seats must have movable armrests on half of the aisle seats.

■ Planes with 100 or more seats must be able to accommodate at least one folding wheelchair on board.

■ Airline personnel may not deny transportation to a passenger with a disability or limit the number of disabled passengers unless it is a matter of safety.

■ You can be required to give two-days' notice and check in an hour ahead of departure if you
  • Are traveling with a power wheelchair on a plane with fewer than 60 seats
  • Require special hookups for equipment such as oxygen or a ventilator
  • Are traveling in a group of 10 or more chair users

■ Except in rare circumstances, airlines cannot require you to travel with an attendant. If they insist, they can choose an attendant but cannot charge for his fare.

■ Your chair must be checked and returned as close to the door of the plane as possible.

Don't ever let airlines check your wheelchair through baggage claim. Having a wheelchair checked this way is more likely to result in the wheelchair disappearing, for greater or lesser periods of time. Some travelers have reported damage to their wheelchair from improper handling. You will also be forced into dependency on airport staff to take you to baggage claim, which you might otherwise be able to reach yourself in your own wheels. You should be able to make the choice.

Airports have many wheelchairs, but they are generally insufficient for a regular chair rider. Some have small wheels that you cannot push yourself. None have heel loops to help your feet stay in place. Airport chairs are generally in poor repair. Their design assumes you will be assisted. Even if airline personnel suggest surrendering your chair well before the flight, you are not required to do so. Such personnel are acting for their convenience, not yours.

Instead, your chair should be a "gate checked." A tag is put on your chair. You get onto the plane from your own chair, and it is brought back to the door of the plane when you get off—even between connecting flights. Make certain that someone on the crew knows your chair is gate checked and ask her to confirm it to the ground crew at your destination:

> Once I let someone convince me to let them have my wheel-
> chair before I boarded the plane. They put me in an airport
> chair that had small wheels so I couldn't push the chair
> myself. Sure enough, the flight was delayed, and I was stuck
> unable to get around. I even had to ask someone to help me to
> the bathroom, since the long wait was enough for nature to
> come calling. Now I absolutely will never give up my chair
> until I'm actually getting on the plane.

You will need to pass through security, like everybody else, but you can't go through the detector because your wheelchair will set off the alarm. You will have to be searched individually. When you approach the security area, be prepared to place any bags—such as a backpack—on the belt to go through the X-ray machine. Usually security personnel will have seen you and will direct you to where they can check you out. You will be searched by hand, which should always be done by a person of the same sex as yourself. They will offer you the option of a private screening and are trained to explain the process to you, including reassuring you that they will not be touching you inappropriately.

Since the attack on the World Trade Center and the Pentagon on September 11, 2001, security has obviously been much more intense at airports, and one could imagine a wheelchair user being more suspect. Yet, the Transportation Safety Administration has made a commitment to reducing the inconvenience as best they can. Using the technology of a small pad to "swipe" for explosive chemical traces, they are able to ensure themselves that the wheelchair is not itself a weapon or containing any dangerous materials.

The better you can accept the necessity of the process, the more efficient—and less frustrating—it will be.

Most airplane aisles are too narrow for a wheelchair to fit through. Sometimes the first-class section is wide enough to allow passage of a narrow wheelchair. In some cases, such as entry through the second door of a DC-10, you can get to certain seats directly from your chair. If you're a regular traveler, it's helpful to get to know some of the specific aircraft, so you can let the reservation agent know what seats would be best for you. Seats in an emergency exit row will not be available to you because of Federal Aviation Administration regulations that such seats can only be occupied by people able and willing to assist in emergencies. That requirement disqualifies people with mobility disabilities. Unfortunately, it also reduces your selection of seats with more leg room—very useful to someone unable to stand during a long flight.

Most times you will enter the plane by means of an aisle chair. This is a narrow seat that fits down the aisle, in which you must be assisted by airport staff. You will have to decide whether it is a safe surface for you to sit on, even for the brief minutes you will spend in it, taking into account that there might be a couple of bumps as the staff get you over the first hump into the door. You might want to travel with another cushion for use on the aisle chair, the airplane seat, or taxicab, for instance.

There are some very tight turns to be made getting into the plane, and the space of the aisle is sometimes just barely wide enough to fit through. You must keep your arms in and watch closely that your clothes don't get caught on a seat arm as you travel down the aisle. The person assisting you might not be patient or attentive enough to prevent collisions with armrests as you travel down the aisle.

The staff that assists people with disabilities are not highly paid or particularly well trained. They are typically employees of the airport or an outside contractor, not the airline itself. You will need to direct them, and, sadly, you should be prepared for the possibility that they will treat you like cargo. Some will be personable and cooperate with you; others will grab at you or start to carry you in without the courtesy of a warning. They will especially need guidance in where you want the aisle chair placed relative to your wheelchair for your transfer and how they should best assist you—or not—during the transfer:

> As a strong paraplegic, I find I am mostly occupied getting
> people out of my way and letting me position things so I can
> do the transfer myself. Invariably, someone will try to push
> me in the chair or will begin to reach under my armpits to lift
> me without asking first.

You might or might not need assistance; the issue is how to maintain control, since others will often not ask what you need. Be prepared to direct the process so it goes smoothly. Try to get to the gate early so you can pre-board ahead of other passengers. Arriving late would mean being carried conspicuously onto the plane through a crowd of occupied seats. You should also arrive early so that the ground crew will not be rushed stowing your chair in time for their scheduled take off. This is especially true if you use a power chair, which might require some disassembly.

Some airlines are better than others about reserving specific seats for people with disabilities. Seats at the bulkhead—structural walls at various points along the fuselage—typically afford more leg room, and there is no passenger in front to recline his seat back and limit your space. Online reservation web sites will often allow you to select seats. You will want to be close to the front to limit your trip down the aisle in the narrow aisle chair. Bulkhead aisle seats are generally your best option. There is also more space for people in the window or middle seat to come and go without stepping on you. See if you can get the reservation agent to guarantee a bulkhead seat for you when you arrange your flight. If the agent cannot do that, you might need to call back a week before your departure for a seat assignment or go to the airport to meet with a ticket agent. The quest for a comfortable seat can be a challenge and, sometimes, comes down to the embarrassment of seeing a gate agent ask someone to surrender his seat on your behalf because airline policy prevented you from getting a commitment from the beginning.

On occasion, you might find yourself upgraded to the first-class section. If there is an open seat, and you can get to it without the need to transfer to an aisle chair, the gate agent has the authority to switch your seat to the front cabin. It makes the airline's life easier—and you get the better food and cloth napkins, too! First-class upgrades are much harder to come by these days, since there are many frequent flyers who have earned upgrades through mileage programs as a bonus.

You will find that you must deal carefully with your bladder needs when you fly. You will not have a wheelchair to use on the plane, and the restrooms are small and inaccessible. Some people prefer to schedule stopovers on long trips so that they can drink more freely on the plane and then have the chance to get off to use a restroom and move around a little. Certainly you should go to the restroom at the last moment before boarding the plane to empty your bladder—though allow for the high likelihood that you'll have to wait for the wide stall while staring at the empty stalls you can't use because they are too narrow.

That means getting there even earlier to check in and making sure that the airline gets an aisle chair for you, with time for your bladder before you preboard. A leg bag is mandatory equipment for most wheelchair-using travelers, especially on long flights. This paraplegic woman typically uses intermittent catheterization:

> It's bad for me to wear an indwelling Foley catheter because it increases my chances of getting an infection. But, if I'm flying a long distance, I wear a Foley and surreptitiously empty it into a tinted bottle.

> Otherwise I always catheterize just before I get on the plane and wear a diaper. Once I got stuck on a plane. It was supposed to be a one-hour flight from Michigan to New York, and they kept saying it would be another half hour, another half hour, so I never got off to go to the bathroom. Then they pulled away from the gate, and I wasn't about to have them go back just to let me go to the bathroom. By the time we landed, I really had to go. I could have flown to Europe in the time I was on the plane.

It's an embarrassing situation, but, if a flight is delayed, you might need to inform a flight attendant that there is a limit to how long you can wait, so you don't find yourself trapped in a similar situation.

Rental Cars

All major car rental agencies provide cars with hand controls. They charge nothing extra, nor do they impose any additional insurance requirements for their use. Since the controls are extra equipment that generally must be installed specifically for your use—agencies don't keep cars on hand with controls always installed—you need to give them sufficient notice. It used to be that agencies needed two weeks advance notice, but now major cities have controls available to accommodate you in a matter of days. In an emergency, you might even get next-day service.

Larger agencies have special offices that handle drivers with disabilities. When you call the general reservation number, explain that you are requesting an adapted vehicle, and ask if they need to transfer you to another extension.

The type of car you rent depends on how you put your wheels into a car. Usually agencies provide a "full-size" model, such as a Toyota Camry or Chevrolet Monte Carlo. They generally assume you will use a four-door vehicle, which works for some people who store their wheels in the front seat, entering through the passenger side, or if you have a companion to stow your chair in the trunk or back seat. Some drivers require a two-door car, stowing the chair in the back seat by reclining the driver's seat all the way back and lifting it over their body and setting the frame in the back seat.

When you reserve the car, reservation operators will ask which side you want the controls on. They will let you provide more detail about the control position, but these are installed at the city where you will pick up the car. If you have exacting needs, it is best to call that local agency and ask to speak to the installer. The central reservation agent can give you the phone number. You may also request a spinner knob, which allows you to easily turn the steering wheel with one hand while maintaining a full grip at all times. Different rental agencies use different types of controls. This might influence with whom you choose to do business:

> The first thing I do when they bring the car is check the position of the controls. Sometimes they are too low, and my leg blocks them from being able to travel enough to get good acceleration, or they are too far back, so I have to extend my arm too far when I brake. It's dangerous to drive when the controls aren't right, so I'd rather take the extra time to make the mechanic adjust them, frustrating as it is to be delayed. Fortunately, it doesn't happen very often.

Typically, a car rental customer at an airport rides a shuttle bus provided by the agency to and from the terminal to the rental car lot. The buses are typically equipped with lifts, and the driver will help you with your luggage if you need it. When you return the rental car, however, go to the normal drop-off lot and ask for someone to ride back with you to the terminal in the car. They will usually consider that easier than transferring your bags from the car to the bus. It's common for someone to be at the lot to check you in as you return the car, so it is not necessary to get out to ask a desk clerk for help.

Rental agencies do not provide permits for disabled parking. You will need to bring one with you. Out-of-state permits are generally accepted throughout the United States and Canada—though you cannot count on this 100% of the time. If you have plates on your vehicle at home, you are entitled to get a placard permit from your Department of Motor Vehicles. Even if you do not drive yourself, you are entitled to a permit to be used by anyone else driving you, including during travel.

Several companies supply adapted vans in many locations across the country, including lift- or ramp-equipped models. Renting a van costs a bit more, but, when you are traveling with a group, it becomes affordable. Vans also accommodate some power-chair users in ways that vehicles from the well-known commercial rental agencies cannot. In any case, contact the local station a day or two before to make sure that they have your details correct. Garage staff have been known to not read the reservation record closely.

Trains

Trains are often less costly than airlines and can sometimes get you to smaller towns and destinations into which you can't easily fly. Despite the ADA, the rail system is not truly accessible to wheelchair riders. It is one thing to get into the car and have your wheelchair secured; it may be quite another if you need a restroom or require electricity to charge your portable ventilator.

The ADA required Amtrak to provide one accessible car per train by July 1995. Accessible in this case means a wide door that can be entered from a level platform and the ability to stay in a wheelchair, secured from movement during the trip. Unfortunately, you cannot count on being able to get assistance with your bags at the station or other needs you might have. Amtrak advertises that they provide assistance in major city stations and give priority to people with disabilities who wish to reserve private rooms with seating for daytime and sleeping provisions for the night.

In May of 1998, Amtrak settled a case brought by the Disability Rights and Education Defense Fund. They agreed to change their reservations policy so that, up until 14 days before departure, accessible bedrooms will be reserved for passengers with mobility impairments. They will also provide written menus and deliver food and snacks that are offered in inaccessible train cars and will take measures to ensure that films can be viewed by all riders.

As with most travel arrangements, you deal with a centralized reservations operator. Always call the local station, in addition, to confirm that an accessible car is on the train for which you are scheduled and that services are available to meet your needs. Since there are a limited number of trains with accessible facilities, you should schedule your travel as early as possible to get what you need.

Intercity Buses

Access to buses is important for long-distance as well as local travel, especially for the many chair riders who live on small, fixed incomes such as Social Security disability payments. The Greyhound Corporation essentially has a monopoly on what is known as "fixed route" transportation by ground in the United States. Greyhound won a waiver allowing them more time to comply with the ADA and, in the meantime, has purchased new buses without lifts. Very few Greyhound buses have lifts, and you will find the same is true of tour buses in major cities.

There are many stories of people injured by drivers or other staff not trained to assist people onto the bus and of wheelchairs damaged by mishandling. The bus will not have an accessible restroom. Even the places they stop might not have a usable bathroom—even if drivers are willing to help you off the bus. The continuing inaccessibility of buses has a severe impact on availability of affordable transportation.

Hotels

Wheelchair accessible rooms are universally available, from bargain-priced motels to the finer hotels. You can generally count on that meaning a bathroom with a wide door, room to turn around, grab bars, a hand-held shower head, and lever controls. Most rooms will have a roll-in shower, so, if you have a preference for a bathtub, you'll need to specifically request one. Some hotels do not have any accessible rooms with a tub. Know exactly what you need, and, if the hotel can't clearly commit to providing those needs, don't choose to stay there.

Beware of consolidators. These are businesses that offer rooms at reduced rates. Hotels sell reservations to a certain number of rooms to consolidators as a way of increasing occupancy rates. Consolidators might tell you the hotel has accessible rooms, but that doesn't mean that the hotel will know you are coming or that such a room will be set aside for you:

> *I had an experience in New York City with a consolidator. The accessible rooms were all taken when I arrived. I had to make do with one of the hotel's normal rooms, which was only usable by the hotel's removing the bathroom door.*

It is generally best to make your reservation by calling the hotel directly to ensure that they know what you need and will guarantee or "block" the room. As hotels fill up, they start to give the accessible rooms to able-bodied guests. Call again a couple of times before you arrive, especially the day before. Ensure that the room will be available when you arrive.

Hotel rooms are often full of chairs you don't need or furniture arranged in a way that limits your movement. Beds are often placed close together or too near a wall, sometimes blocking your ability to reach curtain controls or the thermostat. That is especially a problem when the bedspread hangs off the side and can get caught in your wheels. Don't hesitate to ask hotel staff to move things around or take furniture out of the room for you.

Typical rooms have more than one phone, although the phone by the bed is sometimes on the side without enough space for wheelchair clearance to get to it. Of course, you need a phone by the bed more than anywhere else because you are less mobile once out of your chair. One traveler uses this solution:

> *I take a portable telephone with me when I travel. I plug the hotel's phone cord into my set, and then I have a phone anywhere in the room.*

A portable phone is particularly useful in the bathroom. Finer hotels often have a phone installed near the toilet—which still doesn't help much if the phone rings while you're in the bath or shower.

The organization Hostelling International-American Youth Hostels (HI-AYH) supplies beds for traveling students in the United States and abroad. They provide a bed, pillow, and blanket in a dormitory setting with a shared bathroom for a very low price, as little as $15 a night. There are now 380 hostels in 34 countries that provide wheelchair access, 38 of those in the US. Some provide family quarters or private rooms. The range of accessible features varies, since HI-AYH does not establish uniform standards. As with any hotel, call ahead and determine whether you can adapt to the facilities.

Camping

Campgrounds around the country increasingly provide accommodations for wheelchair users. They create level campsites with a firm earth surface that is easy to roll on. There is usually a paved surface for parking near the campsite. Sites are located near bathroom facilities that often include stall showers with fold-down seats. Sometimes the accessible restroom/ shower unit is restricted to qualified users who get a key from the park ranger.

Some parks reserve accessible sites until later in the day before giving them out to able-bodied campers. The most desirable parks take reservations in advance, and you are well advised to plan your itinerary and make your arrangements before arriving. There may be some accessible trails, but many of them are short "nature trails." The most scenic hikes are on rough terrain with more slope. Strong manual chair users or those with power will have more options. Recreational vehicles (RVs), which you can take onto certain campgrounds, are available for rent with lifts and accessible bath facilities. Some parks are primarily outfitted for RVs, with electricity and water hookups at individual camp sites. Pristine locations are less likely to allow RVs because of a desire to limit pollution and noise.

Traveling with a Ventilator

If you rely on assisted breathing, travel need not be off limits to you, though it might involve a bit more planning and coordination, like this woman who uses a ventilator found:

> *My husband and I are driving to Florida. This is something that we are greatly looking forward to. I have been ill for two and a half years. We need this time together away from doctors, hospitals, and therapists. Every hotel that we have reservations at is an accessible one. We worked closely with AAA and have everything all worked out. We have it in writing that we will be assisted with loading and unloading the car. My portable ventilator runs off the cigarette lighter in the car and has a backup 12-hour battery. My suction machine runs on AC or DC power. My oxygen supply company has made arrangements for liquid tank fill-ups at each motel stop.*

Similarly, you can make arrangements with airlines and train carriers in some cases to provide electricity for a ventilator. Naturally, you should be prepared with backup approaches should there be an emergency.

Assistive Technology

While political advocacy is removing barriers, designers and engineers are expanding your potential. Technology is enhancing the lives of people with disabilities by:

- Increasing employment opportunity
- Providing tools for pursuits such as writing, software design, or graphic arts
- Increasing independence for people with limited upper body strength through dramatic evolution of power wheelchairs and remote-control technology
- Promoting participation in online communities of people with shared interests—disability-related or not
- Accelerating participation in the political process

There are considerable resources available. Rehab centers and independent living centers increasingly offer training programs and support groups on computing. Exposition events are widely held, from small local fairs to large conferences put on by groups such as United Spinal or RESNA, Abilities Expo, and the World Congress and Expo on Disabilities.

Even if you can't easily use your fingers or hands or can't see or hear, you can still use the technology. There is enough demand for alternative methods of using computers to encourage designers and companies to develop new accessible methods of interaction with the computer. These input alternatives include software that reduces keystrokes, adaptive keyboards, voice dictation, voice synthesis, eye movement and head controllers, switches, and puff-and-sip controls.

Assistive technology reduces frustration. You might be able to press keys to type, but the process might be so slow, or you might make so many mistakes in the process, that you will want to give up. Your creativity and thought process are interrupted if you cannot easily interact with the computer. Many features of assistive technology are now commonly found in both Microsoft and Macintosh operating systems.

Software Solutions for Text Entry

If you have limited use of your hands, two software approaches help reduce the number of actual keystrokes required for text entry: word abbreviation and word prediction.

Abbreviation software allows you to enter a small number of letters that are enough for the computer to know what the whole word should be—a sort of shorthand. Pressing the space bar typically initiates expansion of the word. Some programs have a defined a set of abbreviations and allow a number of customizable words. Other programs allow the user to define the shortcuts:

> I really love my abbreviation software. It probably saves me a quarter to a third of the keystrokes I would have to make otherwise. At first it was a little awkward, but now using the abbreviations is totally natural. If I have to type at a computer that doesn't have it, I feel like I'm pressing way too many keys for the amount of text I'm entering.

Word-prediction software puts up a numbered list of words on the screen as soon as a letter is pressed, suggesting what the program "thinks" the desired word might be. You select a word by typing its number. If the word you want has not appeared, you type more letters until it does appear. The software learns by remembering the words that you use the most, making them more likely to appear sooner on the list. With experience, you will usually only need to type a few characters per word.

Macro software lets you define keystrokes (usually in combination with the Control, Alt, or Option modifier keys) to enter blocks of standard text—for example, the closing for a letter. Many programs also allow you to automate command functions and sequences. You might enter a single keystroke to open your email program, tell it to check for mail, and enter a password. Macro software has been available for some time and is incorporated into the Microsoft Windows operating system. The Macintosh operating system also includes many powerful shortcut tools.

Some users are unable to hold down two keys simultaneously. Functions that use the Control key, for instance, become inaccessible. "Sticky Keys" allows you to press one key then the other, and the computer will react to them as if they had been pressed together. This is another standard feature of both Windows and Macintosh system software.

Hardware Solutions

The standard computer keyboard is a set of small keys that you press with your fingertips. The standard keyboard requires dexterity and accuracy beyond the capacity of many people, whether paralyzed by injury or stroke, restricted by arthritis, missing fingers or limbs, and so on. There are keyboards available with large pads sensitive to touch; it is not necessary to press down on a key. Another design allows you to rest your hands directly on the keyboard and apply a slight additional pressure to select a key. There are also keyboards designed for one-handed use.

Most adaptive keyboards work in combination with abbreviation or word-prediction software or allow you to use macros to define keystroke shortcuts. Designers try to make use of all available features to ease the physical demands of computing.

Other Input Devices

Once it is possible to position a pointer on the screen and initiate a "click" that transfers your intent to the machine, you can do quite a lot. An onscreen keyboard allows you to click on letters and commands by simply allowing the cursor to rest on a button for a user-determined pause. A physical keyboard is no longer necessary.

The cursor can be manipulated using a standard mouse, trackball, or pen and pad. For those with no hand use, a "head cursor" can be used, of which there are two types. One senses an object, such as a small, sticky dot placed on your forehead or eyeglasses. Another calibrates to your pupil, whereby you move the cursor with your eyeball, rather than the movement of your head.

Augmentative Speech

People whose speech is impaired now have access to augmentative communication devices that function as the person's voice. These increasingly powerful and portable devices allow the user to piece together sentences with a variety of buttons on the fly or to preprogram sentences or whole speeches. Many people have great difficulty speaking but have enough dexterity with their hands to operate the device. People can have conversations or make public presentations using this technology. Originally the size of a small desktop computer, augmentative speech products now come in sizes as small as your hand.

The Trace Center at the University of Wisconsin at Madison was established in 1971 to address communication needs of people who cannot speak. In the early 1980s, they began to receive funds from the federal government for research in adaptive technology. The Trace Center has worked with computer companies to promote and integrate disability access features. They coordinate conferences and provide publications, such as a 900-page resource book. They continue to pursue research on a variety of computer platforms, including Macintosh and UNIX. Many staff members have advanced science and engineering degrees and play a significant role in the development and promotion of adaptive technology.

Environmental Control

People with quadriplegia lose a substantial degree of independence and, naturally, want to regain as much independence as possible. They necessarily employ personal assistance for dressing and other personal matters, but they also need help operating a light switch, opening a door, answering the telephone, or turning the television on or off.

Computers to the rescue. Systems are available that allow almost complete control of the electrical systems in your house, even for people with no use of their arms. Such systems can be controlled by puff-and-sip control, voice command, or switches—of which there are many types that require minimal dexterity and accuracy.

An example of how such systems work is that a menu, shown on a small display, shows programmed options, such as telephone, lights, bed, and television. You rotate through the choices and choose one, for example, lights. Another set of choices appears, for example, main bedroom fixture, bedside lamp, and hallway light. Once again you scroll through the choices and choose. For a telephone, commonly called numbers can be programmed into a speaker phone that requires no hand use. The menu will also include the operator. Some local phone systems provide special services to disabled customers, such as free operator assistance to dial numbers. Chapter 7, Home Access, further discusses environmental control systems.

Ergonomics—Safety and Computers

People can get hurt using computers. Injuries are typically referred to as cumulative trauma or repetitive strain injuries. Computer users with disabilities need to pay special heed, since the primary locations of computer-related injuries are in the upper extremities—hands, wrists, elbows, and shoulders. For people with a disability, the additional impairments of injured arms or hands are the last thing that they need.

Although having computer skills and using them in the workplace improves your ability to work full time and earn the same pay as nondisabled workers, be vigilant about protecting yourself from overusing your arms, wrists, hands, or shoulders. Learn something about ergonomics—the science of how to relate your body to your work—and develop a work style that does not exceed your body's ability to remain healthy:

> For six years, I have been living with chronic pain in my wrists and elbows from excessive computing and poor working posture. Despite periods of relative comfort and freedom, I remain prone to flare-ups that require me to limit my activities or else risk more severe pain and lasting effects. It has already cost me the ability to perform as a musician. I write by voice dictation.

> I have often told people that my chronic pain problems have been more disabling than my paralysis. I could adapt very well with a wheelchair, hand controls in my car, and refinements at home. Losing the freedom—or ability—to use my arms pushes things to a very different level and demands more intensive adaptations.

There is much available information about ergonomics now—in books, on the Internet, from consultants, and from people assigned to the job in larger companies. There is no reason for someone today to develop the chronic pain that has already struck many thousands of computer users and has forced some to give up or change careers.

Ergonomics means being comfortable and using the body efficiently. Ergonomic skills at the computer or workplace are similar to the ergonomic skills you learn for using a wheelchair—conserve energy, move smoothly, and take care not to overexert and overstrain your tissues. Be aware of what you feel, and don't accept discomfort. Fatigue and discomfort are messages from your body telling you to slow down or make a change in how you use your body. When you are in pain, there is always a cause. Ergonomics as a discipline is about identifying that cause and making changes to the physical setting or work habits to prevent pain.

Muscles—even small ones—are not made to be held in continuous contraction. The flow of blood is substantially reduced when a muscle is in a fixed, "static" exertion—even at a low degree of effort. Particularly for people with limited muscle capacity, being able to make the most of what you have is an even higher priority. When you lean in toward a computer screen, work with arms extended to reach a mouse or keyboard, continuously hold a mouse button, or keep your head in a fixed position for a long period of time, you are making those muscles contract without rest. A computer screen that is too high or low will make your neck and shoulder muscles work constantly. Low-level, continuously held exertions eventually become a source of pain as you exceed the limits of muscle tissues and they begin to send out messages to cease and desist!

Sit as upright as possible without effort, letting your skeleton carry you so your muscles don't have to. Good posture becomes more complicated when fewer muscles are working in your body or if you have a spinal curvature or other asymmetry of the body. The higher a spinal cord injury (SCI), for instance, the less of the trunk muscles are working and the greater the tendency to have to sit in rounded postures for stability. A person with such an injury using a computer needs to take care not to encourage increasingly rounded postures.

Wheelchair users sitting at desks have extra challenges. Able-bodied workers sit in chairs that rotate on a stem, so that they can turn to other areas of the desk or workstation without twisting their bodies. Wheelchairs don't rotate sideways, so you must twist your body to reach to the side. To compensate, keep objects you use most—keyboard, mouse, telephone, paperwork, stapler, and so on—close to you, within easy reach, and more in front of you than to the side. If you turn from the computer to work on some papers or make a phone call, first take the time to turn your wheelchair so that you can still sit straight.

Take advantage of shortcuts and efficiency tools built into your system and applications to help address the problem of cumulative trauma injuries. Why press any more keys or click any more buttons than you have to? Make an art of finding how few clicks it takes to do your work. You will be protecting yourself in the process.

Ergonomics is really about common sense: listening to your body and taking care of yourself. If you eat a balanced diet and drink less coffee and more water, you will lower your risk of injury. If you make a point to breathe, relax, and let go of muscle tension, you lower your risk of developing a repetitive strain injury. If you mix tasks and take regular, small breaks from computing, using your body in a variety of ways throughout the day, you further lower your risk. If you make comfort a high priority, you can safely take advantage of the power and creativity possible through computing.

Education

Any school in the US that receives federal funding falls under provisions of the Rehabilitation Act of 1973 and, therefore, has been required for some time to make facilities accessible. In 1975, the Individuals with Disabilities Education Act was passed, which helps ensure that children with disabilities get access to public education according to their abilities. These children have historically been placed in "special ed" and fallen far short of their intellectual abilities—and so have been denied the chance to aspire to higher achievements. With more children moving through public schools, more students with disabilities are arriving on college campuses, where this growing demand has helped foster the availability of services for students with disabilities.

Education is a definite advantage when it comes to employment. A study by economists Douglas Kruse from Rutgers University—a wheelchair user with spinal cord injury—and Alan Krueger at Princeton University found that more than half of college graduates with SCIs were employed in the study sample of nearly 6,000 persons; only one-sixth of high school graduates were employed. Those with a college education earned 60% to 75% more than those with a high school diploma.[2]

College Campuses

Your first priority is getting an education at the school you prefer, rather than choosing the most accessible school. Identify what you want and then see what it will take to make it work. Contact the school you are considering and ask for the disabled students' services office. They will have staff available to help you with a variety of needs, from housing to financing and transportation to personal assistance services, or ensuring that appropriate furniture is in the classroom.

Some older campuses are a little harder to get around. Older buildings are not so easy to adapt. In some cases, access to a course might necessitate its relocation to another classroom. If you are a manual-chair user on a hilly campus, you might consider using a power chair to get around.

Sheldon Ginns was a staff architect at the University of Michigan in Ann Arbor. In the early 1970s, he was the first to investigate what it would take to provide access on the campus. At the time, there were very few wheelchair riders. He found:

> Many of the changes they needed to make were not very expensive. We could add grab bars, adjust door closers, relocate certain classes, install some basic ramps, or grade up to some entrances to replace steps. The first reaction of the administration was, "Why should we do this? There aren't any students who need it." Now, of course, there are hundreds of chair users here.

Educating children with disabilities

Despite passage of the Individuals with Disabilities Education Act, ensuring true access to education for children with disabilities remains a challenge. There continue to be reports of educators who resist full accommodation, frustrated by lack of training or demands on their time, particularly when communication or learning disabilities are involved.

When parents complain that the school nearest home does not offer needed programs, the school district often urges parents to send children farther away. However, the extra distance means extra travel time and prevents children from developing strong social networks with neighborhood children:

> I have four children: Sarah, Collin, Laura, and Emma Rose. Two of my children have cerebral palsy. My son Collin's CP is more significant than my daughter Laura's. Our local school system is insisting Collin go to another school forty-five minutes from home in a segregated program. My husband and I disagree and insist his needs and development are best served staying in our own neighborhood.
>
> My husband and I are aware that Collin has physical differences. We are also aware of how much he is like other five-year-old kids. Collin thinks that ice cream is the perfect food. He laughs when his sisters get in trouble. Like any other kid, Collin has his strengths and weaknesses. And, like any other parents, we know that we must "raise the bar," so to speak, to challenge him. A "separate but equal" setting has never been, and never will be, an acceptable option for the education of our son.

Children find themselves at a disadvantage in other ways in school. For example, they might miss the sex education often offered in physical education classes, which they do not attend. Accommodation is sometimes lacking in drivers' education.

What matters is that children with disabilities are educated so that they can find their full potential and compete for good jobs. At present, many well-paying jobs are in the technology sector. Tony Coehlo, former-chairman of the President's Committee on Employment of People with Disabilities (now the Office of Disability Employment Policy), once noted:

> The top three occupations for young people with disabilities
> are laborers, operatives, and craft workers. Unless changes
> are made in the education and training of youth with disabilities, we will fall further and further behind.

Success Stories

On the whole, education is opening wider all the time. From major universities to local community colleges to evolving Internet-based home study options, there are ways for you to learn, gain degrees or certifications, and pursue internships.

Even if you have to put up a bit of a fight, you can reach your goals, as James Post did to finish medical school. Medical educators doubted his ability to perform as a physician with spinal cord quadriplegia. They questioned his ability to feel a pulse or palpate organs during an exam without sensation in his fingertips. However, thanks to modern diagnostic equipment and the support of a mentor—a neurologist and polio survivor who faced similar obstacles in becoming a doctor—James Post graduated with honors from the Albert Einstein College of Medicine in 1997.[3]

Employment

> Vast numbers of people with disabilities remain unemployed.
> The 2006 data from the U.S. Census Bureau found a substantial gap in employment for those with disabilities—37%
> employed—compared to nondisabled workers—80%
> employed. These numbers are for noninstitutionalized people,
> age 21 to 64.

Some people are truly unable to handle full-time work because of physical issues such as pain, spasticity, limited energy, or communication difficulties. But, if you feel that your disability precludes being able to work, pause to fully consider whether this is true.

Assistive technologies, discussed earlier in this chapter, have made dramatic gains, and the momentum remains strong. In this modern information economy, the capacity for physical labor is not an issue for a very large portion of the jobs to be filled. With advanced education more widely accessible than ever, jobs that are based on computer skills rather than lifting capacity can be performed by a worker with a disability just as well as one without.

If you feel that your health limits you, perhaps you have more potential for a pain-free, higher-energy lifestyle than you've fully explored. Before giving up on the notion of productive and profitable work, be sure to study all possible options for diet, exercise, and medical strategies that could extend your capacity to put in a full day on the job.

The very possibility of employment for people with disabilities expanded with the passage of Section 504 of the Rehabilitation Act of 1973. The key provision almost went unnoticed. According to Joseph Shapiro in *No Pity*, it was "no more than a legislative afterthought," stating that no federal agency, public university, federal contractor, or entity that received federal funding could discriminate "solely by reason of handicap." As a result, the government and some of the nation's largest employers and places of higher education found themselves required to provide wheelchair accessibility in their buildings.

For many people, the only reasons they could not perform certain jobs was because they simply couldn't get in the front door or there was no restroom that they could use. With passage of the ADA in 1990, accessibility became a requirement in the private sector as well, unless "undue hardship" could be proven. The ADA should not force anyone out of business.

The ADA does not guarantee you a job. It simply protects you from discrimination based on your disability, allowing you to compete fairly with any other qualified workers for a job—or to stay in the one you had when you acquired your disability. You are entitled to "reasonable accommodations" to allow you to perform the "essential tasks" of the job (this being the language of human resources professionals). Ultimately, you have to do the job and accept your own responsibility for the commitments you make to an employer. There is a big difference between asking for the tools and environment you need to work and thinking that your disability allows you special status. That is a mistaken view of disability rights: these laws are not consolation prizes. The ADA is there to allow you to compete fairly. It also gives you the chance to fail if you do not commit to the same standards of performance and behavior as everyone else. That is what inclusion truly is.

Perhaps most of all, challenge your thinking if it is trying to tell you that having a disability equals not being able to work. It could be that fear and doubt are stopping you, not your disability itself. The proof is in the number of people with disabilities of all kinds and degrees who are out there doing it. Don't pass yourself over without giving yourself every possible chance.

Unfortunately, there also appears to be some discrimination on the part of employers, overt or not. Journalist John Hockenberry—a wheelchair user—produced an investigative report shown in 1997 on *Dateline NBC*. He sent two young men to various employers asking for work. One was quadriplegic; the other walked. The resume of the chair rider was intentionally slightly better than the other decoy. Witnessed by hidden cameras, several potential employers used tactics to discourage the man with the disability. In one case, he was told that there were no application forms, although forms were produced for the walking applicant. In another case, the able-bodied man was invited into a preliminary training session not offered to the chair rider.

These prospective employers are at the least guilty of prejudgment without taking the time to ask how the applicant would adapt to the tasks of the job. In most cases, resistance is not a matter of hateful prejudice, but of simple ignorance. When you apply for a job, try to know something ahead of time about the tasks involved and be prepared to explain how you will perform them. You could also point a potential employer to resources such as the Job Accommodation Network, described below.

There are some tax incentives for employers who spend money on accommodations for disabled employees. The Disabled Access Credit (IRS Section 44) allows companies with gross receipts under one million dollars or with fewer than 30 full-time employees to take a tax credit of 50% of their expenditures for access, up to $5,000 a year. The Architectural and Transportation Barrier Removal Deduction (IRS Section 190) can be as large as $15,000. You might improve your chances if you arrive at your job interview equipped with information of this sort.

One of the greatest challenges to the ability to work is the current structure of the benefits system. Social Security disability benefits, for instance, are tied to a person's income—and you are not allowed to make very much without risking the end of your checks or the loss of health and assistance coverage under Medicare. Similar income limits apply to state-administered programs like Medicaid (MediCal in California), which serve people with low incomes. Some people with the skills and desire simply cannot afford to work. Changes are being proposed to reform Social Security to increase incentives for people with disabilities to work.

Social Security Reform/Ticket to Work

Deep disincentives are built into the way the Social Security disability system works, keeping people trapped in the system because it doesn't make sense financially them to go off the program and work. The effort to resolve this issue resulted in the last piece of federal law signed by the president (Bill Clinton, in this case) in the 20th century: the Work Incentives Investment Act, also known as "Ticket to Work."

The Ticket to Work program functions through employment networks—private organizations or government agencies—to provide a variety of services to workers with disabilities. People receive vouchers for vocational rehabilitation, help with job seeking, and possibly job-accommodation assistance. The program allows

- Cash benefits to continue beyond previous limits
- Medicaid and Medicare coverage to remain (possibly with a degree of "buy-in" depending on income
- Coverage for some work-related expenses due to your disability

There is a nationwide network of One Stop Centers where people can access an array of assistance. Learn about their services and locate one nearest you at http://www.dol.gov/dol/topic/training/onestop.htm or by calling 877-US-2JOBS.

WIIA and Ticket to Work have gotten off to a slow start. Just getting the word out is a challenge; only 42% of Americans with disabilities had heard of WIIA as of the 2004 N.O.D./Harris poll, and only 26% knew of the existence of the One Stop Centers. There is some complexity and confusion in the actual implementation, and many people with disabilities are entirely unaware of the existence of the program.[1] Plus, these services do not address the lack of accessible and affordable housing or the challenges with transportation that many people with disabilities face. Social Security reform remains in its infancy.

Office of Disability Employment Policy

Formerly The President's Committee on Employment of the Physically Handicapped and formed by President John Kennedy in the early 1960s, the Office of Disability Employment Policy (ODEP; www.dol.gov/odep) in the US Department of Labor assists the business community in hiring people with disabilities. Each year a conference is held that attracts people around the country, from both government and the private sector. Seminars and lectures at the conference help corporate executives, human resources specialists, disability advocates, union representatives, and other interested parties in promoting employment of people with disabilities.

ODEP helps employers assess whether someone is capable of performing a job. Job-analysis materials help the employer determine employment issues such as:

- What functions are essential to the job
- What physical tasks—climbing, kneeling, lifting, carrying, and so on—are necessary
- How the job would be altered if certain physical requirements were removed or changed
- What movements through the office or field site are necessary
- What social conditions and interaction with colleagues are required
- What general skills are necessary for the job
- How previous experience might be substituted for lack of specific training or education
- What equipment, spatial arrangement, or job redesign measures can accommodate a person's ability to perform the job

ODEP is active on the political front. In March 1998, President Clinton established a task force the mission of which is to bring levels of employment for people with disabilities up to par with the general population.

The Job Accommodation Network

Also a service of the United States Department of Labor, the Job Accommodation Network (JAN) provides information to employees and employers to support the hiring and accommodation of workers with disabilities. An employer can call 800.526.7234 to take advantage of an immense array of resources, including:

- Information on adapting a job for a person with a disability
- Information on accommodating an employee with minimal expense
- Support for mobility, sensory, and neurologic disabilities
- Access to a large library of material about strategies and products
- Services in English, Spanish, and French

JAN promotes the message to employers that hiring people with disabilities expands the pool of qualified employees and that learning how to accommodate disability reduces workers' compensation and other insurance costs. JAN stresses that accommodations do not cost what employers generally expect—88% of accommodations suggested by the JAN cost less than $1,000.

They offer educational conferences around the country and a wide range of web-based interactive seminar programs and manage an exceptionally information-rich web site at www.jan.wvu.edu, where you can learn about any and all types of disability and read profiles of sample job accommodations for each.

Computers and Employment

Technology is creating new opportunities for working with a disability. People can work in offices or at home with an Internet connection in this modern economy that is substantially based on the flow of information rather than on physical labor. Adaptive technology will continue to provide entry points to employment for people with disabilities.

An encouraging note was reported by economists Douglas Kruse and Alan Krueger. They found that people with SCIs with sufficient computer skills were able to earn the same level of income as an able-bodied worker. The disability was completely transparent where pay was concerned—unlike the overall population of people with disabilities who earn less for the same work than the general population. The study reports:

> *Current computer use at work appears to significantly enhance the earnings power of people with SCIs and of the general population, even after controlling for the effects of education, experience, job seniority, union status, gender, and race. Those with SCIs who use a computer at work tend to work substantially more hours per week, and are more likely to hold full-time jobs than are SCI workers who do not work with computers.*[2]

There is a tremendous need for people with computer and technology skills. Jobs in programming, data analysis, or database administration are waiting for qualified candidates. The situation is severe enough that, in 1998, one of the top news stories in California's Silicon Valley was about the desire of the computer industry to allow more immigration of people with these skills because of the industry's claim that there are not enough qualified candidates in the United States. How much could the currently untapped resource of people with disabilities fill the void?

A positive result of the labor shortage is that barriers of discrimination are beginning to fall. Businesses of all sizes are looking at people with disabilities to fill their needs. This burgeoning demand creates an enormous opportunity for people with disabilities who have the skills and experience employers seek.[4]

The study by Kruse and Krueger[2] found that people with quadriplegia, college graduates, and younger people were more likely to use a computer, and this correlated with higher levels of employment. Companies did not have to invest in training people or risk hiring someone without proven skills. Other findings include:

- Only 17% of workers with SCIs returned to their previous job following injury.
- Another 10% said they could have returned to their previous work if they had been provided training and adaptive devices.
- Pay per hour was only slightly lower for people reemployed after injury, but hours—and weekly pay—fell by 25%.
- Fifty-one percent of people in white collar jobs returned to work.
- Thirty-two percent of people in blue collar jobs returned to work.

Larger corporations tend to be more willing to invest in hiring people with disabilities and in the equipment they need. They have the resources to commit to searching for people, sending staff to conferences such as those put on by The Office on Disability Employment Policy or Cornell University's Employment and Disability Institute, and supporting accommodation needs of an employee. Ultimately, these efforts are worth the investment.

Starting Your Own Business

Technology has made it easier to operate a business from home. A computer, a telephone, and a fax machine put you in contact with the world—including clients.

The United States Small Business Administration (SBA) helps some people seeking financing for a small business startup. They don't make direct loans, but, if your bank turns you down, you might qualify for an SBA loan guarantee under the Handicapped Assistance Loan program. If your application is accepted, SBA essentially promises to pay the bank if you default on the loan, removing the bank's risk. The SBA puts certain limits on the interest the bank may charge and also restricts the type of business they will approve. Gambling and real estate investment, for instance, are excluded from its list of approved businesses.

The SBA also provides information to help you start your business. Local offices provide advisers through the Service Corps of Retired Executives program, in which retired business executives review your plans and consult with you to help ensure success.

Temporary Work

The modern workplace has witnessed a notable shift toward contract and part-time workers. Corporations want to reduce full-time staff in order to save fixed overhead expenses of wages and benefits. More work projects are of shorter duration, with rapidly changing marketplaces and technologies. It can be difficult to predict what skills a company will need at any one time. Part-time and contract workers give companies flexibility.

Manpower Incorporated is an example of a temporary employment agency that has grown to be one of the largest corporations in the world. It maintains a list of people with specific skills and refers them to companies that call looking for those skills. Wages are paid by Manpower, which is paid a fee by the employer. Temporary job referrals can result in full-time jobs, since some companies see the service as a way of getting to know a potential employee without having to make a commitment to hire them full time from the start.

Many people question the impact of part-time and contract work on employees and communities. Workers can wonder where the next job will come from, not earn as much as they need, or lose security by not having health or retirement benefits. However, many people like being a contract worker. They get to work on a variety of projects, meet more people, and gain a variety of skills. They also get to experience the employer before making a full-time commitment, if that is an option. If they can perform some work at home, they might be able to gain a tax benefit from deducting the costs of a home office. The flexibility of contract work can be a good employment solution for a person with a disability.

Some companies are experimenting with flex time, in which jobs are shared and—to the degree possible—people set their own hours. This— along with part-time contract opportunities—opens up possibilities for people who have trouble committing to a full-time job because they are unable to predict physical problems, such as severe infections, pressure sores, or exacerbations of multiple sclerosis, for instance, or for people who require extra time in the morning to get clean, dressed, and mobile—possibly with the support of a personal assistant.

The Right to Work

Title I of the ADA requires equal opportunity for people with disabilities, affecting all employers in the private sector with 15 or more employees, as of July 26, 1994. The ADA protects you from being discriminated against for employment solely based on your disability. It does not guarantee you a job. You still have to qualify based on your abilities.

Federal agencies and any business receiving federal contracts of $10,000 or more were already banned from discriminating based on disability by Section 504 of the Rehabilitation Act of 1973. Sections 501 and 503 called on the government and its contractors to take affirmative action to hire people with disabilities. The Vietnam Veterans Readjustment Assistance Act of 1974 similarly requires government contractors to take affirmative action on behalf of covered veterans.

Advocacy and Volunteering

Many people with disabilities are not employed but still have time and skills to contribute. There are satisfying and productive options available. They might even prove to be vehicles to achieving full-time work.

There is plenty of work to do to advance the opportunities—or remove the barriers—for people with disabilities. There is no shortage of groups and associations that need help with advocacy. You can volunteer time at your local independent living center or a disability-specific group like United Cerebral Palsy to advance the inclusion of people with disabilities in our culture.

ADAPT (American Disabled for Attendant Programs Today) is probably the most militant of disability advocacy groups. It has taken direct action in order to achieve access to transportation and personal assistance services so that people's rights are preserved to live in the community rather than nursing homes. There are local chapters of ADAPT in many cities around the country.

You can volunteer time and experience to a local rehabilitation hospital. They typically welcome volunteers in a peer-support role for people facing a new disability. You might be surprised how much you have to offer from your own experience.

There are always issues of importance to the disability community that require people to express support or concerns about pending legislation of public policies. Organizations such as ADAPT or The American Association of People with Disabilities' (AAPD) Justice for All regularly notify people about such activities, as do politically oriented publications such as *The Ragged Edge* or *Mouth*. Tremendous amounts of information flow on the Internet, including calls to action that arrive via your inbox.

There are many other volunteer options to choose from. Visits to a local elementary school are often welcome by teachers, either to support their programs or as a way of offering children positive models of people with disabilities. Many libraries are looking for tutors to help teach adult reading courses. Local churches or agencies need help in serving many people in need, such as those who are homeless. Especially if you are feeling frustrated with your life, devoting time to your community is a wonderful way to forget your own problems and gain meaning and gratification.

The fact is that no one has the right to tell you that you can't work because of your disability. If you have the motivation, a desire to learn and develop a profession or skill, and some notion of how you would adapt your disability to that work, then go do it. Even people who should know better—like rehab staff—might discourage you for fear that you are hoping for too much. But the case has been made many times over. People with disabilities of all sorts are working as doctors, lawyers, activists, writers, publishers, artists, musicians, inventors, business owners, athletes, and almost any other pursuit you can imagine. If you want to work, then get out there and find out on your own terms what it takes.

Athletics

Sports benefit all people. Sports are fun, good for your health, and a way to meet people and feel connected. Wheelchair users participate—and excel—in a long list of sports, sometimes by means of recently designed adaptive devices. There are many sports to choose from and many organized events structured for disabled athletes. Leagues exist for wheelchair basketball, billiards, bowling, quad rugby, archery, and others. In some cases, competition is not only among people with disabilities, as in billiards, shooting, or certain classes of archery.

The National Veterans Wheelchair Games takes place each summer and includes athletes from the United States, Puerto Rico, and Great Britain. The 15 competitive sports include archery, basketball, quad rugby, swimming, track and field, table tennis, and weightlifting. An equestrian event is included as an exhibition.

The most substantial gathering of disabled athletes is the Paralympics, held every two years following the Olympic Games, and on the same site. At the 2006 games in Athens, Greece, 3,800 competitors from 136 countries took part in the games. The Olympic village where the athletes stay goes through a major accessibility update, including installing 750 handheld shower heads, changing bathroom doors, and putting transfer benches in showers. Those who compete in the Paralympics are world-class athletes, as committed to the highest standards of achievement as any Olympic athlete—with equally exciting entertainment and astonishment for attendees.

Associations

Many associations, national and local, promote and provide opportunities for disabled athletes. Following are a few examples:

- BORP is the Bay Area Outreach Program based in Northern California. The organization leads kayaking, rafting, camping, and handcycle outings. (www.borp.org)
- Disabled Sports USA sponsors clinics and events in snow and water skiing, rafting, and camping, among others, and operates an adaptive ski school at Lake Tahoe in California. It holds workshops to train instructors in adaptive fitness programs. (www.dsusa.org)
- The Handicapped Scuba Association trains and certifies people in scuba diving—both divers with disabilities and trainers. The association also sponsors trips; some trips use a luxury yacht adapted for chair users. (www.hasscuba.com)
- The National Center on Accessibility provides information on access to parks, operated in cooperation with the National Parks Service. It also promotes full participation in parks, recreation, and tourism and conducts research in trail design, wilderness policy issues, and the design of beach surfaces for assistive devices. (www.ncaonline.org)
- Wilderness Inquiry provides outdoor adventures for people of all ages and abilities. Rafting, kayaking, camping, canoeing, and horseback trips are held in the United States and Canada. Wilderness Inquiry encourages participation of people with disabilities and recommends manual chairs with knobby tires. (www.wildernessinquiry.org)
- Wheelchair Sports USA oversees local groups in a range of sports and is a clearinghouse of information. (www.wsusa.org)

The Sport Wheelchair

Wheelchairs for sports such as tennis, basketball, hockey, or rugby are adjusted—or specially designed—for the sport. The chairs are invariably rigid because of the need for great agility and responsiveness. Sport chairs use wheel camber, in which the top of the wheel is angled in toward the body to expand the wheelbase at the floor, to minimize tipping. Hockey and rugby chairs have metal guards at the base because of the frequency of collisions. The racing wheelchair is a sleek, precision device with its large third wheel extending well out in front of the chair and its rider.

Archery

People with disabilities can compete equally with nondisabled participants in archery. However, some classifications specific to wheelchair users are used in events sponsored by Wheelchair Archery, USA. One class is for quadriplegic archers who use adapted equipment or might need assistance placing the arrow on the bow. Another class is for chair riders who use equipment that conforms to international rules.

People with limited use of their fingers can wear a cuff with a hook device that allows them to grasp and release the bow. The string is released by extension of the wrist, without any action in the fingers. Archers with quadriplegia may also use support straps. A compound bow is a design that reduces the amount of force required to pull back on the string.

Billiards or Pool

Many people shoot pool from a wheelchair. The table is low and equipment is lightweight. Billiards is a sport easily played with nondisabled competitors. Some quadriplegic players can use a cuff to hold the thick end of the stick, while having enough dexterity in their arms to position the cue and accurately strike the ball. There is a slight disadvantage in reaching balls that are quite some distance away, but pool players have always had access to a device called a bridge, which allows them to reach the cue ball anywhere on the table. Just as a standing player must keep one foot on the floor, a wheelchair player must keep one "cheek on the seat." The sport is promoted by the National Wheelchair Poolplayers Association, www.nwpainc.org, which notes that pool is one of few sports in which chair users can compete on par with able-bodied players.

Bowling

Some wheelchair bowlers grip and throw the ball like a standing bowler. This is more difficult in a wheelchair because of the need to keep the arm away from the wheel as you roll the ball. Since a walking bowler is using the momentum of his body to propel the ball, a wheelchair bowler must either do much more work with his shoulder (with the potential for causing tendinitis) or choose a slower style.

There are metal or wood ramps available for bowlers to use from a wheelchair. The ramp has a level surface at the top. The ball is pushed forward and down the ramp once you have pointed the ramp where you want the ball to go. Another option is a bowling stick, which allows you to direct the ball from the ground. A bowling stick, such as the Bowl-A-Cue, is a pole with four prongs conforming to the shape of the ball and used to push the ball. Another device you can use is a snap handle—a gripper that fits in the three holes and lets go of the ball when you place it down to roll it. Most wheelchair bowlers use a 10-pound ball, rather than the 15 or 16 pounds used by most standing bowlers. The IKAN bowling ramp was designed so that people with high quadriplegia could bowl (www.ikansportsfoundation.org).

The American Wheelchair Bowling Association was formed in 1962. Competitors are required to use brakes, and ramps are not allowed in competition. The Association offers a videotape and book to help you learn how to bowl from a wheelchair (www.awba.org).

Field Events

Field events include throwing javelins, discuses, shot puts, and clubs. The club is a special adapted prop that resembles a bowling pin. It is weighted at the end and can be thrown by people with quadriplegia (Figure 8-3). There are rules about where the legs must be placed and how much contact with the seat is maintained as you position yourself to gain the best possible leverage. Gloves or assistive devices are not allowed in competition.

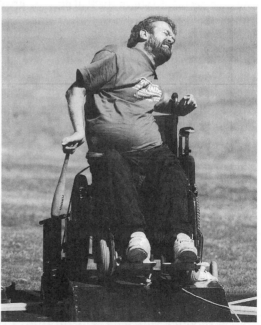

Figure 8-3 The club is a special adapted prop that resembles a bowling pin. It is weighted at the end and can be thrown by people with quadriplegia.

Juggling

Juggling can be learned with practice. You need to be willing to drop things and be patient with failure. It is worth enduring the initial awkwardness to discover how well your body can learn complex tasks and to enjoy feelings of competence and joy.

Most juggling options are limited to people with the ability to grasp with their hands, although a quadriplegic could get involved in plate spinning by putting a cuff on the sticks. You will probably start by learning how to juggle three balls. This is easily done sitting down and does not require a great deal of upper-body balance. There are hundreds of possible patterns you can throw with three balls, so there is endless opportunity for exploration. A ball-juggling routine can become an excellent source of aerobic exercise:

> There are not many juggling wheelchair users, but that need not be true. At the summer International Jugglers' Association events, I am typically the only chair rider. Yet I know an occupational therapist who uses juggling in her work. Juggling could be an excellent option for many other chair riders. I have had the pleasure of advancing to the level of passing clubs in group patterns. When I began, I doubted I would ever achieve that level.

Juggling is a growing amateur sport. Many cities have weekly get-togethers. Experienced jugglers are happy to teach the basics to anyone who shows up and asks for a lesson (www.juggling.org).

Quad Rugby

People with quadriplegia are generally unable to play basketball because of the grip needed to shoot the ball and the greater arm strength usually needed to loft the ball to the hoop 10 feet above. In the 1970s, a group of Canadians developed quad rugby as an alternative sport. The United States Quad Rugby Association was formed in 1988 (www.quadrugby.com).

Quad rugby is a very physical game, a blend of basketball, hockey, and football. It is played with a volleyball, which is lighter than a basketball. The object is to carry the ball across goal lines marked at the ends of the court, usually a basketball court. Players may push their wheels any number of times but are allowed to keep possession of the ball for only 10 seconds. There are many collisions, thus the rugged design of specialized rugby chairs offered by some wheelchair makers. Spoke guards are common for protection of both the spokes and the players' hands.

Brought to greater public fame by the movie, *MurderBall*, quad rugby is one of the most popularly attended events at the Paralympics. It is a very dramatic, entertaining game, where any notion of sympathy for the disabilities of the players cannot survive.

Shooting

Target shooting with a pistol or air rifle can be done from a sitting position and is available to anyone with the visual ability to sight the target. There are puff-and-sip devices for firing the gun for people with quadriplegia who cannot squeeze the trigger with a finger. Competitive shooting is a sport that does not need separate events for people with disabilities—there is no advantage or disadvantage. You may set the rifle on a table using a tripod support and must support the rifle without placing your arms on armrests or other supports. Shooting equipment for wheelchair users can be found at www.beadaptive.com.

Snow Skiing

There are several adaptive devices for both downhill and cross-country skiing. The sit ski is like a sled, with two tracks on the base of a shell in which you sit, strapped in. There is a roll bar at the back to prevent the ski from bearing down on top of you when you fall and roll over. Sitting close to the ground, you hold small poles or grips with metal disks to plant in the snow when you make a turn, just as you would use a pole on normal skis. The sit ski behaves like skis, responding to turns of your body.

Getting onto a chair lift with a sit ski requires the assistance of two lifters, who pick you up and place you on the lift. One lifter rides with you. A buckle is attached to the back of the chair lift during the ride. Getting off the lift is the exciting moment, since you must shimmy forward to the edge and jump off to the ground while the chair is still moving. Operators slow down the lift as you approach, as when you board.

You must be certified to ski unaccompanied on a sit ski. Until you are certified, an instructor will ski with you, holding a tether rope attached to the rear of the sit ski. Since it is possible to slide out of control down the hill, someone must be there to take control until you are sufficiently trained and experienced. The art of being a sit ski instructor is to shadow the skier's movements, with no tension on the tether. You don't even feel her presence unless she needs to help you gain control.

Another version of adaptive snow skiing uses a seat on two skis. It requires minimal upper-body strength and dexterity to control and sits close enough to the snow that you don't fall or roll over as you can on a sit ski.

The mono-ski is the peak experience for disabled snow skiers. It is made of a seat set atop a single regulation ski. Since you are sitting higher up, you use outrigger poles that have small skis on the end. It is possible to fall over in a mono-ski, which is why instructors do not need to use a tether. When you fall, you stop. The mono-ski requires greater dexterity and balance because it relies so much more on the use of your upper body for steering and control. The supporting mechanism is hinged or built in an X-shape, which allows you to elevate the seat to a level at which you can board a chair lift unassisted. It collapses to its lower setting as soon as you are on the lift, back in ski mode:

> *The mono-ski is really cool because it is so responsive, and it*
> *is much better being able to ski without having to be lifted*
> *onto the chair lifts. It's a lot harder to learn, though. I fell over*
> *a lot during my first lessons and really trashed my shoulders*
> *at first!*

A dual-ski design allows people with less upper-body strength to ski downhill. Adaptive cross-country skis rely on the use of poles to propel the skier. A sling seat with a back is mounted on two regulation-sized long skis. Ski Central, www.skicentral.com, is an extensive resource site for skiers with disabilities.

Adaptive skis have also been developed for water skiing. Visit www.usa waterski.org and type "disability" in the search field for more information.

Swimming

Swimming is a popular and excellent exercise option for many people, almost regardless of how severe the disability. It is a full-body exercise with significant cardiovascular benefits. Because you are essentially weightless in water, you are able to move more easily. The natural resistance of the water gives muscles a meaningful, though gentle, form of workout. Even for those able to float only with assistance, it is a relief to be freed of your body weight in the buoyancy of a pool. This woman with paraplegia enjoys swimming:

> *I swim three times a week. There's a pool in my building. I*
> *really love it. I do the crawl and the backstroke. It's a real*
> *sense of freedom to be able to move without the wheelchair. At*
> *first I felt self-conscious in public in my bathing suit with my*
> *bony butt sticking up in the air. But I got over it. I wear a*
> *Speedo, and also biking shorts to cover more of my legs. There*
> *are all of these 20-somethings with perfect bodies, but I just*
> *don't care anymore.*

Your local hospital, rehab center, or recreation center might offer special opportunities or programs for disabled swimmers.

Wheelchair Basketball

Wheelchair basketball is a team sport played on a regulation basketball court with the net at the normal 10-foot height. Two pushes of the chair are allowed before the ball must be dribbled, passed, or shot. You are allowed to push one wheel as you dribble the ball.

There is a "physical advantage" foul. People able to use their legs may not use them to gain an advantage, such as to brake the wheelchair. Since a player can't jump or get up close to the net, those with the ability to shoot from a distance have an advantage. A trick unique to wheelchair basketball involves picking up the ball from the floor. You press it against a wheel as you are moving, and let it come up as the wheel turns.

Players are rated according to physical capacity. For example, a single-leg amputee would get a higher rating than a low-level quadriplegic with slightly limited hand use. The purpose of the rating system is to even out the competitiveness of the teams. No team may have more than a given number of total points when you add up the ratings of the players on the floor at any time.

Wheelchair basketball is played by many people unable to run well enough for able-bodied play, not only those with paralysis (Figure 8-4). It is a rough game, in which players often end up on the floor. There is a significant wheelchair basketball league, with competitive play around the country. Many players practice weekly and travel to games. Wheelchair basketball is sometimes seen as exhibition play before professional games. Get information from the National Wheelchair Basketball Association at www.nwba.org.

Wheelchair Racing

One of the more well-known examples of wheelchair athletics is marathon racing. The riders train hard for the event, which involves hours of continuous racing. Wheelchair racers are the first out of the gate at major marathons, such as the Boston Marathon. The times of the wheelers are faster than the able-bodied runners.

Figure 8-4 Wheelchair basketball is played by many people unable to run well enough for able-bodied play, not only those with paralysis.

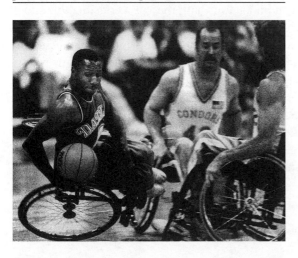

Racing wheelchairs are extremely lightweight and finely balanced and use a three-wheel design in which the third wheel extends out ahead of the chair. Many racers sit in a tucked posture, feet under their bodies for optimal leverage. The push rims are small so that the chair can be propelled by the upward motion of the arms as well as the normal downward push.

In the late 1990s, a downhill wheelchair appeared. The front casters are very large. You lean forward and grip handles attached to the front wheels, which rotate to steer the chair. Hand brakes are mounted on these handles, using cable brakes similar to those on bicycles. You sit low to the ground. It is a bouncy ride, with speeds as high as 30 miles per hour down a mountain hillside.

Wheelchair Tennis

The basic rule of wheelchair tennis is that you get two bounces of the ball on your side of the net before you have to hit it back, as compared to one bounce in the able-bodied version. Since the advent of high-level wheelchair designs for tennis that are remarkably fast and nimble, world-class players rarely require the second bounce, and there is talk of removing the two-bounce rule in upper-level competition.

The art of tennis is to get into the right position, relative to the ball, so that, as you swing the racket, you get the most power and control. It is quite a surprise to discover you can push the chair in just the right direction and speed to be in position to hit the tennis ball, which is moving quite fast. You typically are in motion while you hit the ball, in contrast to a standing player, who tries to plant his feet when taking a shot.

You will need to do a tremendous amount of upper-body movement and have sufficient balance in the chair. Although increased seat dump (the downward angle toward the rear) increases your stability, it also sets you lower down. Being lower is a disadvantage in being able to hit the ball accurately into the opposing side of the court. Many players use seat belts for increased stability.

Chair riders must take care to play in a way to avoid tennis elbow, a form of tendinitis. When you hit a tennis ball, there is a considerable shock sent through the arm to the tendons that attach at the elbow. Proper technique and swing—using the body as much as possible rather than using the arm alone—help minimize the impact. New tennis racquet designs reduce vibration sent through the racquet into your arm when you hit the ball. A firm grip is important and reduces the risk of forming blisters on the hands. Some people with low quadriplegia with sufficient arm strength play tennis by using bandages or cuffs to help grip the racquet. Wheelchair tennis has found great support in the general tennis community, thanks to the International Tennis Federation (www.itftennis.com).

Other Options

This is by no means a complete description of athletic options for chair riders. Other options include:

- Boxing
- Climbing
- Dancing
- Fencing
- Fishing
- Flying
- Golf
- Hand cycling
- Hang gliding
- Hiking
- Hockey
- Horseback riding
- Hunting
- Kayaking/canoeing
- Lawn bowling
- Motorcycling
- Parachuting
- Ping-Pong
- Racquetball
- Sailing
- Softball
- Trap shooting
- Water skiing
- Weight lifting

Many, if not all, of these sports are represented by an organization that disseminates information, sponsors events, and supports development of adaptive methods and equipment. The most comprehensive ongoing source of information on athletics is *Sports 'N Spokes*, a bimonthly magazine published by the Paralyzed Veterans of America. See the Appendix for more resources.

Out There

The more you get out there, the more you learn. Even unpleasant experiences can point toward a better approach for the next time, so that you can better enjoy your life on wheels.

References

1. Risher P, Amorosi S. *The 1998 N.O.D./Harris Survey of Americans with Disabilities*. New York: Louis Harris; 1998.
2. Kruse D, Krueger A. *Disability, Employment, and Earnings in the Dawn of the Computer Age—Executive Summary*. National Bureau of Economic Research Working Paper #5302;1995.
3. Modern medics. *Mainstream Magazine*. 1997; August:18-20.
4. Coelho T. *Opening Remarks*. President's Committee on Employment of People with Disabilities. 51st Annual Technology Symposium. May 7, 1998. New Orleans, Louisiana. Available at: http://www.benderconsult.com/people/speech/coelho.html. Accessed on: March 10, 2008.

Resources

Disability-Specific Organizations

Amputee Coalition of America
900 East Hill Ave., Suite 205
Knoxville, TN 37915
888-AMP-KNOW
www.amputee-coalition.org

Amyotrophic Lateral Sclerosis Association
27001 Agoura Rd., Suite 150
Calabasa Hills, CA 91301
818-880-9007
www.alsa.org

Arthritis Foundation
PO Box 7669
Atlanta, GA 30357
800-283-7800
www.arthritis.org

Brain Injury Association of America
1608 Spring Hill Rd., Suite 110
Vienna, VA 22182
703-761-0750
www.biausa.org

Center for Research on Women with Disabilities
One Baylor Plaza
Houston, TX 77030
713-798-5782
www.bcm.edu/crowd

The International Polio Network
4207 Lindell Blvd., #110
St. Louis, MO 63108
314-534-0475
www.post-polio.org

The International Ventilator Users Network
4207 Lindell Blvd., #110
St. Louis, MO 63108
314-534-0475
www.ventusers.org

The Muscular Dystrophy Association
3300 E. Sunrise DR
Tucson, AZ 85718
800-FIGHT-MD
800-572-1717
www.mdausa.org

National Amputation Foundation
40 Church St.
Malverne, NY 11565
516-887-3600
www.nationalamputation.org

National Family Caregivers
Association
10400 Connecticut Ave., Suite 500
Kensington, MD 20895
800-896-3650
www.nfcacares.org

National Multiple Sclerosis Society
733 Third Ave.
New York, NY 10017
800-FIGHT-MS
www.nmss.org

National Organization for Rare
Disorders
55 Kenosia Ave.
PO Box 1968
Danbury, CT 06813-1968
203-744-0100
www.rarediseases.org

The National Spinal Cord Injury
Association
1 Church St. #600
Rockville, MD 20850
800-962-9629
www.spinalcord.org

The National Stroke Association
9707 E. Easter LN
Building B
Centennial, CO 80112
800-787-6537
www.stroke.org

Spina Bifida Association of America
4590 MacArthur Blvd. NW
Washington, DC 20007
800-621-3141
www.sbaa.org

TASH-Disability Advocacy
Worldwide
1025 Vermont Ave. NW, Floor 7
Washington, DC 20005
202-263-5600
www.tash.org

Osteogenesis Imperfecta
Foundation
804 W. Diamond Ave., Suite 210
Gaithersburg, MD 20878
800-981-2663
www.oif.org

United Cerebral Palsy Association
1660 L St. NW, Suite 700
Washington, DC 20036
800-872-5827
www.ucp.org

United Spinal
75-20 Astoria Blvd.
Jackson Heights, NY 11370
www.unitedspinal.org

Disability Advocacy Groups

AHEAD — Association on Higher
Education and Disability
107 Commerce Center Drive,
  Suite 204
Huntersville, NC 28078
704-947-7779
www.ahead.org

Consortium for Citizens with
Disabilities
1660 L Street, NW, Ste. 700
Washington, DC 20036
202-783-2229
www.c-c-d.org

Disability Rights Education &
Defense Fund
2212 6th St.
Berkley, CA 94710

510-644-2555
www.dredf.org

National Organization on Disability
910 16th St. NW, Suite 600
Washington, DC 20006
202-293-5960
www.nod.org

World Institute on Disability
510 16th St., Suite 100
Oakland, CA 94612
510-763-4100
www.wid.org

Hospitals

Veterans Administration Hospitals
800-827-1000
www.va.gov

Model System Rehabilitation Hospitals

CARF, Commission on
Accreditation of Rehabilitation
Facilities
4891 E. Grant Rd.
Tucson, AZ 85712
520-325-1044
www.carf.org

Boston University Medical Center
1 Boston Medical Center Place
Boston, MA 02118
617-638-8000
www.bumc.bu.edu

Craig Hospital
3425 S. Clarkson St.
Englewood, CO 80113
303-789-8000
www.craighospital.org

The Institute for Rehabilitation and
Research
1333 Moursund
Houston, TX 77030
713-799-5000
http://www.memorialhermann.org/lo
cations/TIRR.html

Kessler Institute
1199 Pleasant Valley Way
West Orange, NJ 07052
973-731-3600
www.kessler-rehab.com

Medical College of Virginia
1250 East Marshall St.
Richmond, VA 23294
804-828-9000
www.vcuhealth.org

MetroHealth Medical Center
2500 MetroHealth DR
Cleveland, OH 44109
216-778-7800
www.metrohealth.org

Mt. Sinai Medical Center
Department of Rehabilitation
    Medicine
One Gustave L Levy PL
New York, NY 10029
212-241-6500
www.mountsinai.org

Rancho Los Amigos Medical Center
7601 E. Imperial Highway
Downey, CA 90242
562-401-7111
www.rancho.org

Rehabilitation Institute of Chicago
345 E. Superior St.
Chicago, IL 60611
800-354-REHAB
www.rehabchicago.org

Rehabilitation Institute of Michigan
261 Mack Ave.
Detroit, MI 48201
313-745-1203
www.rimrehab.org/

Santa Clara Valley Medical Center
751 S. Bascom Ave.
San Jose, California 95128
408-885-5000
www.scvmed.org/portal/site/vmc

Shepherd Center
2020 Peachtree Rd. NW
Atlanta, GA 30309
404-352-2020
www.shepherd.org

Spine Rehabilitation Center
University of Alabama
619 19th St. S.
Birmingham, AL 35249
205-934-4011
www.health.uab.edu/12615/

Thomas Jefferson University Hospital
111 South 11th St.
Philadelphia, PA 19107
215-955-6000
www.jeffersonhospital.org

University of Michigan Medical Center
Department of Physical Medicine & Rehabilitation
1500 E. Medical Center DR
Ann Arbor, MI 48109
734-936-4000
www.med.umich.edu/pmr

University of Missouri-Columbia
Department of Physical Medicine & Rehabilitation
315 Business Loop 70W
Columbia, MO 65203
573-882-3101

som.missouri.edu/PMR

University of Washington School of Medicine
Department of Rehabilitation Medicine
1959 NE Pacific St., Box 356490
Seattle, WA 98195
206-543-3600
depts.washington.edu/rehab

Personal Assistance Services

Center on Human Policy
Syracuse University
805 South Crouse Ave.
Syracuse, NY 13244
315-443-3851
thechp.syr.edu

The Independent Living Centers
www.ilusa.com/links/ilcenters.htm

Rehabilitation Research and Training Center on Aging with a Disability
Rancho Los Amigos National Rehabilitation Center
7601 E. Imperial Hwy, 800 West Annex
Downey, California 90242
562-401-7402
www.agingwithdisability.org

Functional Electrical Stimulation

FES Information Center
10701 East Blvd.
Cleveland, OH 44106
216-791-3800
fescenter.case.edu

Sigmedics, Inc.
335 North Broad St.
Fairborn, OH 45324
937-439-9131
www.sigmedics.com

Service Animals

Assistance Dogs of America
Education and Training Facility
8806 State RTE 64
Swanton, Ohio 43558
419-825-3622
www.adai.org

Canine Companions for Independence
PO Box 446
Santa Rosa, CA 95402-0446
866-224-3647
www.cci.org

Freedom Service Dogs
PO Box 150217
Lakewood, CO 80215
303-922-6231
freedomservicedogs.org

Loving Paws Assistance Dogs
PO Box 12005
Santa Rosa, CA 95406
707-569-7092
www.lovingpaws.org

Service Animal Registry of America
PO Box 607
Midlothian, TX 76065
206-333-6861
www.affluent.net/sara

Wheelchairs and Cushions

Colours
860 E. Parkridge Ave.
Corona, CA 92879
951-808-9131

www.colourswheelchair.com

Crown Therapeutics/Roho
100 N. Florida Ave.
Belleville, IL 62221
800-851-3449
www.therohogroup.com

ErgoAir
9 Riverside DR
Pine Bush, NY 12566
845-744-5216
www.ergoair.com

Grant Airmass
PO Box 3456
Stamford, CT 06905
800-243-5237
www.grantairmass.com

Invacare Corporation/PinDot
1 Invacare Way
Elyria, OH 44035
www.invacare.com

Lasher Sport
PO Box 112044
Anchorage, AK 99511
907-529-8833
www.lashersport.com

OrthoRehab, Specialty Rehab Services by Otto Bock
14630 28th Ave. N
Minneapolis, MN 55447
800-328-4058
www.ottobockus.com

Permobil
6961 Eastgate Blvd.
Lebanon, TN 37090
800-736-0925
www.permobilusa.com

Quickie Designs/Sunrise Medical/Jay Medical
2382 Faraday Ave., Suite 200
Carlsbad, CA 92008

800-333-4000
www.sunrisemedical.com

Supracor
2050 Corporate CT
San Jose, CA 95131
800-787-7226
www.supracor.com

Teftec
12450 Network Blvd.
San Antonio, TX 78249
888-234-1433
www.teftec.com

Wheelchairs of Kansas
204 W.2nd St.
PO Box 320
Ellis, KS 67637
800-537-6454
www.wheelchairsofkansas.com

Home Access/Accessibility Design

AARP
601 E St. NW
Washington, DC 20049
888-OUR-AARP
www.aarp.org

Altro Safety Floors
80 Industrial Way Wilmington
MA 01887
800-377-5597
www.altrofloors.com

Architectural and Transportation Barriers Compliance Board
1331 F St. NW, Suite 1000
Washington, DC 20004
800-872-2253
www.access-board.gov

The Center for Universal Design
North Carolina State University
Campus Box 8613
Raleigh, NC 27695
800-647-6777
www.design.ncsu.edu/cud

Dor-O-Matic
2720 Tobey DR
Indianapolis, IN 46208
800-543-4635
www.doromatic.com

Enerlogic Systems
PO Box 3743
Nashua, NH 03061
603-880-4066

Essex Electronics, Inc.
1130 Mark Ave.
Carpinteria, CA 93013
800-539-5377
www.keyless.com

Hafele America Co.
3901 Cheyenne DR
Archdale, NC 27263
336-434-2322
www.hafele.com

L.E. Johnson Products
2100 Sterling Ave.
Elkhart, IN 46516
800-837-5664
www.johnsonhardware.com

Paralyzed Veterans of America
801 18th St. NW
Washington, DC 20006
800-424-8200
www.pva.org

ProMatura Group
19 County Rd. 168
Oxford, MS 38655
800-201-1483
www.promatura.com

The Ramp Project
Metropolitan Center for Independent
  Living
1600 University Ave.
St. Paul, MN 55104
651-603-2029
www.wheelchairramp.org

Ultraflo
#8 Trautman Industrial DR
Ste. Genevieve, MO 63670
800-950-1762
www.ultraflovalve.com

US Department of Housing and
Urban Development
451 7th St. S.W.
Washington, DC 20410
202-708-1112
www.hud.gov

X-10 USA, Inc.
PO Box 420
Closter, NJ 07624
800-442-5109
www.x10.com

Sexuality

CLEO Living Aids
3957 Mayfield Rd.
Cleveland, OH 44121
800-321-0595

Sexuality Reborn: A Video about
Sexuality and SCI
Kessler Institute for Rehabilitation
1199 Pleasant Valley Way
West Orange, NJ 07052
800-248-3221
www.kessler-rehab.com

The Xandria Collection
Lawrence Research Group
5375 Procyon St., Suite 102
Las Vegas, NV 89118

800-242-2823
www.xandria.com

Parenting Resources

Through the Looking Glass
2198 Sixth St., Suite 100
Berkeley, CA 94710
800-644-2666
www.lookingglass.org

DisAbled Women's Network
Box 1138 North Bay
ON P1B 8K4 Canada
dawn.thot.net

Research Support Organizations

The Miami Project to Cure Paralysis
1095 NW 14th TER
Miami, FL 33136
1-800-St.ANDUP
www.miamiproject.miami.edu

Canadian Spinal Research
Organization
120 Newkirk Rd., Unit 2
Richmond Hill, ON L4C 9S7 Canada
800-361-4004
www.csro.com

People for the Ethical Treatment of
Animals (PETA)
501 Front St.
Norfolk, VA 23510
757-622-PETA
www.peta.org

PVA Spinal Cord Research
Foundation
801 18th St. NW
Washington, DC 20006
800-424-8200
www.pva.org

**Christopher and Dana Reeve
Foundation**
636 Morris Turnpike, Suite 3A
Short Hills, NJ 07078
800-225-0292
www.christopherreeve.org

Adaptive Technology

Don Johnston Incorporated
26799 West Commerce DR
Volo, IL 60073
800-999-4660
www.donjohnston.com

Nuance
1 Wayside Rd.
Burlington, MA 01803
781-565-5000
www.nuance.com

DynaVox Technologies
2100 Wharton St., Suite 400
Pittsburgh, PA 15203
1-866-DYNAVOX
www.dynavoxtech.com

Closing the Gap
526 Main St.
PO Box 68
Henderson, MN 56044
507-248-3294
www.closingthegap.com

Human Ability and Accessibility Center

IBM Corporation
1 New Orchard Rd.
Armonk, New York 10504
800-IBM-4YOU
www-03.ibm.com/able

Neil Squire Society
2250 Boundary Rd., Suite 220

Burnaby, BC V5M 3Z3 Canada
604-473-9363
www.neilsquire.ca

**Trace Research and Development
Center**
University of Wisconsin-Madison
2107 Engineering Centers Bldg.
1550 Engineering DR
Madison, WI 53706
608-262-6966
trace.wisc.edu

Athletics and Recreation

**American Wheelchair Bowling
Association**
PO Box 69
Clover, VA 24534
434-454-2269
www.awba.org

Disabled Sports USA
451 Hungerford DR, Suite 100
Rockville, MD 20850
301-217-0960
www.dsusa.org

Handicapped Scuba Association
1104 El Prado
San Clemente, CA 92672
949-498-4540
www.hsascuba.com

Motorcycle Riding
www.ridemyown.com/links/nolimits.
   shtml

National Disability Sports Alliance
25 West Independence Way
Kingston, RI 02882
401-792-7130
www.ndsaonline.org

**National Wheelchair Basketball
Association**
6165 Lehman DR, Suite 101

Colorado Springs, CO 80918
719-266-4876
www.nwba.org

National Wheelchair Poolplayers Association, Inc.
c/o Bob Calderon
9757 Mount Lompoc CT
Las Vegas, Nevada 89178
702-437-6792
www.nwpainc.org

North American Riding for the Handicapped Association, Inc.
PO Box 33150
Denver, CO 80233
800-369-7433
www.narha.org

Paralyzed Veterans of America
801 18th St., NW
Washington, DC 20006
800-424-8200
www.pva.org

United States Quad Rugby Association
5593 Cedar Oak Blvd.
Sarasota, FL 34233
941-924-1804
www.quadrugby.com

Wheelchair Sports USA
1236 Jungermann Rd., Suite A
St. Peters, MO 63376
636-614-6784
www.wsusa.org

Wilderness Inquiry, Inc.
808 14th Ave. SE
Minneapolis, MN 55414
800-728-0719
www.wildernessinquiry.org

Employment

AgrAbility Project
University of Wisconsin -
  Cooperative Extension
460 Henry Mall
Madison, WI 53706
866-259-6280
www.agrabilityproject.org

Electronic Industries Alliance
2500 Wilson Blvd.
Arlington, VA 22201
703-907-7500
www.eia.org

Job Accommodation Network
PO Box 6080
Morgantown, WV 26506
800-526-7234
www.jan.wvu.edu

Office of Disability Employment Policy
US Department of Labor
200 Constitution Ave NW
Washington, DC 20210
1-866-633-7365
www.dol.gov/odep

President's Committee on Employment of People with Disabilities
1331 F St., NW, Suite 300
Washington, DC 20004
202-376-6200

U.S. Small Business Administration
800-827-5722
www.sba.gov

Travel

Access-Able Travel Source, LLC
PO Box 1796
Wheat Ridge, CO 80034

303-232-2979
www.access-able.com

Accessible Vans of America, LLC
888-AVA-VANS
www.accessiblevans.com

Hosteling International USA
National Administrative Office
8401 Colesville Rd., Suite 600
Silver Spring, MD 20910
301-495-1240
www.hiusa.org

Wheelchair Getaways
PO Box 1098
Mukilteo, WA 98275
800-536-5518
www.wheelchairgetaways.com

Disability Magazines

Accent on Living
PO Box 700
Bloomington, IL 61702
800-787-8444

Emerging Horizons
C & C Creative Concepts
PO Box 278
Ripon, CA 95366
emerginghorizons.com

Exceptional Parent Magazine
551 Main St.
Johnstown, PA 15901
814-361-3860
www.eparent.com

Mouth Magazine
Free Hand Press, Inc.
4201 SW 30th St.
Topeka, KS 66614
www.mouthmag.org

New Mobility
No Limits Communications Inc.

PO Box 220
Horsham , PA 19044
888-850-0344
www.newmobility.com

Paralegia News
PVA Publications
2111 E. Highland Ave., Suite 180
Phoenix, AZ 85016
888-888-2201
www.pvamagazines.compnnews/

Quest Magazine
PO Box 3602
Glendale, CA 91221
www.questmagazine.com

Sports 'N Spokes
PVA Publications
2111 E. Highland Ave., Suite 180
Phoenix, AZ 85016
888-888-2201
www.pvamagazines.comsns/

The Ragged Edge
www.raggededgemagazine.com

Disability Books

101 Accessible Vacations: Travel Ideas for Wheelers and Slow Walkers
Candy B. Harrington
Demos Medical Publishing
ISBN 1932603433 / 9781932603439
$24.95
www.demosmedpub.com

Barrier-Free Travel: A Nuts and Bolts Guide For Wheelers and Slow Walkers, 2nd Edition
Candy B. Harrington
Demos Medical Publishing
ISBN 1932603093 / 9781932603095
$19.95
www.demosmedpub.com

Health Insurance Resources
Dorothy E. Northrop
Demos Medical Publishing
ISBN 1932603344 / 9781932603347
$26.95
www.demosmedpub.com

The Disabled Woman's Guide to Pregnancy and Birth
Judith Rogers
Demos Medical Publishing
ISBN 1932603085 / 9781932603088
$24.95
www.demosmedpub.com

The Personal Care Attendant Guide
Katie Rodriguez Banister
Demos Medical Publishing
ISBN 193260328X / 9781932603286
$16.95
www.demosmedpub.com

There is Room at the Inn: Inns and B&Bs for Wheelers and Slow Walkers
Candy B. Harrington
Demos Medical Publishing
ISBN 1932603611 / 9781932603613
$21.95
www.demosmedpub.com

Online Disability Product Sites

Allegro Medical
800-861-3211
www.allegromedical.com

Care Medical Equipment
800-741-2282
www.caremedicalequipment.com

Sammons Preston—Rehabilitation products
800-323-5547
www.sammonspreston.com

SpinLife.com—Wheelchairs and accessories
800-850-0335
www.spinlife.com

SportAid—Wheelchairs and accessories
800-743-7203
www.sportaid.com

Web sites

360 magazine
www.360usainc.com

ABLEDATA
www.abledata.com

Apparelyzed
Disability discussion forums
www.apparelyzed.com

Care/Cure Community
SpineWire
sci.rutgers.edu/forum/index.php

Cure Paralysis Now
www.cureparalysisnow.org

Disability Benefits 101
www.disabilitybenefits101.org

Disability History Museum
www.disabilitymuseum.org

Disability Information and Resources
www.makoa.org/index.htm

Independent Living Research Utilization Program
www.ilru.org/

MyPleasure.com
www.mypleasure.com/education/sexed/disabilitylist.asp

National Rehabilitation Information
Center
www.naric.com

Sexual Health Network
www.sexualhealth.com

Society for Disability Studies
www.uic.edu/orgs/sds

Spinal Cord Injury, Stroke, and
Paralysis Guide to Support
Organizations
neurosurgery.mgh.harvard.edu/Trau
    ma/paral-r.htm

Spinal Cord Injury Information
Network
www.spinalcord.uab.edu

The Wheelchair Junkie
www.wheelchairjunkie.com

WheelchairNet
www.wheelchairnet.org

$\mathcal{A}ppendix$

Disability Advocacy

In 1977, a group of protestors occupied the San Francisco offices of the US Department of Health, Education, and Welfare, an action that was to last for 25 days. As of publication of this book, this protest remains the longest occupation of federal property on record. The protestors were people with disabilities and, in some cases, their attendants.

Section 504 of the Rehabilitation Act of 1973 had been passed in the US Congress. It included a simple statement that no federal agency, public university, federal contractor, or entity that received federal funding could discriminate "solely by reason of handicap."

Afraid that the Act would commit the government and its contractors to billions of dollars of expense for access, the Secretary of Health, Education, and Welfare, who was responsible for implementation of the legislation, resisted signing the accompanying regulations into action. By the end of the San Francisco occupation, the regulations were signed into law, unchanged.

This was a tremendous victory, achieved by people with disabilities on their own behalf. It emboldened a modern disability movement for independence and inclusion that has since only grown in its power and sophistication. Although there has been tremendous progress made, the maldistribution of disability spending toward care rather than independence continues, and some rights and coverage have been lost.

Every one of us with a disability, those who care about us, and those who want to see our tax dollars spent wisely have a direct interest in disability advocacy issues. And every one of us can at any time find ourselves members of the family of people with disabilities—or facing higher levels of disability impairment. Disability advocacy is a universal political and social issue that continues to be viewed through the lens of caretaking and

449

charity. It is, rather, a lens itself into the core values of democracy and principles of how to assert the power of government for the broader good, both for quality of life and for fiscal responsibility.

If you have a recent disability, you are the beneficiary of an incredible historic saga of modern advocacy. And your awareness and participation are needed in the ongoing process of removing obstacles and opening possibilities that will allow you to have the same immense potential available to you that exists for any other person, taking into account your authentic objective abilities and limitations, unimpeded by artificial external barriers.

Someday the only barrier will be your own choice to go for it or not.

With the above in mind, *Life On Wheels* offers a brief timeline on advocacy accomplishments of the modern disability movement and a list of legislative and policy issues at hand as of this publication.

The Americans with Disabilities Restoration Act of 2007

The US Supreme Court has not been kind to the Americans with Disabilities Act (ADA). In a number of significant decisions, it has dramatically narrowed the range of who qualifies as having a disability.

With the ADA being diluted to the point of near meaninglessness for many people clearly at risk of discrimination, the disability community recognized the need for the original intent of the US Congress to be restored in the view of the judicial system. Thus, the ADA Restoration Act of 2007, which, as Representative F. James Sensenbrenner, Jr., Republican of Wisconsin, a cosponsor of the bill in the House of Representatives, said:

> ... will force courts to focus on whether a person has experienced discrimination "on the basis of disability," rather than require individuals to demonstrate that they fall within the scope of the law's protection.

Representative Steny Hoyer, Democrat of Maryland, introduced the ADA Restoration Act in the House along with 235 cosponsors, including Representative James Langevin, Democrat of Rhode Island, who also happens to be a man with quadriplegia.

On October 4, 2007, Representative Hoyer testified before the House Judiciary Committee, saying:

> When we wrote the ADA, we intentionally used a definition of disability that was broad, borrowing from an existing definition from the Rehabilitation Act of 1973. We thought using established language would help us avoid a potentially divisive

Advocacy Accomplishments Timeline		
1968	Architectural Barriers Act	Requires that, from 1969 onward, any building receiving federal funding has to be accessible.
1973	Rehabilitation Act	Specifically addresses disability access in terms of civil rights and discrimination—the first law to do so.
1975	Education for All Handicapped Children Act	Provides that children with disabilities are entitled to education and services in the public school system.
1984	Voting Rights for the Elderly and Handicapped Act	Requires polling places to be accessible.
1986	Air Carrier Access Act	Protects people from discrimination by commercial air carriers, provides that service animals be allowed on board, and disallows measures such as requiring advance notice of travel for people with disabilities or limiting the number of persons with disabilities on a given flight.
1990	Americans with Disabilities Act	Provides civil rights protections in the realms of employment, transportation, telecommunications, public accommodations, and state and federal government services.
1990	Individuals with Disabilities Education Act	Extends the 1975 law and provides federal funds for schools to assist with accommodations.
2001	First Visitability Ordinance	Requires one-level entrance, wheel chair passage, and a usable ground-floor bathroom—instituted in Pima County, Arizona; other cities and counties soon followed suit.
2005	Money Follows the Person	Shifts the emphasis in the Medicaid program, an initiative of the federal government in which states are given funds, from institutional care to programs that allow people to live in their own homes in the community.

political debate over the definition of "disabled." Therefore,
we could not have fathomed that people with diabetes,
epilepsy, heart conditions, cancer, and mental illnesses would
have their ADA claims kicked out of court.

Track the status of the ADA and the ADA Restoration Act at www.aapd
.com or adarestoration.blogspot.com.

Emergency Preparedness

When Hurricane Katrina struck the Gulf Coast and decimated the city of
New Orleans, the woeful state of emergency preparedness for people with
disabilities was revealed. People with disabilities were trapped in their
homes; some died. Those evacuated were not allowed to bring service animals or prescription medicines and arrived in locations that had no provisions for access. Some were simply turned away from emergency shelters,
finding themselves suddenly imprisoned in nursing homes.

Federal programs are being established as emergency preparedness
rises higher on the priority list in disability advocacy. You are encouraged
to inquire about emergency planning for people with disabilities in your
own community; chances are you will find that little thought has been
given the topic.

Competitive Bidding for Mobility Equipment

As goes Medicare, so goes the insurance industry. The Centers for Medicare
& Medicaid Services (CMS) is a branch of the US Department of Health and
Human Services. In an effort to control the substantial money it spends on
mobility equipment (durable medical equipment), CMS has been pursuing
a policy of competitive bidding, in which the lowest-price provider gains
large contracts for wheelchairs and scooters.

This raises huge concerns for disability advocates. A low-price
provider is not going to provide the up-front consultation and follow-up
services that are necessary for a person to get the right wheels and for the
wheels to be properly configured. Manufacturers are also concerned because
their profit margins will go down as large providers pressure them to cut
prices. This will cut into research and development funding and very likely
force production offshore—resulting in lower-quality chairs overall.

Follow this issue at Advancing Independence: Modernizing Medicare
and Medicaid (www.aimeee.com/aimmm).

The Community Choice Act

Originally known as MiCASA—the Medicaid Community Assistance and Supports Act—the Community Choice Act is the newest incarnation of federal legislation geared to ensure that people with disabilities get the option to live in their own communities rather than be forced into, and essentially imprisoned in, skilled nursing facilities.

The Supreme Court did the right thing in this instance, supporting the Olmstead case on the ADA's provision that services be provided in the "least restrictive setting." The government has a long way to go to implement all of the regulations that are potentially affected by the decision, and the Community Choice Act would go a long way toward achieving that end.

It is well demonstrated that providing services in the community costs less than providing institutionalized care—often dramatically less. There is also frightening evidence of the poor level of care in some of these settings where, at best, people must live according to the institutions' schedule and boundaries, limiting the people's life quality and options. Yet, a very strong nursing home industry lobby resists this reform for obvious reasons: the more than $63 billion spent annually on these services. Follow its progress at www.adapt.org.

The Christopher and Dana Reeve Paralysis Act

This three-pronged piece of legislation was introduced in March 2007 and was designed to

- Expand research at the National Institutes of Health to foster collaboration among scientists.
- Support rehabilitation research to measure the effectiveness of certain rehabilitation to optimize mobility, reduce secondary complications, and further develop assistive technologies.
- Develop unique programs with the Centers for Disease Control and Prevention to improve the quality of life and long-term health for people with disabilities.

Index

455